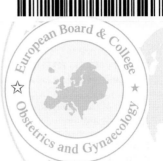

The
Menopause

Edited by

Risto Erkkola

Professor
Department of Obstetrics and Gynaecology
University Central Hospital of Turku
Turku
Finland

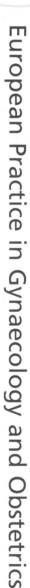

European Practice in Gynaecology and Obstetrics

ELSEVIER

Edinburgh   London   New York   Oxford   Philadelphia   St Louis   Sydney   Toronto 2006

ELSEVIER

© 2006, Elsevier Limited. All rights reserved.

First published 2006

ISBN-13 9 780444 518309
ISBN-10 0 444 51830 4
ISSN 1625-1180

British Library Cataloguing in Publication Data
A catalogue record for this book is available from the British Library

Library of Congress Cataloging in Publication Data
A catalog record for this book is available from the Library of Congress

Notice
Knowledge and best practice in this field are constantly changing. As new research and experience broaden our knowledge, changes in practice, treatment and drug therapy may become necessary or appropriate. Readers are advised to check the most current information provided (i) on procedures featured or (ii) by the manufacturer of each product to be administered, to verify the recommended dose or formula, the method and duration of administration, and contraindications. It is the responsibility of the practitioner, relying on their own experience and knowledge of the patient, to make diagnoses, to determine dosages and the best treatment for each individual patient, and to take all appropriate safety precautions. To the fullest extent of the law, neither the Publisher nor the Editor assumes any liability for any injury and/or damage to persons or property arising out or related to any use of the material contained in this book.

The Publisher

your source for books, journals and multimedia in the health sciences
www.elsevierhealth.com

The Publisher's policy is to use **paper manufactured from sustainable forests**

Printed in China

Contents

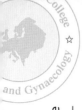

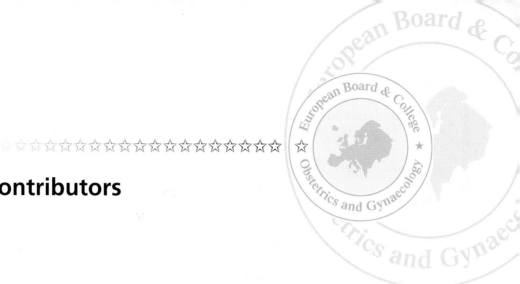

Contributors

Peter Alexandersen MD
Centre for Clinical and Basic Research
Ballerup
Denmark
*The effect of hormone replacement
therapy on bone*

Iñigo Azcoitia PhD
Associate Professor, Departamento de
Biología Celular
Facultad de Biología
Universidad Complutense
Madrid
Spain
The action of oestrogens in the brain

Yu Z Bagger MD
Centre for Clinical and Basic Research
Ballerup
Denmark
*The effect of hormone replacement
therapy on bone*

Barbara Cappagli MD
Department of Reproductive
  Medicine and Child Development
Unit of Obstetrics and Gynaecology
 'P Fioretti'
University of Pisa
Italy
Endocrinology of the menopause

Linda Cardozo MD, PhD, FRCOG
Professor, King's College Hospital
London
UK
Oestrogens and the lower urogenital tract

Claus Christiansen MD, PhD
Centre for Clinical and Basic Research
Ballerup
Denmark
*The effect of hormone replacement
therapy on bone*

Massimo Ciaponi MD
Department of Reproductive
  Medicine and Child Development
Unit of Obstetrics and Gynaecology
  'P Fioretti'
University of Pisa
Italy

Endocrinology of the menopause

George Creatsas MD, PhD
Professor and Chairman, 2nd
  Department of Obstetrics
  and Gynaecology
Alexandra Hospital
Athens
Greece

Alternatives to oestrogen

David Crook PhD
Senior Research Fellow, Division of
  Primary Care and Public Health
Brighton and Sussex Medical School
Brighton
UK

Interpreting the plasma lipoprotein profile
of the postmenopausal woman

Bruno de Lignières MD
Professor, Service d'Endocrinologie et
  Médecine de la Reproduction
Hôpital Necker
Paris
France

Androgen replacement therapies for
postmenopausal women

Risto Erkkola MD, PhD
Professor, Department of Obstetrics
  and Gynaecology
University Central Hospital of Turku
Turku
Finland

Oestrogens, cognitive functioning and
dementia;

Female sex hormones, sleep and mood

Marco Gambacciani MD, PhD
Assistant Professor, Department
  of Reproductive Medicine
  and Child Development
Unit of Obstetrics and Gynaecology
  'P Fioretti'
University of Pisa
Italy

Endocrinology of the menopause

Luis M Garcia-Segura PhD
Research Professor, Instituto Cajal
CSIC
Madrid
Spain

The action of oestrogens in the brain

Andrea R Genazzani MD, PhD
Professor, Department of
  Reproductive Medicine and Child
  Development
Unit of Obstetrics and Gynaecology
  'P Fioretti'
University of Pisa
Italy

Endocrinology of the menopause

Else Høibraaten MD, PhD
Department of Haematology
Ullevål University Hospital
Oslo
Norway

Hormone replacement therapy and
coagulation

Johannes Huber MD, PhD
Professor, Department of
  Gynaecological Endocrinology
  and Reproductive Medicine
Medical University of Vienna
Vienna
Austria

Alternative management of the female
menopause

Jorgen Jespersen MD, DSC
Department of Clinical Biochemistry
Ribe County Hospital
University of Southern Denmark
Esbjerg
Denmark

*The effects of ageing and hormone
replacement therapy on glucose
metabolism*

Olof Johnell MD, PhD
Professor, Department of
  Orthopaedics
UMAS
Malmö
Sweden

*The biology and consequences of
osteoporosis*

Peter Kenemans MD, PhD
Professor, Department of Obstetrics
  and Gynaecology
University Medical Centre
Amsterdam
The Netherlands

*Postmenopausal hormone replacement
treatment and the breast*

Irene Lambrinoudaki MD
Lecturer, 2nd Department of
  Obstetrics and Gynaecology
Alexandra Hospital
Athens
Greece

Alternatives to oestrogen

Petri Lehenkari MD, PhD
Department of Surgery
University of Oulu
Finland

The prevention of osteoporotic fractures

Anette Løken Eilertsen MD
Department of Haematology
Ullevål University Hospital
Oslo
Norway

*Hormone replacement therapy
and coagulation*

Kathrin Machens VMD, PhD
Schering AG
Berlin
Germany

*Economic aspects in the management
of the menopause*

Christian Matthai MD
Department of Gynaecological
  Endocrinology and Reproductive
  Medicine
Medical University of Vienna
Vienna
Austria

*Alternative management of the female
menopause*

Lars-Åke Mattsson MD, PhD
Professor, Department of Obstetrics
  and Gynaecology
Sahlgrenska Academy
Göteborg University
Göteborg
Sweden

Endometrial effects and bleeding patterns

Markus Metka MD, PhD
Assistant Professor, Department
  of Gynaecological Endocrinology
  and Reproductive Medicine
Medical University of Vienna
Vienna
Austria

*Alternative management of the female
menopause*

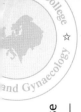

The menopause

Ian Milsom MD, PhD
Professor, Department of Obstetrics
and Gynaecology
Sahlgrenska Academy
Göteborg University
Göteborg
Sweden
*Menopause-related symptoms and their
treatment*

Rossella E Nappi MD, PhD
Assistant Professor, Department
of Obstetrics and Gynaecology
IRCCS Policlinico San Matteo
University of Pavia
Italy
Sexuality and the menopause

Manuel Neves-e-Castro MD
Professor, CFH-Clinica de Feminalogia
Holistica
Lisbon
Portugal
*Hormone replacement therapy:
when to start, when to stop?*

Santiago Palacios MD, PhD
Professor and Director, The Instituto
Palacios of Women's Health
Madrid
Spain
*How to select progestin for hormone
replacement therapy*

Päivi Polo-Kantola MD, PhD
Department of Obstetrics and
Gynaecology, and Sleep Research
Center Dentalia
University Central Hospital of Turku,
and Department of Public Health
University of Turku
Turku
Finland
*Female sex hormones, sleep and mood;
Oestrogens, cognitive functioning
and dementia*

Margaret Rees MA, DPhil., FRCOG
Reader in Reproductive Medicine,
Honorary Consultant in Medical
Gynaecology, John Radcliffe Hospital
Oxford
UK
*The use of hormone replacement therapy
in Europe and around the world*

Dudley Robinson MD, MRCOG
King's College Hospital
London
UK
Oestrogens and the lower urogenital tract

Göran Samsioe MD, PhD
Professor, Department of Obstetrics
and Gynaecology
Lund University Hospital
Lund
Sweden
*Current views on hormone replacement
therapy and cardiovascular disease*

Rafael Sànchez Borrego MD
Medical Director, Diatros, Clinica de
Atencion a la Mujer
Barcelona
Spain
*How to select progestin for hormone
replacement therapy*

Per Morten Sandset MD, PhD
Professor, Department of
Haematology
Ullevål University Hospital
Oslo, Norway
*Hormone replacement therapy
and coagulation*

Karin Schmidt-Gollwitzer MD, PhD
Professor, Obstetrics and Gynaecology
Schering AG
Berlin
Germany
*Economic aspects in the management
of the menopause*

Hermann P G Schneider MD, PhD
Professor, Department of Obstetrics
 and Gynaecology
University of Muenster
Germany

*Menopause, hormone replacement therapy
and quality of life*

Sven O Skouby MD, DSC
Professor, Department of Obstetrics
 and Gynaecology
Frederiksberg Hospital
University of Copenhagen
Copenhagen
Denmark

*The effects of ageing and hormone
replacement therapy on glucose
metabolism*

Heikki Kalervo Väänänen MD, PhD
Professor, Institute of Biomedicine
University of Turku
Finland

The prevention of osteoporotic fractures

Marius Jan van der Mooren MD, PhD
Associate Professor, Department
 of Obstetrics and Gynaecology
University Medical Centre
Amsterdam
The Netherlands

*The administration and dosage
of oestrogens;*

*Postmenopausal hormone treatment
and the breast*

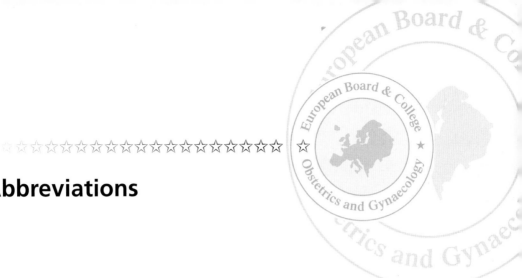

Abbreviations

The abbreviations used in this book are adapted from those accepted by the European Menopause and Andropause Society (Maturitas 2005 51:8–14).

AT	androgen therapy
CCEPT	continuous combined oestrogen–progestogen therapy
CSEPT	continuous sequential oestrogen–progestogen therapy
EPT	oestrogen–progestogen therapy
ET	oestrogen therapy
HRT	hormone replacement therapy (incorporating ET and EPT)
local ET	therapy has a predominantly local (vaginal), not systemic, effect
progestogen	progesterone or progestin
systemic ET/EPT/HRT	therapy has a systemic, not solely local, effect.

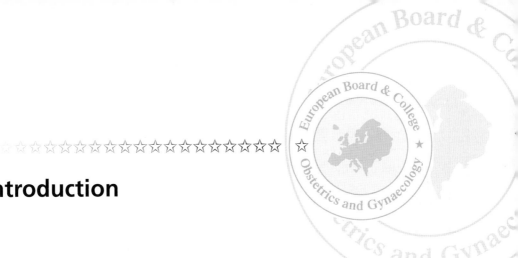

☆☆☆☆☆☆☆☆☆☆☆☆☆☆☆☆☆☆☆ ☆

Introduction

In the past 10 years a turbulent and confusing atmosphere has dominated the field of female menopause care. Since the first publication of the Heart and Estrogen/Progestin Replacement Study (HERS) project in 1998, numerous publications appeared that were totally in opposition to the existing observational studies, some of which had lasted for decades with huge numbers of participants, and which had shaped our understanding of the effects of postmenopausal hormone replacement therapy (HRT) until then. The medical profession was honest and sincere when interpreting the new findings.

After the first HERS study came the first Women's Health Initiative (WHI) study in July 2002, then the Million Women Study (MWS) in August 2003 and finally the WHI oestrogen arm study in April 2004. These basic publications were followed by several in-depth analyses of the primary data and by publications on some subgroups of the huge prospective WHI project, as well as results from the extensive observational MWS. These publications were all important in raising new issues in menopausal medicine, and they also required a lot of closer analysis and brainwork to be fitted to the wealth of earlier and concurrent literature in this field.

These results, however, impacted hugely on the medical profession. Before the profession had had time for a thorough interpretation of the data, it was also publicized widely in the media (as expected), creating great confusion among millions of postmenopausal patients throughout that part of world where HRT was widely available and used. The official statements of US, European and national agencies supervising medical care expressed a very critical view of HRT; this was also quickly publicized. The consequence of this was a sudden discontinuation of HRT. In many countries 20–50% of users stopped the treatment abruptly. Many of those women have since returned to HRT or have tried to find alternative treatments such as phyto-oestrogens, sleep medication or antidepressants. However, many of these women still suffer from menopausal symptoms.

This book in the EBCOG series was initiated in 2000 and it was originally due to be published in 2002. Fortunately this did not happen. In the very beginning, an extremely prominent group of writers was recruited to participate in the preparation of the book. Initially, the attitude to the EBCOG project was very positive – some early contributions even arrived. Then the new information about the alarming effects of HRT started to appear and the flow of typescripts slowed down. This was very understandable.

Now, with the added perspective of a few years, as well as closer and in-depth analysis of the strengths and weaknesses of new publications, a clearer picture of the menopause and its treatment has started to emerge. As a consequence, many of the contributors to this book volunteered to rewrite their chapters. The result has been a book on menopause which is very much up to date, and where all the latest available information has been included.

This is a comprehensive review of the female menopause. Aspects of ageing and treatment, are described. There are chapters on the development of the female menopause, and of menopause-related symptoms and changes in the quality of life. Furthermore, important metabolic and biochemical changes in lipid and carbohydrate metabolisms and in changes in the coagulation system are presented in their clinical context. Important chapters on the effects of ageing and HRT on various clinical issues are included – they deal with the influence on circulation, bone, brain function, behavioural and mental changes and, of course, on the risks of malign neoplasms. Some chapters deal with practical guidelines for selecting the appropriate treatment, including alternative medicine. We incorporate a fascinating review of the current use of HRT in Europe as well as predictions, and we provide a final extensive analysis of health economics of the treatment of menopause.

I am extremely grateful to the internationally renowned contributors to this book. They include high-level researchers, opinion leaders and authorities in the field of the female menopause. They have helped EBCOG to achieve the goal of publishing a state-of-the-art, applied resource on this very important aspect of gynaecology. I am also grateful to the representatives of Elsevier, Tina Carrington, Greyling Peoples and, in the final stage especially, to Lulu Stader, who all have given their strong support toward the preparation of this book.

I suspect that following the hasty reactions of many agencies, doctors and users of HRT, a new and more balanced view on menopause and HRT is now emerging. The clearer indications and contraindications, the more precise individualization and dosing of the HRT, and the improved communication with our patients, are all the result of the extensive discussion and new guidelines concerning menopausal medicine. I hope that this EBCOG volume will help us be better doctors in treating our patients more efficiently and more safely. This is our ultimate aim.

1

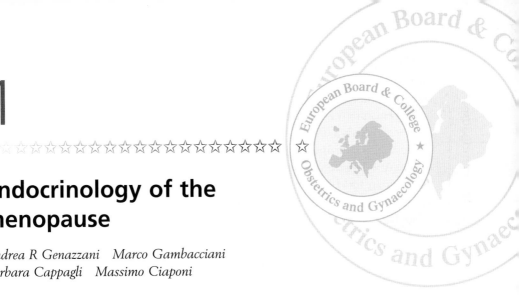

Endocrinology of the menopause

Andrea R Genazzani   Marco Gambacciani
Barbara Cappagli   Massimo Ciaponi

ABSTRACT

The menopause occurs in all women by the middle of their sixth decade. Ovulation starts to decrease in frequency by the age of 40, and reproductive ovarian function ceases within the following 15 years. Under gonadotrophic stimulation, the gonads produce and secrete several steroidal and non-steroidal factors, which in turn regulate the function of the hypothalamic–pituitary axis in different ways. However, ovarian sex steroid production is profoundly modified with the onset of the menopause. Women, at menopause, not only lack oestrogens but have also been progressively deprived of androgens and some oestrogens originating from adrenal androgen precursors. Thyroid anomalies are more frequent in women than men. There is an increasing prevalence of high levels of thyroid-stimulating hormone with age, particularly in postmenopausal women. About 25% of postmenopausal women show clinical or subclinical thyroid disease, and, unfortunately, the symptoms can be similar to postmenopausal complaints.

KEYWORDS

Adrenal, hypothalamus, menopause, pituitary, thyroid

INTRODUCTION

Physiological systems have substantial reserves in younger individuals but the process of ageing and the associated pathological processes gradually eliminate these reserves. Changes in endocrine systems, which include the menopause in women, androgen deficiency in men, loss of skeletal mass, decrease in growth hormone serum concentrations and an increased incidence of type 2 diabetes are all more common or certain in older individuals.[11] Improvements in medical care

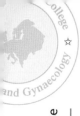
have dramatically increased women's average life expectancies in developed countries, thus women spend at least one-third of their lives in a state of hypo-oestrogenism.

Menopause is a universal finding in women by the middle of their sixth decade. Interestingly, later menopause (as compared with early) is associated with earlier mortality.[16] The frequency of ovulation decreases by the age of 40, and reproductive ovarian function ceases in the vast majority of women during the following 15 years.[4,18] The components of the reproductive axis communicate with each other through endocrine signals. Under gonadotrophic stimulation, the gonads produce and secrete several steroidal and non-steroidal factors, which, in turn, regulate the function of the hypothalamic–pituitary axis in different ways. An episodic and pulsatile mode of secretion of hormonal signals characterizes the function of the reproductive axis, particularly that of the hypothalamic–pituitary part. The target cell response, and consequently the harmonic function of the corresponding gland, will depend on the adequate dynamics of this pulsatile secretion. The function of each component of the reproductive axis is strongly influenced by locally produced signals acting either in a paracrine or autocrine manner. These particular signals represent the fine-tuning of the regulating systems that eventually amplify or reduce the magnitude of response to a particular endocrine signal, providing additional mechanisms for tissue homeostasis and a better functional plasticity of the target gland.[19] A new understanding of the endocrinology of menopause is that women, at menopause, not only lack oestrogens (due to the cessation of ovarian activity) but have also been progressively deprived for a few years of androgens and some oestrogens originating from adrenal androgen precursors. Other endocrine systems may also be affected by menopausal transition and/or the ageing process.

Thyroid anomalies are more frequent in women than men. There is an increasing prevalence of high levels of thyroid-stimulating hormone (TSH) with age, particularly in postmenopausal women. About 25% of the postmenopausal population show clinical and/or subclinical thyroid disease; also, the rate of thyroid cancer increases in this population. Unfortunately, the symptoms of thyroid disease can be similar to postmenopausal complaints and are difficult to differentiate clinically.[14]

THE HYPOTHALAMIC–PITUITARY AXIS

The female reproductive axis includes the hypothalamic–pituitary part and the ovaries. The physiology of the hypothalamic–pituitary–gonadal axis includes endocrine interactions between the hypothalamic–pituitary system and the gonads, as well as paracrine interactions within the various endocrine glands of the reproductive system (pituitary; ovary).[3] Sexual maturation and the subsequent development of reproductive competence, as well as menopausal physiopathology, depend on the precise and coordinated function of this axis. The neuroendocrine components of this axis, including the hypothalamus and the pituitary gland, are central to this system. The menstrual cycle is now thought to be determined mainly by the ovaries themselves, which send various signals to the pituitary and hypothalamus. The hypothalamus is an autonomous pacemaker with a pulse frequency modulated by ovarian signals; in turn, it is indispensable to ovarian function.

In women, the ovarian cycle produces a single mature oocyte every month from puberty to menopause. The hypothalamus synthesizes gonadotrophin-releasing hormone (GnRH), which stimulates the synthesis and secretion of the pituitary gonadotrophins, follicle-stimulating hormone (FSH) and luteinizing hormone (LH) via the portal circulation. Within the hypothalamus, the special-ized neuronal system responsible for synthesizing and secreting GnRH is itself modulated by peptide and neurotransmitters that mediate feedback signals of ovarian origin. The pulsatile secretion of GnRH by the hypothalamus stimulates the pulsatile secretion of gonadotrophins from the pituitary. LH and FSH regu-late the hormonal production of the gonads as well as gametogenesis but are themselves modulated by the ambient gonadal hormone concentrations. The ovarian follicles and the interstitial and Sertoli cells of the testis are the targets for these pituitary signals. The steroid hormones – oestradiol (E_2), progesterone, testosterone and peptides (inhibins) – produced by the gonads in turn – regulate hypothalamic–pituitary secretions. While changes in the brain may contribute to reproductive ageing, the major focus of current research is on the ovaries, where the progressive loss of follicles ultimately leads to an absence of follicular func-tion and the consequent permanent cessation of menstruation: the menopause. The serum patterns of pituitary and ovarian hormones throughout the menstrual cycle alter as the menopause approaches. The increase in follicular phase of the FSH prior to menopause is attributed to an early decline in the ovarian hormone inhibin B (INH-B), which negatively regulates FSH secretion. Serum INH-B is believed to reflect the age-related decrease in ovarian follicle reserve, as this is the primary source of serum INH-B. The later rise in serum LH during the menopause transition is due to the cessation of ovarian follicle development. During this time in most women, ovarian follicles function less well,[15] serum E_2 concentrations are lower than in younger women and FSH concentrations are higher.[15] LH is reported to be unchanged. Eventually follicular activity ceases, oestrogen concentrations fall to postmenopausal values, and concentrations of LH and FSH rise above premenopausal levels.[7,9,18]

THE OVARIES

The ovaries are the organs that play a key role in the endocrinological changes of menopause. Follicular growth and maturation from primordial to antral follicles are mostly independent of gonadotrophins.[8] A complete intraovarian paracrine system is implied in this gonadotrophin-independent follicular growth and in the modulation of the action of gonadotrophins in the ovary. FSH allows a small number of follicles to avoid atresia; it is only indispensable for the final matura-tion of the preovulatory follicle during the follicular phase of the cycle. LH is responsible for the final growth of the dominant follicle in the late follicular phase, of ovulation during the LH peak, and for the survival of the corpus luteum during the luteal phase. The cyclical variations of gonadotrophins are under the control of ovarian steroids and peptides.[8] The cycle length is determined by the duration of terminal follicular growth and by the fixed lifespan of the corpus luteum. The serum patterns of pituitary–ovarian hormones throughout the menstrual cycle alter as menopause approaches. The increase in follicular-phase FSH prior to menopause is attributed to an early decline in the ovarian hormone INH-B, which negatively regulates FSH secretion.[12] These changes begin subtly with reductions of fecundability being observed after 25 years of age. The transition from reproductive to postreproductive life is characterized by menstrual irregularity including anovulation or short luteal phases. The pituitary gonadotrophins FSH and LH stimulate the ovarian secretion of E_2 and the inhibins from follicular granulosa cells, and androgens from interstitial cells, including theca cells.

A primary event in the ageing of the reproductive axis appears to be a decline in the secretion of INH-B as follicle numbers decrease.[10] This leads to a slow rise in FSH in women who continue to cycle regularly, particularly in the last decade of reproductive life. As the menopause approaches, decreasing concentrations of both E_2 and INH-B lead to more marked increases in the gonadotrophins, which reach their postmenopausal peak 2 to 3 years after final menses.[1] Observing from the ovarian point of view, the elevation of gonadotrophins and the reduction of inhibin levels reflect the loss of folliculogenesis and ovulation. There are also accompanying decreases in ovarian androgen secretion. However, the postmenopausal gonad directly secretes more testosterone after the menopause than before. During reproductive life, ovarian steroid biosynthesis is gonadotrophin-dependent and occurs in theca and granulosa cells. In the menopausal ovary, there is atresia of ovarian follicles, with sparing of the androgen-producing theca-interstitial cell component. The ageing ovary therefore produces significantly reduced amounts of oestrogen, with continued, though decreased, androgen production. The most prominent hormonal changes at the menopause are drastic reductions of E_2 and progesterone secretion by the ovaries. In fact, in fertile women, the primary component of circulating oestrogen is E_2, which is produced by the granulosa cells of the developing ovarian follicles. About 95% of E_2 is produced by the ovaries with the remaining 5% created by the conversion of oestrone (E_1), testosterone and androstenedione in peripheral tissue. During menopause, the majority of the circulating E_2 in plasma is derived from the peripheral conversion of E_1. After menopause, ovarian E_2 biosynthesis is negligible, and direct glandular secretion of E_1 by either the ovaries or the adrenal glands is minimal during the postmenopausal years.[13] It is currently believed that the postmenopausal ovary remains a gonadotrophin-driven, androgen-producing gland.[5] Thus circulating oestrogens in postmenopausal women are derived principally from the peripheral aromatization of ovarian and adrenal androgens, i.e. the aromatization of androstenedione to E_1 increases in postmenopausal women. Adipose tissue is the most important source of the peripheral aromatization of androstenedione into E_1.[13] Androgen biosynthesis from the adrenal gland, in addition to that from the ovaries, decreases with age. However, although ovarian androgen production

levels at the time of menopause. The biological activity of these steroids, either
before or after menopause, depends on the amount of steroid available in the
unbound fraction. To this end, sex hormone-binding globulin (SHBG) levels are
an important determinant of hormone action. Not only does the concentration of
SHBG influence the biological effect of testosterone and E_2 but these steroids also
regulate SHBG concentrations. Older women, who have a higher body mass index
than younger women, also have the lowest SHBG levels and more circulating free
hormones.[13]

THE ADRENAL GLANDS

In normal menstruating women, the ovaries and the adrenal cortex contribute
nearly equal amounts of testosterone, dihydrotestosterone (DHT) and androstenedione in the peripheral circulation. Alternatively, dehydroepiandrosterone sulphate
(DHEAS) is almost exclusively produced by the adrenal cortex.[6] During perimenopause transition, a phase of elevated androgen action is found in early
menopause. Ultimately, in late menopause, ovarian androgen production decreases
while androgen production in the adrenal glands is maintained. In particular, the
adrenals produce prohormones which are metabolized peripherally to active androgens and oestrogens. Also in late menopause, adrenal androgen production
decreases. Quantitatively, women secrete greater amounts of androgen than oestrogen. The major circulating steroids generally classified as androgens include
DHEAS, DHEA, androstenedione, testosterone and DHT, in descending order of
serum concentration, though only the latter two bind to the androgen receptors.
The other three steroids are better considered as pro-androgens.[6]

DHEA is primarily an adrenal product, regulated by adrenocorticotrophic
hormone (ACTH) and acts as a precursor for the peripheral synthesis of more
potent androgens. DHEA is produced by the ovaries and the adrenal glands as
well as being derived from circulating DHEAS. There is a relatively constant
decline in circulating DHEA and DHEAS in adults, of approximately 2% per
year. DHEA and DHEAS decline with age, without any specific influence of the
menopause. In effect, serum DHEA decreases by about 60% between the maximal levels seen at 30 years of age to the age of menopause. This decreased secretion of DHEA and DHEAS by the adrenals is responsible for a parallel decrease
in androgen and oestrogen formation in peripheral tissues by the steroidogenic
enzymes specifically expressed in each cell type in individual target tissues.[6] The
decline is well documented in both men and women, and it is more consistent in
older men than in older women. This postmenopausal gradual decline in DHEAS
is thought to be the result of attenuated adrenal 17,20-desmolase activity in later
life and not related to gonadal function in the adult. As a result, the adrenal
glands' ability to convert C21 progestins into C19 androgen is diminished. In
postmenopausal women, the site of progesterone production is controversial but
it seems that 17-hydroxyprogesterone (17-OHP), detectable in postmenopausal
women, is secreted by the adrenal glands.

In postmenopausal women, androstenedione is also secreted, almost exclusively by the adrenal glands. The levels of androstenedione decrease by almost 40 to 50% after the menopause and remain constant even when the ovaries are removed. From a biological point of view the most significant active androgen is testosterone, which circulates bound tightly to SHBG and loosely to albumin. It is generally held that the non-SHBG-bound fraction is the bioavailable moiety. Hence, clinically useful testosterone measurements require data on total concentrations as well as SHBG level. Clinical symptoms of androgen insufficiency include loss of libido, diminished well-being, fatigue and blunted motivation; patients have been reported as responding well to testosterone replacement, generally without significant side-effects.[2] Thus the climacteric is not only characterized by a decrease in oestrogens levels, but in the late phase also by a decrease of androgen levels. During this time there is no critical source of androgens. The postmenopausal ovaries, as well as the adrenal glands, are androgen-secreting organs, and the levels of testosterone are not directly influenced by the menopausal transition or the occurrence of menopause. The scarce amount of postmenopausal oestrogens originate primarily from the peripheral conversion of androgens, which are produced by the adrenal glands and the ovaries.

THE THYROID GLAND

Thyroid anomalies are more frequent in women than men. Oestrogen fluctuations modify thyroxine carrier protein levels but they hardly influence thyroid function, particularly if hyperthyroidism occurs in menopause. In the same way, thyroidal pathology actually interferes very little with ovarian function. There is an increasing prevalence of high levels of TSH with age – particularly in postmenopausal women – which are higher than in men.[14] In middle-aged women in a German study, there was a 9.6% prevalence of TSH values outside the euthyroid range. About 2.4% of the population of postmenopausal women show clinical thyroid disease, while 23.2% show subclinical thyroid disease. Among the group with subclinical thyroid disease, 73.8% are hypothyroid and 26.2% are hyperthyroid. The rate of thyroid cancer increases with age and therefore increases in the postmenopausal population. Unfortunately, the symptoms of thyroid disease can be similar to postmenopausal complaints and are difficult to differentiate clinically. It is important that even mild thyroid failure can have a number of clinical effects such as depression, memory loss and cognitive impairment, and a variety of neuromuscular complaints. There is also an increased cardiovascular risk, caused by increased serum total cholesterol and low-density lipoprotein cholesterol as well as a reduced level of high-density lipoprotein. Therefore, routine screening of thyroid function in the climacteric period to determine subclinical thyroid disease is recommended. Hormone replacement therapy (HRT) in women with hypothyroidism treated with thyroxine causes changes in free thyroxine and TSH. Increased binding of thyroxine to elevated thyroxine-binding globulin causes an elevation of TSH by feedback. Since adaptation is insufficient, there is an increased need for thyroxine during HRT, and TSH levels should be controlled at 12 weeks after the beginning of therapy.

Thyroid hormones play a dominant role in bone metabolism. While there are only marginal differences between hypothyroid patients and euthyroid controls, there are large differences for hyperthyroid patients. Previous thyrotoxicosis and subsequent long-lasting L-thyroxine treatment are together associated with a reduction in femoral and vertebral bone density in postmenopausal women. In these cases HRT is important for the prevention of bone loss.[14] TSH concentrations seem not to be correlated with FSH, SHBG, DHEA-S, testosterone, and E_2 concentrations. Although TSH was associated with bleeding length and self-reported fearfulness, it was not associated with indicators of the menopausal transition, including menopausal stage defined by bleeding regularity, menopausal symptoms or reproductive hormone concentrations.[17] Thus, since women are more subject to thyroid pathologies, and hypothyroidism is particularly prevalent in the postmenopausal population, they should be routinely studied for thyroid disease by a screening test (TSH) and neck palpation annually from the age of 40.

References

1. Burger H G, Dudley E, Mamers P et al 2002 The ageing female reproductive axis I. Novartis Foundation Symposium; 242:161–167; discussion 167–171

2. Davis S R, Burger H G 2003 The role of androgen therapy. Best Practice & Research. Clinical Endocrinology & Metabolism 17:165–175

3. Genazzani A D, Petraglia F, Sgarbi L et al 1997 Difference of LH and FSH secretory characteristics and degree of concordance between postmenopausal and aging women. Maturitas 26:133–138

4. Johnson S R 1998 Menopause and hormone replacement therapy. Medical Clinics of North America 82:297–320

5. Jongen V H, Sluijmer A V, Heineman M J 2002 The postmenopausal ovary as an androgen-producing gland; hypothesis on the etiology of endometrial cancer. Maturitas 43:77–85

6. Labrie F, Luu-The V, Labrie C et al 2001 DHEA and its transformation into androgens and oestrogens in peripheral target tissues: intracrinology. Frontiers in Neuroendocrinology 22:185–212

7. McKinlay S M, Brambilla D J, Posner J G 1992 The normal menopause transition. Maturitas 14:103–115

8. Macklon N S, Fauser B C 2001 Follicle-stimulating hormone and advanced follicle development in the human. Archives of Medical Research 32:595–600

9. Meldrum D R, Davidson B J, Tataryn I V et al 1981 Changes in circulating steroids with aging in postmenopausal women. Obstetrics and Gynecology 57:624–628

10. Muttukrishna S, Sharma S, Barlow D H et al 2002 Serum inhibins, estradiol, progesterone and FSH in surgical menopause: a demonstration of the ovarian pituitary feedback loop in women. Human Reproduction 17:2535–2539

11. Perry H M, III 1999 The endocrinology of aging. Clinical Chemistry 45:1369–1376

12. Prior J C 1998 Perimenopause: the complex endocrinology of the menopausal transition. Endocrine Reviews 19:397–428

13. Schindler A E 2003 Thyroid function and postmenopause. Gynecological Endocrinology 17:79–85

14. Sherman B M, West J H, Korenman S G 1976 The menopausal transition: analysis of LH, FSH, estradiol, and progesterone concentrations during menstrual cycles of older women. The Journal of Clinical Endocrinology and Metabolism 42:629–636

15. Shifren J L, Schiff I 2000 The aging ovary. Journal of Women's Health & Gender-Based Medicine 9 (Suppl 1):S3–S7

16. Snowden DA 1990 Early natural menopause and the duration of postmenopausal life. Findings from a mathematical model of life expectancy. Journal of the American Geriatrics Socidty 38:402–408

17. Sowers M, Luborsky J, Perdue C et al 2003 Thyroid-stimulating hormone (TSH) concentrations and menopausal status in women at the mid-life: SWAN. Clinical Endocrinology 58:340–347

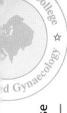

18. Speroff L 1993 Menopause and hormone replacement therapy. Clinics in Geriatric Medicine 9:33–56
19. Ulloa-Aguirre A, Timossi C 2000 Biochemical and functional aspects of gonadotrophin-releasing hormone and gonadotrophins. Reproductive Biomedicine Online 1(2):48–62

2

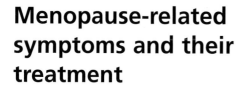

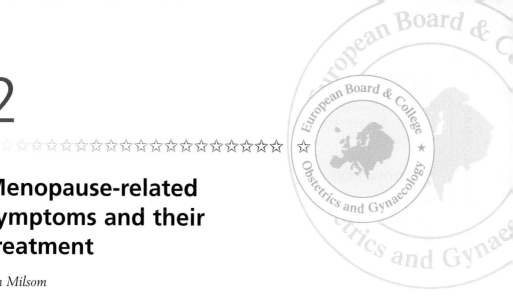

Menopause-related symptoms and their treatment

Ian Milsom

ABSTRACT

The menopause is a physiological event that occurs in all women who reach midlife. Symptoms shown to be associated with oestrogen deficiency after the menopause are hot flushes and night sweats, insomnia and vaginal dryness. However, many other symptoms and conditions (irregular menstrual bleeding, osteoporosis, arteriosclerosis, dyslipidaemia, depressed mood, irritability, head-ache, forgetfulness, dizziness, deterioration in postural balance, palpitations, dry eyes, dry mouth, reduced skin elasticity, restless legs, and muscle and joint pain) have also been implicated as associated with the menopause but are not necessarily correlated to oestrogen levels.

Oestrogens are effective in treating vasomotor symptoms, urogenital atrophy symptoms and irregular menstrual bleeding that occurs in the perimenopausal period. Conjugated oestrogens are given orally, and oestradiol may be given orally as tablets or transdermally as a patch or gel for a period of 3 weeks or longer. Perimenopausal women and women during the first 1 to 2 years after the menopause who have an intact uterus must be treated with a gestagen for at least 12 to 14 days every month in order to prevent endometrial hyperplasia and possible endometrial cancer. With this regimen the woman will have a withdrawal bleeding every month.

When the woman is 2 to 3 years postmenopausal then she can be recommen-ded continuous administration of a fast combination of oestradiol and a gestagen that normally does not induce bleeding. Tibolone is an alternative substance (whose metabolites have both oestrogenic and gestagenic effects) that can also be used for the same indications as oestrogen preparations, the difference being that no additional gestagen is required.

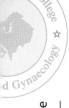
KEYWORDS

Climacteric, gestagens, hormone replacement therapy (HRT), hot flushes, menopause, oestrogens, progestogens, urogenital symptoms, vasomotor symptoms

INTRODUCTION

The phenomenon of the menopause was known to the ancient Greeks; Aristotle (384–322 BC) described the cessation of menstruation at the age of 40. In the nineteenth century, the menopause was believed to be directly responsible for madness and even in more modern times it has still been believed to cause certain psychiatric illnesses.[1] The word 'menopause' is derived from *men* and *pausis* and is a direct description of the physiological event in women where menstruation ceases to occur. The word 'climacteric' is a Greek derivation of the 'ladder' or 'steps of a ladder'. Over the years, the view of middle-aged women has varied from the extremes of either climbing up or down that ladder.[58] Symptoms associated with the menopause have also been known for a long time but it was not until the 1930s that climacteric symptoms could be effectively treated with oestrogens isolated from the urine of pregnant women.[5] However, treatment was not very widespread until after the publication of Robert A Wilson's best-selling book *Feminine Forever*,[60] after which treatment became more popular among physicians and women.

Symptoms that have been shown to be associated with oestrogen deficiency after the menopause are hot flushes and night sweats, insomnia and vaginal dryness.[6,11,27,43] Many other symptoms and conditions (irregular menstrual bleeding, osteoporosis, arteriosclerosis, dyslipidaemia, depressed mood, irritability, headache, forgetfulness, dizziness, deterioration in postural balance, palpitations, dry eyes, dry mouth, reduced skin elasticity, restless legs, and muscle and joint pain) have also been implicated as associated with the menopause[4,24,43] but are not necessarily correlated to oestrogen levels.[45,51] An overriding issue regarding the biology and symptomatology of the menopause is its relationship to the underlying ageing process.

VASOMOTOR SYMPTOMS

Hot flushes are defined as transient, recurrent periods of heat sensation and redness, often concomitant with sweats. An increase in peripheral vasodilatation, skin temperature and skin moisture has been demonstrated during such episodes by the registration of skin conductance, thermograms or plethysmography in the affected areas of the face, neck, head or breast.[54] The duration is often 2 to 3 minutes but with a range from a few seconds up to one hour[55,59] and there is a wide variety in frequency. Vasomotor symptoms are probably caused by changes in the temperature centre in the hypothalamus via different neurotransmitter systems as a result of fluctuations in oestrogen levels. The effect may also be mediated by β-endorphins, since low oestrogen levels after the menopause result in a more labile gonadotrophin-releasing hormone (GnRH) secretion which may induce a sudden resetting of the thermoregulatory centre.[56] No direct correlation has been found between the severity of vasomotor symptoms and serum levels of sex steroids.[45,51]

Vasomotor symptoms have been reported as occurring among women from different countries and societies but with varying prevalence. For example Mayan women[35] experience no hot flushes whereas in most western countries there is general agreement from both cross-sectional and longitudinal studies that 50–75% of postmenopausal women report hot flushes and night sweats of varying severity.[14,16,33,34,47,52,57] This difference may be explained by genetic differences, different ways of identifying symptoms, different lifestyles and dietary habits.[8,31,40,41,49] Vasomotor symptoms have been reported as most frequently experienced around the menopause but even 30–50% of women over 60 years of age experience symptoms.[3,52,57] Women with a surgically induced menopause often have more severe symptoms compared to women with a natural menopause.[11,50] However, it should also be noted that 10% of regularly menstruating women experience vasomotor symptoms[33] and 15–50% still report complaints 15 years or more after the menopause.[3,30,43,52,57]

UROGENITAL SYMPTOMS

Vaginal atrophy and urogenital complaints such as vaginal discomfort, dysuria, dyspareunia and recurrent lower urinary tract infections are more common in women after the menopause.[38] Epidemiological studies[26,38] have demonstrated that more than 50% of postmenopausal women suffer from at least one of these symptoms. Symptoms cause not only discomfort for the afflicted individual but may also negatively influence sexual health.[1,30] Many women are so embarrassed by their 'hidden problems' that they are unable to discuss their dilemma with other women or their doctor.[38]

Embryologically, the female genital tract and urinary systems develop in close proximity, both arising from the primitive urogenital sinus. Animal and human studies have shown that the urethra is oestrogen-sensitive, and oestrogen receptors have been identified in the human female urethra, urinary bladder, the vagina and the pelvic floor muscles.[25] Symptomatic and cytological changes have been demonstrated in the genitourinary tract during the menstrual cycle, in pregnancy and following the menopause.[44] In addition, factors influencing vaginal cytology, vaginal pH and the vaginal bacterial flora in elderly women have been identified.[37]

Several features of the vaginal microenvironment change with increasing age, mostly in response to alterations in oestrogen and progesterone concentrations (Table 2.1).

The histology of the vagina changes extensively after the menopause, when the mucosa often becomes quite thin, and heavily infiltrated with neutrophils. Associated hormonal changes have also been shown to induce changes in the bacterial colonization of the vagina. After the menopause the vagina is colonized

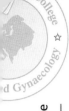

Table 2.1 Signs and symptoms of postmenopausal vaginal atrophy

Signs	Symptoms
Thinner epithelium	Dryness
Loss of rugae	Irritation
Reduced secretion	Burning
Reduced elasticity	Itching
Reduced width and length of vagina	Discharge
Altered bacterial flora	Dyspareunia

with a predominantly faecal flora in contrast to the dominance with lactobacilli encountered during the fertile period of life.[37,44] The presence of lactobacilli in fertile women provides protection against vaginal and periurethral colonization by Gram-negative bacteria, which have been implicated in the pathogenesis of cystitis and urethritis. The diagnosis of vaginal atrophy can be simply made by taking a careful history complemented by a vaginal speculum inspection.

OTHER MENOPAUSE-RELATED SYMPTOMS

Many other symptoms and conditions (irregular menstrual bleeding, osteoporosis, arteriosclerosis, dyslipidaemia, depressed mood, irritability, headache, forgetfulness, dizziness, deterioration in postural balance, palpitations, dry eyes, dry mouth, reduced skin elasticity, restless legs, and muscle and joint pain) have also been implicated to be associated with the menopause[43] but are not necessarily correlated to oestrogen levels.[45,51] Endometrial effects and bleeding patterns are dealt with in Chapter 22. The biology and consequences of osteoporosis (Ch. 8) as well as the prevention (Ch. 10) and treatment of osteoporosis (Ch. 9) are dealt with in this book. The influence of ageing and HRT on carbohydrate (Ch. 5) and lipid metabolism (Ch. 4) as well as cardiovascular diseases (Ch. 7) are also dealt with.

Sleep disturbance and insomnia during the climacteric have been recognized by some authors as directly caused by oestrogen deficiency.[6,11,14,16,27,43] Some support for this opinion was provided in a randomized double-blind trial of the effect of transdermal oestrogen therapy on sleep. In this trial, short-term treatment with oestrogen replacement therapy improved objective sleep quality by alleviating the frequency of nocturnal movement arousals. However, other investigators have considered sleeping problems to be secondary to the occurrence of night sweats.[18,33]

Several studies have indicated a possible correlation between depression and the menopause but most investigators have found no association between overt endogenous depression and oestrogen deprivation.[12,15,19,29,32] However, milder mood changes and irritability are often related to severe climacteric symptoms.[20,22,23,28] Women with previous premenstrual tension report more frequent severe vasomotor symptoms and depressed mood after the menopause.[9,18,23,43]

THE TREATMENT OF MENOPAUSAL SYMPTOMS

Oestradiol and conjugated oestrogens are effective in treating the vasomotor symptoms, urogenital atrophy symptoms and irregular menstrual bleeding that occur in the perimenopausal period. Conjugated oestrogens are given orally and oestradiol may be given orally as tablets, transdermally as a patch or gel, or intranasally for a period of 3 weeks. Subdermal pellets or long-acting oestrogen injections have also been used. Perimenopausal women and women during the first 1 to 2 years after the menopause who have an intact uterus must be treated with a gestagen for at least 12 to 14 days every month in order to prevent endometrial hyperplasia and possible endometrial cancer. With this regimen the woman will have a withdrawal bleeding every month.

It is also possible to choose a preparation with a fast combination of oestrogen and gestagen using a sequential dosage regimen. Cyclical addition of the gestagen can with time be successively reduced to every other month or every third month in order to reduce the number of bleeding episodes. When the gestagen is not administered every month the possibility of endometrial hyperplasia must always be considered. If the woman desires a bleed-free regimen then the gestagen can be administered by means of an intrauterine system releasing levonorgestrel, which provides endometrial protection.

When the woman is 2 to 3 years postmenopausal she can be recommended continuous administration of a fast combination of oestradiol and a gestagen which normally does not induce bleeding. Tibolone is a substance whose metabolites have both oestrogen and gestagen effects, and which can also be used for the same indications as oestrogen preparations, the difference being that no additional gestagen is required.

There is a wealth of evidence to support the efficacy of hormone replacement therapy (HRT) in the treatment of climacteric symptoms such as vasomotor symptoms, urogenital symptoms and irregular bleeding in perimenopausal women. During the last two decades a debate has continued regarding the possible pros and cons of HRT. A large number of observational studies have shown that long-term use of oestrogens has prophylactic effects against coronary heart disease (CHD)[13,53] and osteoporosis.[10] However, recently randomized controlled studies such as the Women's Health Initiative trial[48] and the Heart and Estrogen/progestin Replacement Study (HERS)[21] could not find evidence for primary or secondary preventive effects of HRT on CHD. An increased risk of breast cancer[2,48] and venous thromboembolism[7,48] among HRT users has also been reported.

Thus, in many countries, guidelines regarding treatment have been modified as a result of this new information. HRT is still recommended for the treatment of vasomotor symptoms but the duration of treatment should be reassessed on a yearly basis as long-term use (>5–10 years) appears to increase the risk of breast cancer. HRT should be continued as long as the benefits are judged to outweigh the risks. The risk of breast cancer appears to be greater when oestrogen is given in combination with gestagen as compared to oestrogen administration alone.

However, it should also be noted that the risk of breast cancer appears to return to baseline 5 years after the cessation of HRT.

Numerous studies have demonstrated a beneficial effect of oestrogen therapy in the management of vaginal atrophy; treatment with the oral, transdermal or vaginal application of oestrogens is also now well-established.[17,36,39,42] Local vaginal application has been shown to be highly effective without inducing the systemic side-effects sometimes associated with oral or transdermal HRT. Oral or transdermal HRT given for the treatment of climacteric symptoms relieves vaginal atrophy symptoms for the majority of peri- and postmenopausal women.[52,57] However, despite systemic therapy some women still experience vaginal symptoms. In these cases HRT can be complemented with local vaginal treatment with oestrogens, which can be given in the form of vaginal tablets or suppositories, vaginal cream or as a vaginal ring. Long-term compliance to HRT has also previously been reported to be a problem[46] and local treatment with oestrogens has been shown to be a simple, acceptable and effective alternative form of treatment for urogenital symptoms in postmenopausal women.

References

1. Barlow D H, Cardozo L D, Francis R M et al 1997 Urogenital ageing and its effect on sexual health in older British women. British Journal of Obstetrics and Gynaecology 104:87–91
2. Beral V 2003 Breast cancer and hormone-replacement therapy in the Million Women Study. The Lancet 362:419–427
3. Berg G, Gottwall T, Hammar M et al 1988 Climacteric symptoms among women aged 60–62 in Linköping, in 1986. Maturitas 10:193–199
4. Brown J C 1976 Psychiatric and psychosomatic aspects of gynecology. The Practitioner 216:153–168
5. Butenandt A 1930 Über die Reindarstellung des Follikelhormones aus Schwangerenharn. Zeitschrift für Physiologische Chemie 191:127
6. Campbell S, Whitehead M 1977 Oestrogen therapy and the menopausal syndrome. Clinical Obstetrics and Gynecology 4:31–47
7. Castellsague J, Perez Gutthann S, Garcia Rodriguez L A 1998 Recent epidemiological studies of the association between hormone replacement therapy and venous thromboembolism. A review. Drug Safety 18:117–123
8. Chompootweep S, Tankeyoon M, Yamarat K et al 1993 The menopausal age and climacteric complaints in Thai women in Bangkok. Maturitas 17:63–71
9. Collins A, Landgren B-M 1995 Reproductive health, use of estrogen and experience of symptoms in perimenopausal women: a population-based study. Maturitas 20:101–111
10. Consensus development conference: diagnosis, prophylaxis, and treatment of osteoporosis. The American Journal of Medicine 1993, 94:646–650
11. Dennerstein L, Burrows G D, Hyman G et al 1978 Menopausal hot flushes, a double-blind comparison of placebo, ethinyl oestradiol and norgestrel. British Journal of Obstetrics and Gynaecology 85:852–856
12. Dennerstein L, Smith A, Morse C et al 1993 Menopausal symptomatology: the experience of Australian women. The Medical Journal of Australia 159:232–236
13. Falkeborn M, Persson I, Adami H O et al 1992 The risk of acute myocardial infarction after oestrogen and oestrogen–progestogen replacement. British Journal of Obstetrics and Gynaecology 99:821–828
14. Hagstad A, Janson P O 1986 The epidemiology of climacteric symptoms. Acta Obstetricia Gynecologica Scandinavica (Suppl) 134:59–65
15. Hällström T, Samuelsson S 1985 Mental health in the climacteric. The longitudinal study of women in Gothenburg. Acta Obstetricia Gynecologica Scandinavica (Suppl) 130:13–18
16. Hammar M, Berg G, Fåhraeus I et al 1984 Climacteric symptoms in an unselected sample of Swedish women. Maturitas 6:345–350

17. Henriksson L, Sternquist M, Boquist L et al 1994 A comparative multicenter study of the effects of continuous low-dose estradiol released from a new vaginal ring versus estriol vaginal pessaries in postmenopausal women with symptoms and signs of urogenital atrophy. The American Journal of Obstetrics and Gynecology 171:624–632

18. Holte A, Mikkelsen A 1991 The menopausal syndrome: a factor analytic replication. Maturitas 13:193–203

19. Holte A 1992 Influences of natural menopause on health complaints: a prospective study of healthy Norwegian women. Maturitas 14:127–141

20. Holte A 1991 Prevalence of climacteric complaints in a representative sample of middle-aged women in Oslo, Norway. Journal of Psychosomatic Obstetrics and Gynaecology 12:303–317

21. Hulley S, Grady D, Bush T et al 1998 Randomized trial of estrogen plus progestin for secondary prevention of coronary heart disease in postmenopausal women. Heart and Estrogen/progestin Replacement Study (HERS) Research Group. The Journal of the American Medical Association 280:605–613

22. Hunter M, Battersby R, Whitehead M I 1986 Relationship between psychological symptoms, somatic complaints and menopausal status. Maturitas 8:217–228

23. Hunter M 1992 The South-East England longitudinal study of the climacteric and postmenopause. Maturitas 14:117–126

24. Hunter M S 1990 Somatic experience of the menopause. A prospective study. Psychosomatic Medicine 52:357–367

25. Iosif C S, Batra S, Ek A et al 1981 Estrogen receptors in the human lower urinary tract. American Journal of Obstetrics and Gynecology 141:817–820

26. Iosif C S, Henriksson L, Ulmsten U 1981 The frequency of disorders of the lower urinary tract, urinary incontinence in particular as evaluated by a questionnaire survey in a gynecological health control population. Acta Obstetricia Gynecologica Scandinavica 60:71–76

27. Jaszman L J B 1976 Epidemiology of the climacteric syndrome. In: Campbell S (ed) The Management of the Menopause and the Postmenopausal Years. MTP Press, Lancaster, p 11–23

28. Kaufert P, Gilbert P, Tate R 1992 The Manitoba project: a re-examination of the relationship between the menopause and depression. Maturitas 14:143–156

29. Kaufert P A, Gilbert P, Hassard T 1988 Researching the symptoms of the menopause: an exercise in methodology. Maturitas 10:117–131

30. Lindgren R, Berg G, Hammar M et al 1993 Hormonal replacement therapy and sexuality in a population of Swedish postmenopausal women. Acta Obstetricia Gynecologica Scandinavica 72:292–297

31. Lock M, Kaufert P, Gilbert P 1988 Cultural construction of the menopausal syndrome: the Japanese case. Maturitas 10:317–332

32. McKinlay J, McKinlay S M, Brambilla D 1987 The relative contribution of endocrine changes and social circumstances to depression in mid-aged women. Journal of Health and Social Behavior 28:345–356

33. McKinlay S M, Brambilla D J, Posner J C 1992 The normal menopause transition. Maturitas 14:103–115

34. McKinlay S M, Jeffreys M 1974 The menopausal syndrome. Journal of the British Society of Preventive Medicine 28:108–115

35. Martin M C, Block J E, Sanchez S D et al 1993 Menopause without symptoms: the endocrinology of the menopause among rural Mayan Indians. American Journal of Obstetrics and Gynecology 168:1839–1843

36. Mattsson L-Å, Cullberg G 1983 A clinical evaluation of treatment with estriol vaginal cream versus suppository in postmenopausal women. Acta Obstetricia Gynecologica Scandinavica 62:397–401

37. Milsom I, Arvidsson L, Ekelund P et al 1993 Factors influencing vaginal cytology, pH and bacterial flora in elderly women. Acta Obstetricia Gynecologica Scandinavica 72:286–291

38. Milsom I, Molander U 1998 Urogenital ageing. The Journal of the British Menopause Society 4:151–156

39. Molander U, Milsom I, Ekelund P et al 1990 Effect of oral oestriol on vaginal flora and cytology and urogenital symptoms in the post-menopause. Maturitas 12:113–120

40. Moore B 1981 Climacteric symptoms in an African community. Maturitas 3:25–29

41. Nagata C, Matsushita Y, Shimizu H 1996 Prevalence of hormone replacement therapy and users' characteristics: a community survey in Japan. Maturitas 25:201–207

42. Nilsson K, Heimer G 1992 Low-dose oestradiol in the treatment of urogenital oestrogen deficiency – a pharmacokinetic and pharmacodynamic study. Maturitas 15:121–127

43. Oldenhave A, Jaszman L, Haspels A et al 1993 Impact of climacteric on well-being.

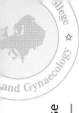

American Journal of Obstetrics and Gynecology 168:772–780

44. Osborne N G, Wright R C, Grubin L 1979 Genital bacteriology: a comparative study of premenopausal women with postmenopausal women. American Journal of Obstetrics and Gynecology 135;195–198

45. Rebar R 1987 The physiology and measurement of hot flushes. American Journal of Obstetrics and Gynecology 156:1284–1288

46. Rees M C P 1997 The need to improve compliance to HRT. British Journal of Obstetrics and Gynaecology 107 (Suppl 16):1–3

47. Rödström K, Bengtsson C, Lissner L et al 2002 A longitudinal study of women in Gothenburg during a quarter of a century. Menopause 9:156–161.

48. Rossouw JE, Anderson G L, Prentice R L et al 2002 Risks and benefits of estrogen plus progestin in healthy postmenopausal women: principal results from the Women's Health Initiative randomized controlled trial. The Journal of the American Medical Association 288:321–333

49. Sharma V K, Saxena M S L 1981 Climacteric symptoms: a study in the Indian context. Maturitas 3:11–20

50. Sherwin B B, Gelfand M M 1985 Differential symptom response to parenteral estrogen and/or androgen administration in the surgical menopause. American Journal of Obstetrics and Gynecology 151:153–160

51. Sherwin B B, Gelfand M M 1988 Sex steroids and affect in surgical menopause: a double-blind cross-over study. Psychoneuroendocrinology 13:345–357

52. Stadberg E, Mattsson L-Å, Milsom I 1997 The prevalence and severity of climacteric symptoms and use of different treatment regimens in a Swedish population. Acta Obstetricia Gynecologica Scandinavica 76:442–448

53. Stampfer M J, Colditz G A, Willett W C et al 1991 Postmenopausal estrogen therapy and cardiovascular disease. Ten-year follow-up from the nurses' health study. The New England Journal of Medicine 325:756–762

54. Sturdee D W, Reece B L 1979 Thermography of menopausal hot flushes. Maturitas 1:201–205

55. Sturdee D W, Wilson K A, Pipili E et al 1978 Physiological aspects of menopausal hot flushes. British Medical Journal 2:79–80

56. Tepper R, Neri A, Kaufman H et al 1987 Menopausal hot flushes and plasma β-endorphins. Obstetrics and Gynecology 70:150–152

57. Thunell L, Stadberg E, Milsom I et al 2004 A longitudinal study of climacteric symptoms and their treatment in a random sample of Swedish women. Climacteric 7:357–365

58. Utian W H 1997 Menopause – a modern perspective from a controversial history. Maturitas 26:73–82

59. Voda A M 1981 Climacteric hot flash. Maturitas 3:73–90

60. Wilson R A 1966 Feminine Forever. M Evans, New York

3

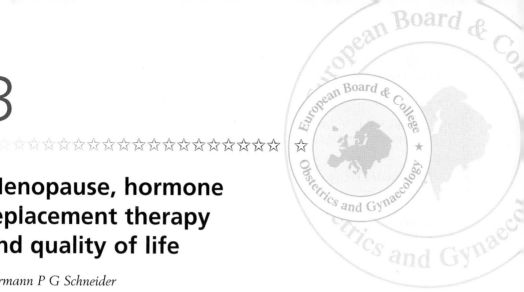

Menopause, hormone replacement therapy and quality of life

Hermann P G Schneider

ABSTRACT

For a complete assessment of the outcomes of any intervention, the impact on patients in terms of health status and health-related quality of life ought to be documented. Unlike conventional medical indicators, individual perceptions of health and illness point to the individual's attitude toward health, doctors and hospital care.

Patient-assessed health outcome measures are classified as disease- or population-specific and may be generic or dimension-specific. Among generic measures, SF-36, Sickness Impact Profile, and Nottingham Health Profile dominate. Menopause with its multiplicity of symptoms has attained standardized specific scales, which satisfy the criteria of factor analysis, subscale structure, sound psychometric properties and standardization using representative populations of climacteric women. According to their chronological order, these are the Greene Climacteric Scale, Women's Health Questionnaire, Menopause Symptom List, Menopause Rating Scale (MRS) and Utian Quality of Life Score.

The MRS, with its three independent factorial dimensions of somato-vegetative, psychological and urogenital symptoms, consists of a total of 11 items, each rated on a five-point scale of severity. The MRS has been validated in eight languages and its construct validity was established by extended practical experience.

European women's perceptions of hormone replacement therapy (HRT), as surveyed in Germany, the UK, France and Spain, point to greater awareness of HRT as a treatment option for menopausal symptoms. HRT users tend to be better informed than non-users. Preventive and therapeutic aspects of HRT remain widely unchallenged by the results of the Women's Health Initiative (WHI). Quality of life is perceived as a major health benefit, which causes women to start or continue HRT.

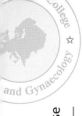

☆ ☆☆☆☆☆☆☆☆☆☆☆☆☆☆☆☆☆☆☆☆☆☆☆

KEYWORDS

Climacteric symptomatology, European women's perception of hormone replacement therapy, menopausal transition, quality of life, standardized menopause-specific scales

INTRODUCTION

Population surveys, clinical trials and other forms of evaluated study increasingly incorporate self-reported measures from patients to help determine if treatments are doing more good than harm, if health and quality of life are improving or worsening, or which particular item may differ.[9] For a complete assessment of the outcomes of any intervention, it is essential to provide evidence of the impact on patients in terms of health status and health-related quality of life. When patient-reported outcomes are assessed, they need to be compared to clinical measurements that remain the primary end-points for most clinical trials and represent important markers for disease, injury and their trajectories. But unlike conventional medical indicators, the broader impacts of illness and treatment need, wherever possible, to be assessed and reported by the patient. Individual perceptions of health and illness influence what people do about their health, whether or not they visit doctors, refer to a hospital, or ignore signs and symptoms. By that token, policy makers are particularly interested in these outcomes.[25]

The literature of patient-assessed health outcome measures comprises some 3921 reports, of which 1819 (46%) were disease- or population-specific measures, 865 (22%) were generic, 690 (18%) were dimension-specific, 409 (10%) were utility and 62 (1%) were individualized.[9] From 1990 to 1999, the number of new reports of development and evaluation rose from 144 to 650 per year; reports of disease-specific measures rose exponentially. Over 30% of evaluations were in cancer, rheumatology and musculoskeletal disorders, and older people's health. The generic measures – SF-36, Sickness Impact Profile and Nottingham Health Profile – accounted for 612 (16%) reports.[9]

Many researchers have been criticized for their failure to use appropriate measures of health-related quality of life when addressing the impact of interventions. Reasons may be inappropriate or poorly validated indicators, the lack of appropriate and widely adopted methods or practical and logistical difficulties in obtaining reliable reports. The recent enthusiasm for the potential of questionnaires to provide accurate evidence of outcomes from the patients' perspectives has generated a realm of less well-developed methods. These may add to the problems of generally agreed definition, theoretical bases, the appropriate use of measures and the recognition of the social basis of definitions and measurements with a resultant confusion as to quality of life and quality of care.[17]

QUALITY OF LIFE CONCEPTS

There is no universally accepted definition of quality of life and it is constantly being redefined.[1] About 50 years ago, the World Health Organization (WHO)

defined health as 'complete physical, mental and emotional well-being'. In 1993, the WHO more specifically defined quality of life as 'individual perceptions of their position of life in the context of the culture and value systems in which they live and in relation to the goals, standards and concerns'.[36] The definition includes six domains: physical health; psychological state; levels of independence; social relationships; environmental features; and spiritual concerns. Quality of life may also be defined as 'the extent to which our hopes and visions are met by experience'.[6] Health status, functional status, well-being, quality of life and health-related quality of life are concepts that are used interchangeably in discourse and measurement.

A new WHO publication of 2001 presented the International Classification of Functioning, Disability and Health (ICF). It was accepted by 191 countries as the international standard to describe and measure health and disability. Using the ICF framework, the WHO estimates that as much as 500 million healthy life-years are lost each year due to disability associated with health conditions. This is more than half the years that are lost annually due to premature death. The ICF takes into account the social aspects of disability and provides a mechanism to document the impact of the social and physical environment on an individual's functioning. It puts all disease and health conditions on an equal footing irrespective of their cause. For example, a person may not be able to attend work because of a cold or angina, but also because of depression. This neutral approach puts mental disorders on a par with physical illness and has contributed to the recognition and documentation of the worldwide burden of depressive disorders, which is currently a leading cause, worldwide, of life-years lost due to disability.[37] In order to provide adequate construct validity, the WHO is carrying out worldwide health surveys to collect data based on the ICF.

MENOPAUSAL TRANSITION

Menopause is a transition in life and therefore differs from illness. Moreover, menopause challenges self-identity, which may be determined by age-related changes, illness, cognitions and symptom attributions. These need to be taken into account when assessing changes that affect quality of life during the menopause.[2]

Contemporary views on the natural history and progress of the menopause have recently been ascertained.[5] The postreproductive longevity of the human female is unprecedented biologically. On the other hand, the end of reproductive capacity signals the end of the possibility of Darwinian adaptation, positive adaptation to the state of oestrogen deficiency may become maladaptive. Our mastery of the environment, public health measures and the availability of antibiotics have led to a doubling of the average lifespan. An adaptation to falling oestrogen levels or oestrogen deficiency occurs on several physiological occasions. The puerperium has been taken as a useful model as this is the time when the mother makes a covenant with her newborn offspring. She might stay alive, keep the newborn alive, and develop the means of nurturing it until puberty. The maladaptive response to the menopause is represented by increased arterial resistance

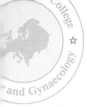

and its cardiovascular consequences, conservation of energy and mobilization of fat from the femoral area, bone loss as a result of calcium mobilization, and neurological consequences such as flushing and diminished sleep. In the absence of postreproductive Darwinian adaptation, the changes that occur in all tissues – in contrast to what women will experience in reproductive years – may be harmful in postreproductive life (F Naftolin, personal communication). The fundamental significance of reproductive versus chronological age becomes apparent. This is why we advocate adequate treatment of women as of their postreproductive phase of life.

According to the Massachusetts Women's Health Study, which provided data from 2577 women, the median age for the onset of menopause is 51.3 years, and the range of menopause is approximately 48 to 55.[22] The perimenopausal transition, for most women, would last for approximately 4 years. Thinner women experience a slightly earlier menopause,[23] obviously related to the contribution of body fat to oestrogen production. Factors of little influence are race, income, geography, parity or height.[22,23] The cessation of menses by most women is perceived to have almost no impact on subsequent physical and mental health.[22] The Massachusetts Women's Health Study has provided information that women would express either positive or neutral feelings about menopause with the exception of those who experience surgical menopause. By that token, the majority of women feel healthy and happy and do not seek contact with physicians. Medical intervention at this point should be regarded as an opportunity to provide and reinforce a programme of preventive healthcare. Such issues for women include stopping smoking, the control of body weight and alcohol consumption, prevention of heart disease and osteoporosis, maintenance of mental well-being (including sexuality), cancer screening and the treatment of neurological problems.

The Melbourne Women's Midlife Health Project has defined the most common symptoms of the menopausal transition as ageing and stiff joints, lack of energy, hot flushes, nervous tension, trouble sleeping and feelings of being sad and downhearted.[5] The only changes in symptom scores that were specifically related to the occurrence of the menopausal transition included hot flushes, dryness of the vagina, night sweats and trouble sleeping, and the disappearance of breast soreness. An increase in central abdominal fat was noted during the transition and was associated with baseline weight, weight increase, baseline free testosterone and an increase in free testosterone. Oestradiol (E_2) was the only specific predictor of change in bone mineral density (BMD). BMD loss was dependent on the final value of E_2 and it was noted that an E_2 level of 240 pmol/L was required for the preservation of BMD. No other hormones or changes in hormone levels had a significant effect. Body mass index, exercise and calcium did not relate to bone loss during the transition. It was also noted that depressed mood declined significantly with age but that the transition accentuated symptoms that tended to foster a depressed mood. The transition may also amplify the mood effects of job loss, poor health and daily hassles, making the menopausal transition a phase of vulnerability.

The change from early to late menopause was also associated with a significant variation in a number of parameters of sexual function. These include decreased feelings for the partner, decreased responsivity, decreased libido, increased vaginal dyspareunia and an increase in partner problems. From late perimenopause to postmenopause, there was a further decline in responsivity and sexual frequency, a small further decrease in libido, an increase in dyspareunia and growing partner problems.

Menopause has also been looked at as a wonderful signal occurring at the right time of life when preventive healthcare is especially critical.[33] This way, menopause is considered a normal stage in development, incorporating biology, psychology, society and culture.

HOW CAN QUALITY OF LIFE BE MEASURED IN THE CLIMACTERIC?

Improvement of quality of life is a primary purpose of health promotion. This can be achieved by preventive health programmes with their greater impact on morbidity rather than mortality.[8] The aim is maximal vigour in life rather than accepting linear senescence. Some linear decline is unavoidable but the slope can be changed by effort and practice.

ADEQUATE ASSESSMENT

To be adequate is an essential minimum but it may not be enough to do justice to an important aspect of healthcare.[1] Assessments of quality of life in the menopause have been inadequate to a large extent.[9] Garratt and co-workers pointed to the low level of development and evaluation in gynaecology, in spite of the psychosocial distress reported in gynaecology clinics. They admit that the selection of measures can be daunting. However, before constructing a new measure for an immediate purpose, validated constructs should be critically reviewed and adopted.

Some examples may illustrate inadequate assessment.[1] The agenda of the medical profession and their women patients may not be the same. Janice Rymer and her colleagues have recently published a clinical review on making decisions about HRT.[28] They illustrate the confusion of current medical advice and the impact of the result of the HERS study[16] and the WHI investigation.[38] Their review includes the benefits and risks of the effects of relief of menopausal symptoms and quotes only one study on the effect of oestrogen on quality of life in which the latter is measured by a utility model. The benefits and risks of osteoporosis, cardiovascular disease, thromboembolic disease, and colorectal, breast, endometrial and ovarian cancer are reviewed. They conclude that for symptomatic perimenopausal women, sequential HRT for one to two years is likely to improve quality of life with minimal risk. It is not clear, however, what the authors mean by 'quality of life' other than a reduction of menopausal symptoms.

Most women during the menopausal transition expect HRT to alleviate their menopausal symptoms and improve their quality of life. The ancillary WHI

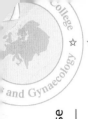

study reported by Hays et al challenges this expectation.[13] The participants of this randomized controlled trial were also assessed at baseline and at one year on a number of quality-of-life measures – the results show that HRT has no benefit in any quality of life measures. In women with moderate to severe vasomotor symptoms at baseline, there was a small benefit in sleep disturbance but no benefit in the other quality-of-life measures. Deborah Grady concludes that there is no role for HRT in the treatment of women without menopausal symptoms.[10] The WHI study used a checklist of menopausal symptoms but no standardized validated measure with accepted psychometric properties. The response categories were summed to give an overall score although previous research has used factor analysis, which shows that symptoms are not independent or of equal weight.[1] The rationale for the choice of the other quality-of-life measure is not apparent. The measure of sexual functioning was a single item and gives no measure of arousal, responsiveness or libido. The Modified Mini Mental State examination is not a sensitive measure of cognitive improvement in healthy, relatively intelligent adults. There was no measure of social functioning or of self-esteem.

ASPECTS OF CLIMACTERIC SYMPTOMATOLOGY

The standard method used for collecting information on the prevalence and severity of menopausal symptoms has been a checklist of symptoms. Symptoms are defined as 'an indication of a disease or a disorder noticed by the patient himself. A presenting symptom is one that leads a patient to consult a doctor.'[24]

In general, symptoms represent a subjective expression or manifestation of some underlying physical, psychological or social dysfunction. Symptoms are, in effect, evidence of disease.[11] Why do women seek medical assistance during the climacteric? Most of the time for hot flushes and sweating, atrophy of the vaginal epithelium, atrophic urethritis with a formation of urethral caruncles, dyspareunia and pruritus due to vulvar, introital and vaginal atrophy; also for urinary difficulties such as stress incontinence, urgency and abacterial urethritis and cystitis. In addition, psychological symptoms such as anxiety, depressive mood, irritability, insomnia and decreased libido are extremely common.

The menopause is associated with a multiplicity of symptoms. Involutional melancholia and depressive mood may appear as psychiatric disturbances. However, a deleterious effect of the menopause on mental health is not supported by psychiatric investigation. Even depression, contrary to general belief, is less common among middle-aged women.[12] Conversely, the menopause may increase minor 'psychological' complaints. Becoming forgetful in their advanced years is a concern of many women, hence the differentiation of the ageing process from pathological memory loss is an important clinical task. There may be gender differences in cognition during the ageing process and in the course of dementia. Sex hormones appear to have a role in neuronal development and act as neuroactive substances. This relates to neuronal outgrowth and protection as well as immune-based metabolic clearance.[7]

Coronary risk factors are highly prevalent among older women. About a third of middle-aged women have hypertension, over a quarter of these are cigarette smokers and the same fraction are also overweight. These risk factors tend to predominate in populations of lower socioeconomic class as well as with lower educational levels. Relative coronary risk is impaired by gender. The relative risk of hypertension is comparable for women and men, at about 1.5; the gender risk for developing hypercholesterolaemia is 1.1 and 1.4, respectively; for diabetes 2.4 and 1.9, respectively; for overweight 1.4 and 1.3, respectively; and for smoking 1.8 and 1.6, respectively.[3] The proposed positive effects of oestrogen on cardiovascular risk were thought to be attributed to improvements in the lipid profile, most notably an increase in high-density lipoprotein cholesterol. The development of a proinflammatory state has been suggested as a possible mechanism whereby oestrogen may exert an early, negative cardiovascular effect. Individual variability of response to oestrogen has led to a search for genetic influences on the cardiovascular effects of oestrogen. Evidence now suggests that the woman's response to oestrogens may vary depending on the presence or absence of one or more common variants of the oestrogen receptor α (ER-α) gene. Furthermore, recently published new preliminary data suggest that postmenopausal women taking HRT (and older men) are at a higher risk for clinical or anatomic manifestations of coronary disease if they have the ER-α IVS1-397 C allele or other closely linked variants in the ER-α gene.[15] The effect of such gene polymorphisms on oestrogen-sensitive clinical events is not yet known. However, if there is indeed an oestrogen-sensitive phenotype defined by the presence or absence of certain ER-α polymorphisms, this would suggest that genetic screening may ultimately assist clinicians and women in making better decisions about use of HRT.[15]

Other longstanding metabolic consequences of the climacteric include osteoporosis and osteoporotic fractures, skin changes, weight gain and obesity as well as degenerative diseases of the central nervous system (CNS). Ongoing research is looking into the action of oestrogen and other sex steroids on the vascular system, immunity, CNS function or musculoskeletal disease, with special emphasis on the cellular level. Detailed knowledge of symptoms, however, and their effects on the daily life of women, will assist the caregiver in providing competent care and generate means of longstanding professional assistance during the ageing process. Objective information about an individual's symptoms is very helpful in providing objective information about the way in which the climacteric may affect quality of life.

STANDARDIZED MENOPAUSE-SPECIFIC SCALES

Reliable and valid measures of multisymptom conditions generally come in the form of scales and subscales, developed on the basis of principles of test construction and scaling.[26] In the field of psychology, the techniques developed to construct such measures became known as psychometrics. The assessment of differences between individuals required the construction of measures sensitive enough to distinguish between subjects and the various items under investigation. This, in turn, led to attempts to construct 'scales'. Scales, by definition, are instruments that measure phenomena on a continuum using ordinal scaling.[11] Scales measuring more complex human characteristics, such as intelligence or personality traits, invariably consist of a number of items which are summated to give an overall score for each person. They usually consist of a number of symptoms, yielding a total score which reflects the degree of severity of a condition along a graded continuum for each individual. Moreover, each symptom is usually rated in terms of its frequency of occurrence or severity.

Scales and subscales

Scales for measuring a complex phenomenon or multifaceted syndromes are generally made up of a number of subscales, each measuring a different facet of the syndrome. However, summating symptoms from apparently different domains is meaningless. In order to understand methodological evaluation better, Greene has pointed to the overall measure of 'size' as the addition of a person's height and waist measurements. Such a measure would fail to distinguish tall and thin from small and obese people, as both would tend to have a similar overall 'size' score.[11] Similarly, the common practice of reporting symptoms individually is bound to fail because such a measure would not assess a condition comprehensively.

Scales for measuring human characteristics or conditions have been categorized into two types: general and condition-specific. Thus the types of questionnaire developed focus on either generic or disease- and treatment-specific aspects. The contents of the different generic scales are similar in many ways, as they all assess the ability of patients to cope with their condition physically, emotionally and socially, including their general performance at work and in daily life. The more commonly used instruments are the Sickness Impact Profile,[4] the Nottingham Health Profile,[18] the Quality of Well-Being Scale[20] or the Short-Form (SF)-36 Health Survey.[21] The generic measures cover the multidimensional aspects of quality of life over a wide range of health problems. The scales may be less responsive to treatment-induced changes and could be considered lengthy and time-consuming.

The disease-specific measures are more likely to be responsive and make sense to clinicians as well as to patients. Their specific measures relate to concepts and domains in patient populations, diagnostic groups or diseases. One of the very first was the Women's Health Questionnaire (WHQ), a menopause-specific instrument.[19] The WHQ consists of a final 32 items, including eight subscales, and assesses, in addition to vasomotor symptoms, important areas such as further somatic symptoms, mood, sleeping problems, cognitive difficulties and sexual functioning.

Factor analysis

Factor analysis is a multivariant mathematical technique traditionally used in psychometrics to construct measures of psychological and behavioural characteristics, such as intellectual abilities or personality traits.[11] It addresses the problem of how to analyse the structure of the interrelationships (correlations) among a large number of variables (test scores, questionnaire responses, behaviour, symptoms) by identifying a set of underlying dimensions known as factors. The overall objective of factor analysis is data summarization and data reduction.

A key aspect of factor analysis is the orderly simplification of a number of interrelated measures. Factor analysis describes the data using many fewer dimensions than the original variables. It is designed to order and give structure to observed variables and, as a result, allows for the construction of instruments in the form of scales and subscales.

The relationship between a symptom and a factor is measured by a correlation coefficient known as factor loading. This way, an instrument can be constructed which consists of separate subscales and will measure different aspects of the symptom picture, based on the way symptoms cluster together within factors and on the size of the factor loadings. This results in a scale which yields a symptom profile for each subject.[11] In the end, by identifying symptoms that cluster together or form groups of factors, one may be able to delineate facets of the symptom picture and identify those symptoms that are an essential part of a syndrome and those which are not.

Menopause-specific instruments

Gerald Greene has formulated the four criteria that standardized menopause-specific scales should satisfy:[11]

1. To be constructed on the basis of a factor analysis.
2. To consist of several subscales, each measuring a different aspect of climacteric symptomatology.
3. To possess sound psychometric properties.
4. To be standardized using representative populations of climacteric women.

The following five enlisted scales fulfil these four criteria. Their subscales correspond to the factors that have emerged in the course of factor analysis. The structure of each of the scales is listed in Table 3.1. The five scales, according to their chronological order of construction, are the:

1. Greene Climacteric Scale;
2. Women's Health Questionnaire;
3. Menopause Symptom List;
4. Menopause Rating Scale;
5. Utian Quality of Life Score.

The characteristics of each of these menopause-specific instruments are listed in Table 3.2. The Greene Climacteric Scale was the first climacteric symptom scale to be constructed on the basis of a factor analysis. After some modifications, the final version of the scale consists of 21 symptoms, each rated on a four-point scale of severity.[11] Test–retest reliability coefficients of the subscales achieved a satisfactory level. Years of usage attained construct validity.

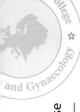

The menopause

and Gynaecology

☆ ☆☆☆☆☆☆☆☆☆☆☆☆☆☆☆☆☆☆☆☆☆☆☆

Table 3.1 Subscale structure of standardized menopause-specific scales

Greene Climacteric Scale	Women's Health Questionnaire	Menopausal Symptom List	Menopause Rating Scale	Utian QoL Score
Vasomotor	Vasomotor	Vasosomatic	Somato-vegetative	Emotional
Somatic	Somatic	General somatic	Urogenital	Occupational
Anxiety	Anxiety	Psychological	Psychological	Health
Depression	Depression	Sexual		
	Cognitive			
	Sleep			
	Sex			
	Menstrual			

Adapted with permission from reference 11.

Table 3.2 Characteristics of standardized menopause-specific scales

Name of scale	Number of items	Rating points	Rating measure	Number of subscales	Reliability of subscales
Greene Climacteric Scale	21	4	Severity	4	0.83–0.87
Women's Health Questionnaire	32	2	Present/ Absent	8	0.78–0.96
Menopausal Symptom List	25	6	Frequency Severity	3	0.73–0.83
Menopause Rating Scale	11	5	Severity	3	0.60 (average)[a]
Utian QoL Score	23	5	Severity	4	Not available

[a] Over a period of 1.5 years.
Adapted with permission from reference 11.

The Women's Health Questionnaire was based on a factor analysis of 36 symptoms reported by a general population sample of climacteric women in south-east England. The final version consists of eight subscales, four of which are identical to those of the Greene Climacteric Scale. The final scale contains 32 symptoms, each rated in a binary fashion (0/1). There is also satisfactory test–retest reliability. This questionnaire has often been used as a comparative measure, thereby demonstrating its construct validity.

The Menopause Symptom List was constructed on the basis of a principle components factor analysis of 56 symptoms presented by a small general population of Australian women.[27] The scale consists of three subscales: vasosomatic; general somatic; and psychological. The latter combines the anxiety and depression subscales of the Greene Climacteric Scale and the Women's Health Questionnaire. The vasomotor subscale, besides two vasomotor symptoms, also includes other somatic symptoms for reasons not quite apparent. The final version of the scale consists of 25 symptoms, each rated on a six-point scale of both frequency and severity. Test–retest reliability coefficients are satisfactory while validation experience is limited.

The Menopause Rating Scale (MRS) was standardized on a large general population sample of German women in which the factor analysis identified three independent factorial dimensions: somato-vegetative; psychological; and urogenital symptoms (Table 3.3). The somato-vegetative subscale contains vasomotor symptoms in addition to other somatic complaints. The psychological subscale is a combination of anxiety and depressive symptoms.

The final MRS consists of 11 symptoms, each rated on a five-point scale of severity (see Table 3.3). According to WHO Standards the degrees of severity are consistent with:

- No problem   none, absent, negligible   0–4%
- Mild problems   slight, low   5–24%
- Moderate problems   medium, fair   25–49%
- Severe problems   high, extreme   50–95%
- Complete problems   total   95–100%

as to symptoms.[37]

The highest MRS score should therefore be relabelled 'total' rather than 'extremely severe'. In its subsample of women retested in a follow-up over a period of 1.5 years, a high degree of stability in all three subscales and total scores was noted.[30] Both the psychological and somato-vegetative subscales were compared with each of the eight multi-item scales from the SF-36, subdivided into quartiles.[31] These subscales did not correlate equally across all dimensions of the

Table 3.3   Validated items of the Menopause Rating Scale

Item	Description
1	Hot flushes, sweating (episodes of sweating)
2	Heart discomfort (unusual awareness of heart beat, heart skipping, heart racing, tightness)
3	Sleep problems (difficulty falling asleep, difficulty in sleeping through the night, waking up too early)
4	Depressive mood (feeling 'down', sad, on the verge of tears, lack of drive, mood swings)
5	Irritability (feeling nervous, inner tension, feeling aggressive)
6	Anxiety (inner restlessness, feeling 'panicky')
7	Physical and mental exhaustion (general decrease in performance, impaired memory, decrease in concentration, forgetfulness)
8	Sexual problems (change in sexual desire, in sexual activity and satisfaction)
9	Bladder problems (difficulty in urinating, increased need to urinate, bladder incontinence)
10	Dryness of the vagina (sensation of dryness or burning in the vagina, difficulty with sexual intercourse)
11	Joint and muscular discomfort (pain in the joints, rheumatoid complaints)

Adapted with permission from reference 32.

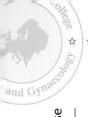
SF-36; there was, however, a pattern of correlations – the highest being with those domains of the SF-36 that are most relevant to women during the menopausal transition. The degree of severity of menopausal symptoms, as measured with the MRS, does reflect the profile of quality-of-life dimensions of SF-36 for postmenopausal women.

The MRS has been validated in eight languages – first into English,[32] followed by French, Spanish, Swedish, Mexican, Turkish, Brazilian and Indonesian.[14] In addition, its construct validity was established in a clinical trial for sequential HRT.[29] This extended practical experience with the MRS leaves no doubt as to the improvement of quality of life as the result of practice-based HRT during menopausal transition.

The Utian Menopause Quality of Life Score was based on a two-stage factorial process. The scale is not exclusively a symptom measure, although it does contain one scale related to emotional well-being. Other subscales refer to occupational, health and sexual aspects of quality of life. The final scale consists of 23 items, each rated on a five-point Likert scale.[35] Reliability and validity data are not yet available. The authors advocate the use of their scale in conjunction with a standardized measure of climacteric symptoms.

EUROPEAN WOMEN'S PERCEPTION OF HORMONE REPLACEMENT THERAPY

In the first quarter of 2003, a cross-sectional survey was conducted in four European countries (Germany, the UK, France and Spain) to ascertain the current profile of menopausal women.[34] A stratified sample of 8012 women, aged 45 to 75 years, was questioned via standardized computer-aided telephone interviewing. Quotas were used as to age, regional distribution and educational level to ensure that a representative sample of women was drawn from four different survey countries.

A total of 73% of all interviewed women were aware of HRT as a treatment option for menopausal symptoms, this percentage varying from 41% in Spain to 90% in the UK. Among non-HRT users, the proportion of women who had heard of HRT was, on average, 60%. Women were well informed about the most widely discussed benefits and risks of HRT, osteoporosis prevention and breast cancer. When it comes to less well-known risk such as uterine or colon cancer, the majority of HRT users, as well as 'never users', do not appear to be adequately informed. Regarding the effect of HRT on heart diseases, the opinion of two-thirds of the women rather reflect uncertainty either due to inadequate counselling or reinforced by the ongoing scientific debate on this topic.

European women do not only start HRT for present symptom relief, although 70% of the users state that this was one of the main reasons to initiate therapy. They also greatly value the possibility of preventing postmenopausal osteoporosis. Both effects of HRT remain unchallenged by the results of the WHI. The maintenance or improvement of general well-being is also closely linked to HRT use (Fig. 3.1). There is some variability in the ranking of the main reasons to start

The three most frequently mentioned HRT benefits and risks

Q: What do you think are the benefits of HRT in general?
Q: What do you think are the risks and disadvantages of HRT in general?

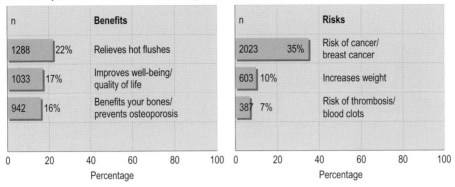

Fig 3.1 The three most frequently mentioned benefits and risks related to HRT. The figure is based on answers to the questions: what do you think are the benefits of HRT in general, and what do you think are the risks and disadvantages of HRT in general? Base n = 5837 women who knew about HRT.

HRT use, e.g. French women put the greatest emphasis on the prevention of osteoporosis instead of the relief of hot flushes, while British women considered relief from depressive mood, anxiety and irritability as highest ranking, then followed by osteoporosis prevention.

In order to further objectify well-being, the MRS had been applied in all countries. Mean MRS scores for individual symptoms were registered. The mean MRS score of HRT never users (n = 2.154) versus ever users (former and current, n = 2596) was 11 versus 9, respectively. However, while these differences are significant in Germany and the UK, the scores in France and Spain are indistinguishable. Of those women who identified themselves as symptom-free when starting HRT, a total of 86% (n = 524) would admit mild symptoms in at least one of the subscales of the MRS. Of the three MRS subscales, somato-vegetative factors scored highest, immediately followed by psychological factors such as irritability, anxiety and depressive mood, as well as physical and mental exhaustion (Fig. 3.2). This dominance of mental health is most apparent in France and Spain, less so in the UK and Germany.

There are major differences in the knowledge of HRT's benefits and risks among women in the four survey countries. Expectations of the therapy vary according to different cultural backgrounds. Among reasons for starting or continuing HRT, items of mental health are high-ranking, and quality of life is perceived as a major HRT benefit.

CONCLUSION

Quality of life is best defined by individual perceptions of physical health, psychological state, level of independence, social relationship, environment and spiritual

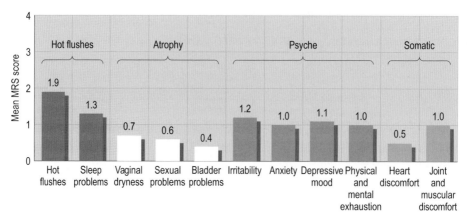

Fig 3.2 Menopause Rating Scale scores in European women before starting HRT.[34] The figure is based on the answer to the question: how severe were the following symptoms before you started HRT? Base n = 2596 current and former HRT users.

concern. Health status, functional status, well-being, quality of life, and health-related quality of life are concepts with interchangeable uses. In the end, quality of life may represent the extent to which our hopes and visions are met by experience.

Menopause – a transition in life – challenges self-identity, which may be determined by age-related changes, illness, cognitions and symptom attributions. The contemporary post-reproductive longevity of the human female, as yet, has not offered the possibility of Darwinian adaptation. Therefore, the state of oestrogen deficiency, in contrast to reproductive age, becomes maladaptive. The maladaptive response to menopause is represented by increased arterial resistance and its cardiovascular consequences, the conservation of energy and the mobilization of fat from the femoral area, bone loss as a result of calcium mobilization, and neurological consequences such as flushing and diminished sleep. All of this is not seen as a result of puerperal and lactational oestrogen deficiency. The fundamental significance of reproductive versus chronological age becomes apparent. This is why the adequate treatment of women as of their postreproductive phase of life is strongly advocated.

European women's perceptions of HRT, as surveyed in Germany, the UK, France and Spain, best represents today's HRT practice. Women are greatly aware of HRT as a treatment option for menopausal symptoms. They are also well informed about the most widely discussed benefits and risks of HRT, osteoporosis prevention and breast cancer. Regarding the effect on rarer cancer or cardiovascular disease, the opinion of two-thirds of the women rather reflects uncertainty, most likely due to inadequate counselling and reinforced by media impact. The main reasons why women start or abandon HRT remain largely unchallenged by recent critical epidemiology.

Menopause-specific instruments like the Greene Climacteric Scale, Women's Health Questionnaire, Menopause Symptom List, Menopause Rating Scale and Utian Quality of Life Score all serve the purpose of objective information about an individual woman's climacteric and the way in which it may affect her quality of life. On the basis of a widely applied MRS, it could be documented that expectations of HRT vary according to different cultural backgrounds. Among reasons for starting or continuing HRT, mental health is ranked highly. Overall, quality of life is perceived as a major health benefit.

References

1. Alder E M 2004 Adequately assessed quality of life. In: Schneider H P G, Naftolin F (eds) Climacteric Medicine: Where do we go? Parthenon, London
2. Alder E M 2002 How to assess quality of life: problems and methodology. In: Schneider H P G (ed) Hormone Replacement Therapy and Quality of Life. Parthenon, London, p 11–22
3. Anda R F, Waller M N, Wooten K G et al 1991 Behavioral risk factor surveillance, 1988. In: CDC Surveillance Summaries. M M W R, Vol 39, No 55-2, US Department of Health and Human Services, Centers for Disease Control, p 1–22
4. Bergner M 1993 Development, use and testing of the Sickness Impact Profile. In: Walker S, Rosser M (eds) Quality of Life Assessment: Key issues in the 1990s. Kluwer Academic Press, Dordrecht, p 201–209
5. Burger H G 2004 Natural history and progress of the menopause. In: Schneider H P G, Naftolin F (eds) Climacteric Medicine: Where do we go? Parthenon, London
6. Calman K C 1984 Quality of life in cancer patients – an hypothesis. Journal of Medical Ethics 10: 124–127
7. Diaz-Brinton R, Chen S, Montoya M et al 2000 The women's health initiative estrogen replacement therapy is neurotrophic and neuroprotective. Neurobiological Aging 21: 475–496
8. Fries J F, Green L W, Levine S 1989 Health promotion and the compression of morbidity. The Lancet 1:481
9. Garratt A, Schmidt L, MacKintosh A et al 2002 Quality of life measurement: bibliographic study of patient-assessed health outcome measures. British Medical Journal 324:1417–1421
10. Grady D 2003 Postmenopausal hormonal therapy for symptoms only. The New England Journal of Medicine 348:1835–1837
11. Greene J G 2002 Measuring the symptom dimension of quality of life: general and menopause-specific scales and their subscale structure. In: Schneider H P G (ed) Hormone Replacement Therapy and Quality of Life. Parthenon, London, p 35–44
12. Hällström T, Samuelsson S 1985 Mental health in the climacteric. The longitudinal study of women in Gothenburg. Acta Obstetricia Gynecologica Scandinavica Suppl 130: 13
13. Hays J, Ockene J K, Brunner R L et al 2003 Effects of estrogen plus progestin on health-related quality of life. The New England Journal of Medicine 348:1839–1854
14. Heinemann L A J, Potthoff P, Schneider H P G 2003 International versions of the Menopause Rating Scale (MRS). Health and Quality of Life Outcomes 1:28–31
15. Herrington D M, Howard T D, Hawkins G A et al 2002 Estrogen-receptor polymorphisms and effects of estrogen replacement on high-density lipoprotein cholesterol in women with coronary disease. The New England Journal of Medicine 34:967–974
16. Hulley S, Grady D, Bush T et al 1998 Randomized trial of estrogen plus progestin for secondary prevention of coronary heart disease in postmenopausal women. The Journal of the American Medical Association 280:605–613
17. Hunt S, McKenna S 1992 Do we need measures other than QALYs? In: Hopkins A (ed) Measures of the Quality of Life and the Uses to Which Such Measures May Be Put. Royal College of Physicians, London
18. Hunt S M, McKenna S P, McEwen J et al 1981 The Nottingham Health Profile: Subjective health and medical consultations. Social Science and Medicine 15A:221–229
19. Hunter M 1992 The Women's Health Questionnaire (WHQ): A measure of mid-aged women's perceptions of their

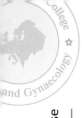
emotional and physical health. Psychology and Health 7:45–54

20. Kaplan R M, Anderson J P, Ganiats T 1993 The Quality of Wellbeing Scale: Rationale for a single quality of life index. In: Walker S, Rosser M (eds) Quality of Life Assessment: Key issues in the 1990s. Kluwer Academic Press, Dordrecht, p 65

21. McHorney C A, Ware J E, Raczek A E 1993 The MOS 36-item short-form health status survey (SF-36). II. Psychometric and clinical tests of validity in measuring physical and mental health constructs. Medical Care 31:247–263

22. McKinlay S M, Brambilla D J, Posner J G 1992 The normal menopause transition. Maturitas 14:102

23. MacMahon B, Worcester J 1966 Age at menopause US 1960–62. Vital Health Statistics 11:1

24. Martin E A 1994 The Oxford Medical Dictionary. Oxford University Press, Oxford

25. Patrick D L 2003 Patient-Reported Outcomes (PROs): An organizing tool for concepts, measures, and applications. Quality of Life Newsletter 31:1–5

26. Peck D, Shapiro C 1990 Measuring Human Problems: A practical guide. Wiley, Chichester

27. Perz J M 1997 Development of the Menopause Symptom Checklist. A factor analytic study of menopause-associated symptoms. Women and Health 25:53–69

28. Rymer J, Wilson R, Ballard K 2003 Making decisions about hormone replacement therapy. British Medical Journal 326:322–326

29. Schneider H P, Rosemeier H P, Schnitker J et al 2000 Application and factor analysis of the menopause rating scale [MRS] in a post-marketing surveillance study of Climen. Maturitas 37:113–124

30. Schneider H P G, Heinemann L A J, Rosemeier H P et al 2000 The Menopause Rating Scale (MRS): reliability of scores of menopausal complaints. Climacteric 3:59–64

31. Schneider H P G, Heinemann L A J, Rosemeier H P et al 2000 The Menopause Rating Scale (MRS): comparison with Kupperman index and quality-of-life scale SF-36. Climacteric 3:50–58

32. Schneider H P G, Heinemann L A J, Thiele K 2002 The Menopause Rating Scale (MRS): Cultural and linguistic validation into English. LAMSO 3

33. Speroff L 1994 A signal for the future. In: Lobo R (ed) Treatment of the Postmenopausal Woman. Raven Press, New York, p 1–8

34. Strothmann A, Schneider H P G 2003 Hormone replacement therapy: the European women's perspective. Climateric 6:337–346

35. Utian W H, Janata J W, Kingsberg S A et al 2000 Determinants and quantification of quality of life after the menopause: the Utian Menopause Quality of Life score. In: Aso T (ed) The Menopause at the Millennium. Parthenon, London, p 141–144

36. WHO Division of Mental Health 1993 WHO-QOL study protocol: The development of the World Health Organization quality of life assessment instrument (MNG/PSF/93)

37. WHO 2001 The WHO international classification of function (ICF). Press Release WHO/48, Geneva, 15 November

38. Writing Group for the Women's Health Initiative Investigators 2002 Risks and benefits of estrogen plus progesterone in healthy post-menopausal women. The Journal of the American Medical Association 288:321–333

4

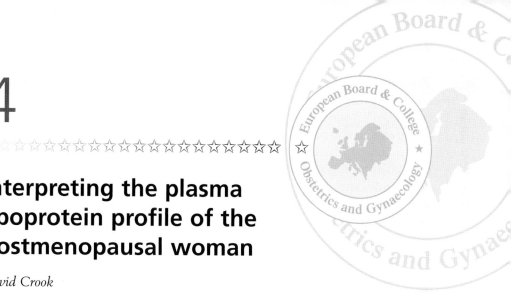

Interpreting the plasma lipoprotein profile of the postmenopausal woman

David Crook

ABSTRACT

Myocardial infarction (MI) and stroke are rare events in young women but emerge as major concerns in later life. There now exists a reasonably strong evidence base to justify measuring plasma cholesterol levels (if other risk factors are present) and using cholesterol-lowering drugs, such as statins, where appropriate. In contrast, the management of plasma triglyceride levels remains controversial – diet, exercise and other lifestyle modifications may be of benefit but are difficult to sustain. Hormone replacement therapy (HRT) can profoundly influence a woman's plasma lipoprotein profile. Interpretation of the extensive database on the effects of different therapies is now problematical as there is no evidence that any form of HRT is better than placebo in preventing arterial disease (and some evidence that it is worse). On *theoretical* grounds non-oral HRT might be safer than oral HRT in terms of arterial diseases, but in the absence of appropriate randomized controlled trials (RCTs) of clinically relevant end-points this remains a speculation.

KEYWORDS

Cholesterol, high-density lipoprotein (HDL), low-density lipoprotein (LDL), lipoprotein (a), myocardial infarction (MI), oestrogen, progestogen, stroke, triglycerides

INTRODUCTION

The development and refinement of HRT during the second half of the twentieth century have seen a constant and at times almost obsessive interest in the effects of these therapies on arterial disease risk markers such as plasma lipoprotein levels.

The initial impetus for this research came from the observation that oestrogens and androgens could influence the plasma lipoprotein profile in ways that were considered 'favourable' or 'unfavourable' in terms of arterial disease.[4] The lipoprotein profile seen in patients treated with oestrogens was noted to be similar to that seen in individuals at low risk of myocardial infarction (MI), whereas the profile induced by androgens was thought to resemble that seen with MI patients. For scientists interested in unraveling the details of plasma lipoprotein metabolism, steroid hormones offered an exciting and ultimately rewarding tool by which to perturb normal metabolism and so understand how the system worked. For those interested in the relationship between plasma lipoproteins and arterial disease these findings offered a new way of testing their hypotheses: if steroid hormones could be shown to have the clinical effects on arterial disease that would be predicted from their effects on the plasma lipoprotein profile then this would be a validation of the clinical usefulness of such measurements.

A third group of investigators contributed to these studies: those whose interests lay primarily in the health of postmenopausal women and specifically in the management of the climacteric. To this group the effects on plasma lipoprotein levels offered a possible insight into the long-term risk–benefit equation of HRT. Plasma lipid and lipoprotein levels rapidly became used as a surrogate for MI and stroke: to study the effects of different HRT formulations on these diseases would take many years and would cost tens of millions of euros. Plasma lipoprotein levels (and to a lesser extent those of glucose, insulin and coagulation factors) became accepted as an affordable way of refining and perfecting HRT in terms of the potential impact on vascular health.

Some researchers were always aware of the limitations of using disease surrogates but as the observational epidemiologists reported 50% less MI in HRT users as compared to non-users, as the studies in monkeys and other animals showed protection from diet-induced atherosclerosis and as the role of oestrogens as regulators of endothelial function emerged, these concerns were rarely voiced.

The main problem has been that our attitudes to risk are changing. The most obvious example is the increased plasma triglyceride levels induced by the oral administration of conjugated equine oestrogens (CEE) and (to a lesser extent) with oestradiol. At the time these were not considered to be a problem but now do cause concern, especially in the context of the triglyceride–coagulation–fibrinolysis axis.[5] The ability of oral (but not non-oral) oestrogens to increase plasma levels of C-reactive protein (CRP) toward those seen in patients at very high risk of arterial disease[8] is a relatively recent finding but one that would cause severe problems for a pharmaceutical company if their HRT product were to be put forward for licensing today.

I contend that the *potentially* harmful effects of certain HRT not only on triglyceride metabolism but also on low-density lipoprotein (LDL) particle size and factor VII coagulant activity were not given adequate consideration primarily because of the intense excitement generated by observational epidemiology, experimental pathology and haemodynamic studies. With few exceptions, there was relatively little in pursuing potentially adverse effects of formulations such as oral CEE/medroxyprogesterone acetate (CEE/MPA) when the consensus view was that this same formulation prevented MI. Instead, a research industry developed in which newer formulations were developed with the objective of being 'even better' than CEE/MPA in terms of arterial disease, a position now simply untenable given the RCT evidence base.

The intention of this chapter is to summarize what we know and, perhaps more importantly, what we do not know, about plasma lipoprotein profiles in postmenopausal women.

THE INFLUENCE OF AGE ON PLASMA LIPOPROTEIN LEVELS

In general, the plasma lipoprotein profile deteriorates with age in women, as it does in men. Total cholesterol levels increase by about 1% per year, mostly due to an increase in those of LDL. Triglyceride levels may show an even greater increase, whereas plasma levels of high-density lipoproteins (HDL) and lipoprotein (a) [Lp(a)] remain remarkably stable. The reasons for these changes in cholesterol- and triglyceride-rich lipoprotein levels are poorly understood but clearly have implications for what we consider to be 'normal'. At various times investigators have proposed age-related changes in the activities of classic determinants of the plasma lipoprotein profile such as apolipoprotein B_{100} (apoB_{100}) receptors or various enzymes. Others suggest a role for age-related oxidative damage or glycosylation, or that these changes are secondary to age-related changes in plasma levels of growth hormone.

An additional factor may lie in the way those of us living in the affluence of industrialized countries drift into bad habits as we age. More and more we eat for personal gratification and social pleasure, not because of hunger. More and more we go for the 'quick fix' of prepared meals and restaurant food; when we do eat, we eat too much. Many of us compound these errors by relishing fatty foods and alcohol, a combination guaranteed to play havoc with the plasma lipoprotein profile. At the same time we drift away from the physical exercise habits of our youth: we drive rather than walk and take the lift rather than the stairs. For most people, the sport of youth becomes solely a voyeuristic pleasure.

THE INFLUENCE OF MENOPAUSE ON PLASMA LIPOPROTEIN LEVELS

Although I contend that the menopause *per se* has not been proven to be a risk factor for arterial diseases (age being a major confounder of most studies), I will concede that there is good evidence for a worsening of the plasma lipoprotein profile associated with this process.[7] Most studies find increases of about 0.5 mmol/L in plasma total cholesterol levels, due to increases in those of LDL. Increases are seen in those of triglyceride-rich lipoproteins and there may be a shift towards the small dense end of the LDL particle spectrum. Contrary to popular belief, HDL levels are not affected by the menopause, consistent with the lack of effect of female puberty on plasma levels of this lipoprotein.[4]

THE INFLUENCE OF HORMONE REPLACEMENT THERAPY ON PLASMA LIPOPROTEIN LEVELS

The basic pattern of change seen with HRT on the plasma lipoprotein profile was established many decades ago. The effects are determined by the dose(s) of component steroids, the dosing schedule and the route of administration, as well as factors such as concomitant medications or disease and tobacco abuse. The massive database of studies underpinning these conclusions has naturally formed the basis of a series of comprehensive reviews. One that is in my view compulsory reading is Ian Godsland's 2001 meta-analysis of all studies published between 1974 and 2000 (Table 4.1).[3]

The effect of combinations of HRT steroids on the plasma lipoprotein profile can usually be predicted if one knows the effects of these steroids when given on their own. The basic pattern of change is as follows. Oral administration of oestrogenic steroids tends to reduce plasma total cholesterol levels (by reducing those of LDL) and increase those of triglycerides and HDL. In contrast, androgenic steroids tend to induce the opposite pattern, i.e. increases in LDL levels and falls in those of triglycerides and HDL. Both oestrogenic and androgenic steroids can lower plasma levels of that most enigmatic lipoprotein Lp(a). The effect of the progestogen on combined therapy varies considerably according to their androgenic/anti-oestrogenic properties: natural progesterone and progesterone derivatives, such as dydrogesterone, are metabolically 'transparent', having little or no effect on plasma lipoprotein metabolism, while steroids such as levonorgestrel can induce 'androgenic' changes if given at a sufficiently high dose.

ORAL OESTROGENS

By far the largest body of data relating to HRT effects on plasma lipoprotein metabolism concerns oral oestrogen monotherapy. Oral oestrogens upregulate $apoB_{100}$ receptors (a similar mechanism of action to that seen with statins), increasing LDL uptake by the liver (and so leading to subsequent elimination of cholesterol in bile) and reducing plasma LDL levels by about 12%. From the start this oestrogen-induced fall in plasma LDL levels has been used to validate the claim of 50% reduction in MI seen with HRT. What is particularly intriguing, as we stand surrounded by the wreckage of studies such as the Heart and Estrogen/progestin Replacement Study (HERS) and the Women's Health Initiative (WHI), is to see the way in which statin effects on LDL are being pushed to one side by the interest in another potential mechanism: the fall they induce in CRP.[6] If this shift continues, then the correct interpretation of oestrogenic effects of reducing LDL levels but increasing those of CRP may well be that oral oestrogens would *not* be expected to reduce the risk of MI or stroke, consistent with the RCTs evidence base.

Claims have been made for an antioxidant effect of oestrogen on LDL but the clinical significance of these laboratory-derived data is not known. Oral oestrogens

Table 4.1 Meta-analysis: effects of selected HRT regimens on plasma lipid and lipoprotein levels[a]

HRT formulation	Total cholesterol	Triglycerides	LDL cholesterol	HDL cholesterol	Lp(a)[b]
Oral CEE (0.625 mg/d)	-2.6 (-3.3 to -1.9)	18.6 (16.3 to 20.9)	-11.7 (-12.5 to -10.9)	14.8 (13.9 to 15.7)	-23.9 (-27.8 to -20.0)
Oral CEE (0.625 mg/d) + MPA (2.5 mg/d continuous)	-4.8 (-6.0 to -3.6)	9.0 (6.3 to 11.7)	-12.0 (-13.1 to -10.9)	9.7 (8.4 to 11.0)	-20.7 (-25.4 to -16.0)
Oral oestradiol 17b(2.0 mg/d)	-4.2 (-5.9 to -2.5)	11.2 (6.4 to 16.0)	-12.4 (-14.8 to -10.0)	11.2 (9.1 to 13.3)	-12.9 (-17.6 to -8.2)
Oral oestradiol 17b (2.0 mg/d) + NETA (1.0 mg/d continuous)	-12.0 (-13.3 to -10.7)	-5.6 (-10.0 to -1.2)	-12.2 (-14.0 to -10.4)	-11.0 (-12.9 to -9.1)	-34.4 (-40.6 to -28.2)
Transdermal oestradiol β (0.05 mg/d)	-3.3 (-4.3 to 2.3)	-8.6 (-12.6 to -4.6)	-3.9 (-5.4 to -2.4)	5.1 (3.6 to 6.6)	5.3 (-2.7 to 13.3)
Transdermal oestradiol β (0.05 mg/d) + NETA (0.17–0.35 cyclically)	-5.0 (-6.0 to -4.0)	-8.1 (-11.4 to -4.8)	-7.0 (-8.4 to -5.6)	0.7 (-0.7 to 2.1)	1.8 (-5.4 to 9.0)
Tibolone (2.5 mg/d)	-7.4 (-8.7 to -6.1)	-25.0 (-29.1 to -20.9)	-0.8 (-2.9 to 1.3)	-22.0 (-24 to -20.0)	-39.2 (-44.7 to -33.7)

CEE, conjugated equine oestrogen; HDL, high-density lipoprotein; LDL, low-density lipoprotein; Lp(a), lipoprotein (a); MPA, medroxyprogesterone acetate; NETA, norethisterone (norethindrone) acetate.
[a] Data are presented as percentages of pretreatment levels (mean and 95% confidence intervals).
[b] Lp(a) data are from relatively few studies and in some cases results of slightly different doses were pooled for the purposes of this analysis.
Adapted with permission from reference 3.

reduce Lp(a) levels by about 20%; again there is no RCT evidence that reducing Lp(a) by any means is of benefit in terms of clinical end-points. The influence of oral oestrogens on LDL particle size is particularly interesting. Not all LDL particles carry the same atherogenic load: a minor population of 'small, dense' LDL particles are thought to be more dangerous. The problem here is that oral oestrogen shifts the LDL size spectrum toward these smaller particles. At the very least this suggests that we should be cautious about the clinical benefit of HRT-induced effects on LDL levels.

How are we to interpret the elevated fasting plasma triglyceride levels seen with oral oestrogens? Various explanations have been suggested for this inconsistency, e.g. the increase is seen in 'safe' triglyceride-rich lipoproteins, or the increase is meaningless if HDL levels are also raised, or that postprandial triglyceride metabolism is the real issue. All one can say is that the extrapolation of HRT-induced changes in triglyceride metabolism to vascular disease risk is more complex than had originally been thought.

Oral oestrogens increase HDL levels by 10–15% by increasing the synthesis of apoA1, a key component, by reducing lipase-mediated catabolism and by down-regulating scavenger receptors B1 (SRB1). The effect on SRB1 receptors would not be expected to confer clinical benefit.

NON-ORAL OESTROGENS

When the hepatic impact of oestrogens is minimized by the non-oral administration of HRT, the influences on plasma lipoprotein levels are less striking. Non-oral oestrogens, such as transdermal oestradiol, induce less of a reduction in LDL levels (typically about 5%) compared to oral therapy and increase HDL levels by a similar degree. Triglyceride levels are reduced, not increased, by non-oral oestrogens. However, the clinical significance of this effect is not known. Is it possible that the adverse vascular effects seen in studies such as HERS and WHI are linked to the increased plasma triglyceride levels seen with CEE? If so, would non-oral therapy have given a different result?[2]

ADDING A PROGESTOGEN

Progestogens oppose the ability of oral oestrogens to increase plasma triglyceride levels. In contrast, the ability of oral oestrogens to lower Lp(a) levels may be strengthened by progestogen coadministration, at least in the case of oral oestradiol. Some progestogens can oppose the increases seen in HDL with oral oestrogens; indeed steroids such as levonorgestrel, if given in high doses, can negate the oestrogenic effects on this potentially important aspect of lipid metabolism. But how do we assess the net effect of combined therapy on MI risk? Clearly this remains an impossible task at present and one of decreasing relevance in the face of the RCT data.

RALOXIFENE

Although not strictly an HRT, raloxifene is worth mentioning due to its oestrogen-like ability to reduce plasma levels of LDL and Lp(a) but utter lack of effect on those of HDL or triglycerides.

TIBOLONE

Tibolone has no effect on plasma LDL levels but reduces those of triglycerides and HDL (typically by 20% in both cases) and induces spectacular (40%) falls in those of Lp(a). This effect on HDL has been a consistent problem in the acceptance of this most idiosyncratic of HRT formulations. In 1998 I speculated that the fall in HDL seen with tibolone may not necessarily be harmful.[1] Our subsequent cholesterol efflux studies,[9] in which tibolone was shown not to impair the removal of cholesterol from cells, support this contention. I continue to maintain that according to current concepts of lipoprotein pathobiology, one can make just as good an argument that tibolone will reduce the risk of MI as one can argue that the drug is atherogenic. What is needed is an adequately powered RCT with MI as the major end-point. It is a matter of considerable personal frustration that such a study does not exist.

CONCLUSION

1. Essentially all aspects of plasma lipoprotein metabolism have been linked to atherosclerosis, either as potential contributors to atherogenesis (LDL, Lp(a), triglyceride-rich lipoproteins) or as potentially protective agents (HDL).
2. Essentially all aspects of plasma lipoprotein metabolism have been shown to be influenced by the steroid hormones used in HRT.
3. Oral oestrogen has traditionally been perceived as having a 'protective' effect against arterial disease due to the increase in HDL and fall in LDL; the increase in triglycerides has tended to be put to one side.
4. Non-oral oestrogens do not increase HDL and have less effect on LDL than do oral oestrogens, but they do reduce triglyceride levels.
5. Some progestogens have been perceived as compromising these protective effects of oestrogen but there is no clinical evidence to support this.
6. The promotion of plasma lipoprotein levels as surrogates for MI risk in HRT users has not kept pace with developments in plasma lipoprotein metabolism (such as lipoprotein heterogeneity) and functional aspects of lipoproteins (such as cholesterol efflux).
7. In the woman with elevated plasma LDL levels, the basis of therapy should be drugs of proven clinical benefit (such as statins) rather than oestrogen.
8. In the postmenopausal woman with elevated triglyceride levels the disorder will most commonly be part of the 'metabolic syndrome' and drug therapy, except in extreme cases, may be of limited benefit. Lifestyle interventions, such as weight loss, smoking cessation and exercise have the potential to correct modest hypertriglyceridaemia but are hard to achieve in practice.

The menopause

and Gynaecology

References

1. Crook D 1998 Effects of estrogens and progestogens on plasma lipids and lipoproteins. In: Fraser I S, Jansen R P S, Lobo R A et al (eds) Estrogens and Progestogens in Clinical Practice. Churchill Livingstone, London, p 787–798

2. Crook D 2001 Do we need clinical trials to test the ability of transdermal HRT to prevent coronary heart disease? Current Control Trials in Cardiovascular Medicine 2:211–214

3. Godsland I F 2001 Effects of post-menopausal hormone replacement therapy on lipid, lipoprotein, and apolipoprotein (a) concentrations: analysis of studies published from 1974–2000. Fertility and Sterility 75:898–915

4. Godsland I F, Wynn V, Crook D et al 1987 Sex, plasma lipoproteins and atherosclerosis: prevailing assumptions and outstanding questions. American Heart Journal 114:1467–1503

5. Miller G J 1999 Lipoproteins and the haemostatic system in atherothrombotic disorders. Baillière's Best Practice & Research. Clinical Haematology 12:555–575

6. Ridker P M, Cannon C P, Morrow D et al 2005 C-reactive protein levels and outcomes after statin therapy. The New England Journal of Medicine 352:20–28

7. Stevenson J C, Crook D, Godsland I F 1993 Effects of age and menopause on serum lipids and lipoproteins in healthy women. Atherosclerosis 98:83–90

8. Stork S, van der Schouw Y T, Grobbee D E et al 2004 Estrogen, inflammation and cardiovascular risk in women: a critical appraisal. Trends in Endocrinology and Metabolism 15:66–72

9. Von Eckardstein A, Crook D, Elbers J et al 2003 Postmenopausal hormone replacement with tibolone lowers high-density lipoprotein cholesterol but not cholesterol efflux capacity of plasma. Clinical Endocrinology 58:49–58

5

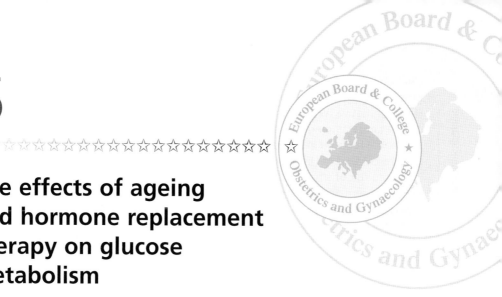

The effects of ageing and hormone replacement therapy on glucose metabolism

Sven O Skouby   Jorgen Jespersen

ABSTRACT

In women, increased body weight and central body fat distribution are often observed throughout the climacteric period, and the prevalence of the metabolic syndrome increases dramatically in the perimenopausal period and beyond. More specifically, insulin sensitivity in middle-aged women seems to be related more to the menopause than chronological age and therefore there is evidence to suggest that as age increases after menopause there is an increasing negative influence on glucose tolerance and an increased risk of impaired glucose tolerance. The metabolic syndrome is defined by a cluster of abnormalities that includes insulin resistance, hypertension, obesity, hypertriglyceridaemia and low HDL cholesterol. Evidence that inflammation is another component of metabolic syndrome raises the possibility that this is an additional process that links the syndrome to coronary heart risk. Also, population studies strongly suggest the existence of a relationship between metabolic abnormalities associated with metabolic syndrome and the development of diabetes and cardiovascular disease. It appears that lifestyle modifications can contribute to the prevention of progression to diabetes and the reduction of individual coronary heart disease (CHD) risk factors, but several conditions also indicate an interaction between sex steroids and insulin sensitivity. One condition is increased insulin resistance during the high oestrogen and progesterone states of pregnancy; another is the luteal phase of the menstrual cycle and another is insulin resistance, which can be observed in women with polycystic ovary syndrome (PCOS). The level of sex hormone-binding globulin (SHBG) seems to be a strong predictor of future type 2 diabetes. Differences exist, however, between the physiological and pharmacological actions of endogenous and exogenous sex steroids. Exogenous sex steroids with oestrogen and progestogen activity represent a wide spectrum of hormones and, therefore, also differences in their pharmacokinetic properties and pharmacodynamic effects. Research examining the effect of hormone replacement therapy (HRT) on the development of diabetes has been inconclusive, and no long-term randomized clinical trial results were available until the recently published Heart and Estrogen/progestin Replacement Study (HERS) and the findings of the Women's Health Initiative (WHI) study. The findings of these trials concur with previous observational findings of the large Nurses' Health Study, where current users of HRT had a reduced incidence of diabetes. Whether these results justify extending the prescription of HRT to diabetic women may be questioned. The reported increased risk of stroke and other cardiovascular risks from the randomized studies are of concern and a search for optimal HRT in relation to type and dose is needed. At the time of writing, the results from the HERS and WHI in diabetic women are encouraging, but more information from existing data needs to be retrieved and more specialized data obtained from new research before definite guidelines on best practice can be defined.

KEYWORDS

Ageing, diabetes, glucose, hormone replacement therapy (HRT), menopause, metabolic syndrome, oestrogen, progestogen

INTRODUCTION

Changes in the human environment and in human behaviour and lifestyle, in conjunction with genetic susceptibility, have resulted in a dramatic increase in the incidence and prevalence of diabetes around the world. From 1995 to 2025 it is expected that there will be a 42% increase (from 51 to 72 million) in the developed countries and a 170% increase (from 84 to 228 million) in the developing countries.[19] The prevalence of the metabolic syndrome in nondiabetic adults in Europe has been reported to be as high as 15%. The subsequent rapid escalation of the number of people with type 2 diabetes and diabetes-related cardiovascular disease demands urgent action on prevention. An important rule of any prevention strategy is the identification of individuals who are at high risk. In women increased body weight and central body fat distribution are often observed throughout the climacteric period, and the prevalence of metabolic syndrome increases dramatically after the age of 40.[18] It has been reported that the decline in insulin sensitivity following the menopause is related more to the menopause than chronological age[33] and a large community-based population survey indicates that in postmenopausal women, as their ages increase after menopause, there is an increasing negative influence on glucose tolerance and an increased risk of impaired glucose tolerance by 6% for each year since menopause started.[35] This chapter discusses the impact of endogenous and exogenous sex steroids on the age-dependent decrease in glucose tolerance in normal women and the glycometabolic control in women with type 2 diabetes.

THE METABOLIC SYNDROME

The metabolic syndrome is also known as insulin resistance syndrome[5] and syndrome X.[28] The cluster of metabolic abnormalities includes glucose intolerance, insulin resistance, central obesity, dyslipidaemia and hypertension, all well-documented risk factors for cardiovascular disease.[16] There is a wide variation in prevalence to gender. In global studies, the prevalence varies in urban populations from 8 to 24% in men, and from 7 to 43% in women. A very consistent finding is that the prevalence of the metabolic syndrome is highly age-dependent. The prevalence in the USA (National Health and Nutrition Examination Survey: NHANES III) increased from 7% in participants aged 20–29 years to 44% and 42% for those aged 60–69 years and at least 70 years, respectively.[9] The metabolic syndrome is associated with an increased risk of both diabetes[14] and cardiovascular disease.[15]

The most accepted and unifying hypothesis to describe the pathophysiology of the syndrome is insulin resistance; a major contributor to the development of insulin resistance is an overabundance of circulating fatty acids. The association of the metabolic syndrome with inflammation is well documented.[31] The increases in proinflammatory cytokines – including interleukin-6, resistin, tumour necrosis factor α (TNFα) and C-reactive protein – reflect overproduction by the expanded adipose tissue mass. Adiponectin is an antiinflammatory cytokine that is produced exclusively by adipocytes. Adiponectin enhances insulin sensitivity and inhibits many steps in the inflammatory process.[32] An alternative concept to explain the metabolic syndrome is leptin resistance.[27]

Several investigative techniques have been devised for the *in-vivo* quantification of resistance to insulin-stimulated glucose uptake. All have limitations and none is suitable for routine clinical use. The euglycemic clamp technique, which involves simultaneous infusions of insulin and glucose, has been used extensively and is regarded as the standard. The method is, however, complex, nonphysiological and resource demanding. A computer (minimal change) modeling of an i.v. glucose tolerance test (IVGTT) is easier when applicable in larger series although the differential equations necessary (from simultaneous changing glucose and insulin concentrations) are complex. An alternative is the Homeostasis Model Assessment (HOMA).[25]

SEX STEROIDS AND CARBOHYDRATE METABOLISM

Several conditions suggest an interrelationship between insulin sensitivity and the effects of sex steroids. Examples include the increased insulin resistance during the high oestrogen and progesterone state of pregnancy, during the luteal phase of the menstrual cycle and in women with high androgen production (in PCOS and stromal hyperthecosis). In the context of sex steroids it is also of interest that during the fertile period insulin sensitivity to glucose is greater in women than in men. The overall association between oestrogen levels expressed as SHBG and glucose metabolism is shown in Box 5.1. Correspondingly, the San Antonio Heart Study demonstrated that SHBG is negatively correlated with fasting insulin, and insulin and glucose responses to oral glucose.[13] Thus, the metabolic effects of endogenous oestrogens suggest that oestrogen replacement therapy would have the potential to reverse the cluster of metabolic changes included in the metabolic syndrome.

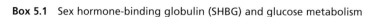
> **Box 5.1** Sex hormone-binding globulin (SHBG) and glucose metabolism
>
> - SHBG is suggested as a strong predictor of subsequent type 2 diabetes in pre- and postmenopausal women.
> - Low concentrations of SHBG are associated with insulin resistance and android obesity.

Some discrepancies may, however, exist between the physiological and pharmacological actions of endogenous and exogenous administered sex steroids. Exogenous sex steroids with oestrogen and progestogen activity represent a wide spectrum of hormones with different molecular structures and therefore also differences in their pharmacokinetic properties and pharmacodynamic effects. The oestrogens may be natural human or equine from genuine sources or artificial with or without steroid structure. The progestogens represent an even wider selection of hormonal compounds with progesterone-like activities and some with partial androgen, antiandrogen, mineralocorticoids or antimineralocorticoid activities.[29] Moreover, patches, gels, implants and 'vagitories' with no first-pass hepatic effect are available as exogenous sex steroids. It has to be born in mind that such differences in pharmacokinetic properties will also influence the metabolic impact of hormonal treatment. In animal studies it has been shown that 17β-oestradiol (E_2) treatment enhances insulin secretion in islet cells and thereby augments the insulin response to glucose, and reduces insulin resistance.[20] Also, natural progesterone may result in an increased insulin response to glucose, but this is probably due to decreased insulin sensitivity in the target tissue resulting in increased beta cell responsiveness.

Much of our knowledge about the effect of the exogenous sex steroids on glucose metabolism in women is derived from the oral contraceptive (OC) area. When administering OCs a decrease in glucose tolerance is often observed concomitant with a hyperinsulinaemic response to the glucose load. The impact on glucose metabolism is shown to be clearly dose-dependent and the low-dose types of combined OCs therefore have less impact on the glucose tolerance. There is usually no deterioration of the glucose curve whereas hyperinsulinaemia and decreased insulin sensitivity can still be observed.[30] Several investigations on the administration of HRT, insulin sensitivity and glucose tolerance have been reported but the conclusions are not uniform. Some discrepancies may be due to the route of administration. Following oral administration the hormones pass directly from the gut to the liver via the portal vein, giving a high local concentration that markedly affects hepatic metabolism. In contrast, transdermal administration avoids first-pass metabolism and it is therefore not surprising to find different effects from oral compared with parenteral administration. Barret-Connor and Laakso have published results from a comparative study on post-challenge glucose and insulin levels in women using no HRT, unopposed conjugated equine oestrogen (CEE) and CEE plus medroxyprogesterone acetate (MPA).[1]

The glucose and insulin values were age and body mass index (BMI) adjusted before comparison was made. Fasting glucose levels were significantly lower in the oestrogen-treated group compared to the untreated group. No difference was seen between the CEE + MPA group and the group with unopposed CEE treatment, but fasting insulin values were lower in the oestrogen-treated group than in the untreated group. This is interesting because fasting insulin is considered to be a fairly good marker for insulin sensitivity.

In contrast, Cagnacci et al found no significant effect on fasting insulin levels or beta cell sensitivity to oral glucose from oral intake of CEE.[2] This group compared the oral intake of CEE with the transdermal administration of E_2. Following the transdermal administration, fasting insulin levels decreased and beta cell response to glucose increased indicating an increase in insulin sensitivity. This study is interesting because it evaluates the significance of the oestrogen effect on the liver for the glucose homeostasis, and in contrast to oral CEE the transdermal oestrogen administration increased hepatic insulin clearance.

Godsland et al have compared insulin sensitivity (IVGTT, 'minimal model') during the sequential intake of oral CEE + levonorgestrel (LNG) with the transdermal administration of E_2 + oral norethisterone (NET).[11] Oral intake of CEE + LNG caused a decrease in glucose tolerance and an increased overall plasma insulin response. Insulin resistance was greater during the combined phase compared with the oestrogen only phase. The transdermal regimen had relatively few effects on insulin metabolism although the first phase beta cell insulin secretion was enhanced. Both regimens increased hepatic insulin uptake. This study therefore indicates that the addition of a progestogen to oestrogen therapy may markedly influence the effect on glucose metabolism in parallel to the observations made during administration of OCs.

Lindheim et al demonstrated the impact of dose via a bimodal effect of oral CEE on insulin sensitivity with an improvement occurring with the lower dose of 0.625 mg but with a deterioration with the dose of 1.25 mg.[21] The authors suggest that this effect may be related to the first-pass hepatic portal effect in that transdermal E_2 (0.1 mg), which may be equated more closely with the larger dose of oral CEE (1.25 mg), improved insulin sensitivity. Progestin, however, appeared to attenuate the beneficial effects of transdermal E_2 and may alter the clearance of insulin.[22] Duncan et al[6] found no beneficial effect of unopposed oral or transdermal E_2 on insulin sensitivity and suggest that the addition of an oral progesterone (NET) confers no clinically important risk or benefit. Gaspard et al.[10] found after 2 years' treatment with oral E_2 combined sequentially with dydrogesterone (DG), a direct progesterone derivative, did not change oral glucose tolerance tests (OGTTs) but decreased areas under the insulin curves and fasting insulin values indicating improvement in insulin sensitivity.

Using transdermal E_2 and the same progesterone, Cucinelli et al demonstrated (with the euglycemic clamp technique) the amelioration of insulin resistance after 12 weeks of treatment.[4] Using both a high-dose (2 mg) and low-dose (1 mg) oral regimen of E_2 combined with DG for 24 months, Godsland et al, when applying the minimal change model, found favourable effects on insulin secretion and elimination in menopausal women.[12] When comparing oral E_2 (2 mg) + DG with tibolone in obese (BMI ≥ 27) women, Morin-Papunen et al found that after

☆ ☆☆☆☆☆☆☆☆☆☆☆☆☆☆☆☆☆☆☆☆☆☆☆☆☆☆☆

12 months of tibolone, the whole-body glucose uptake decreased contrasting the effect of oral $E_2 + DG$ using the euglycemic technique.[26] Comparing oral tibolone with oral CEE (0.625 mg) + MPA (5 mg) Wiegratz et al found no significant changes with either treatment in the results obtained from OGTTs performed baseline and after 6 months in non-obese women.[34]

We have examined the impact on glucose metabolism and insulin sensitivity during oral administration of 2 mg E_2 in combination with the intrauterine delivery system of LNG (Mirena®) and compared the results with data obtained with a continuous combined HRT (CCHRT) with 2 mg E_2 plus 1 mg NETA. After 6 months no changes were observed in the OGTTs or insulin sensitivity using the minimal change model (Table 5.1). The largest randomized comparative study on HRT and risk markers for a deterioration of glucose metabolism is the Post-menopausal Estrogen/Progestin Intervention (PEPI) study, a 3-year trial to assess the effect of four hormone regimens on cardiovascular risk factors.[7] In 788 women the impact of the hormone regimens was determined on insulin and glucose concentrations measured during a standard OGTT. When compared with women taking placebo, those taking CEE at 0.625 mg daily with or without a progestational agent had mean fasting insulin levels that were lower, a mean fasting glucose level that was lower and mean 2-hour glucose levels that were higher. No significant differences were apparent between women taking CEE only versus the three progestin regimens: MPA (2.5 mg daily), continuous MPA, MPA at 10 mg on days 1 to 12 MPA, and micronized progesterone (MP) cyclically at 200 mg on days 1 to 12. The impact of HRT on insulin and glucose depended on baseline levels of fasting insulin and 1-hour glucose. However, the treatment effects on carbohydrate metabolism appeared to be consistent across participant subgroups by lifestyle, and clinical and demographic characteristics. The interpretation was that oral HRT involving 0.625 mg daily CEE may modestly decrease fasting levels of insulin and glucose. Post-challenge glucose concentrations are increased, which may indicate delayed glucose clearance.

HORMONE REPLACEMENT THERAPY AND DIABETES

Only a few studies have evaluated the effect of HRT on the incidence of diabetes. The influence of HRT on the subsequent development of diabetes was examined

Table 5.1 The Danish Collaboratory Climacteric Study. Glucose disposal rate (Si per minute per pU per ml) following continuously combined HRT and oral oestrogen combined with the Mirena system®

	Baseline	6 months	P
EE + NET (n = 35)	0.9	0.8	Not significant
E2 + LNG (n = 30)	1.8	1.3	Not significant

E2, oestradiol; EE, equine oestrogen; LNG, levonorgestrel; NET, norethisterone in a prospective cohort of 21 028 postmenopausal US women aged 30 to 55 years and who were free of diagnosed diabetes in 1976.[23] During 12 years of follow-up it was confirmed that current HRT users had a relative risk of diabetes of 0.80 (95% CI; range 0.67–0.96) as compared with never users, after adjustments for age and BMI. In the HERS, 2763 postmenopausal women with documented CHD were randomly assigned to daily oestrogen plus progestin therapy (EPT) or to placebo.[17] The effect of HRT on fasting glucose levels and incident diabetes over 4 years of follow-up was evaluated. A total of 2029 women without diabetes were included. Incident diabetes was defined by self-report of diabetes or disease complication, a fasting glucose level of 6.9 mmol/L or greater (126 mg/dL) or the initiation of therapy with diabetes medication. Fasting glucose levels increased significantly among women assigned to placebo but did not change among women receiving HRT. The incidence of diabetes was 6.2% in the HRT group and 9.5% in the placebo group (hazard ratio 0.65; 95% CI; range 0.48–0.89) corresponding to a 35% lower incidence among HRT users. The number needed to treat for benefit to prevent one case of diabetes was 30; changes in weight and waist circumference did not mediate this effect. Obviously, evaluation of the preventive effect of HRT on the occurrence of type 2 diabetes was not the primary objective of the HERS and only one combination (0.625 mg CEE + 2.5 mg MPA) taken continuously was considered, but the described effects are strong. Previous research examining the effect of HRT on development of diabetes has been inconclusive, and no long-term randomized clinical trial results were available. The findings, however, are in accordance with the observational findings of the Nurses' Health Study (n = 21 028) where current users of HRT had a reduced incidence of diabetes (relative risk 0.80; 95% CI; range 0.67–0.96) when compared with past users and women who had never used HRT and whose values were adjusted for age and BMI.[23]

In addition, the WHI also offers new insights into how diabetes may be prevented in women.[24] The study was designed to examine the effect of postmenopausal HRT on a number of health outcomes, with a primary end-point of CHD, death or nonfatal myocardial infarction (MI). In the EPT arm, more than 15 000 women were randomized to receive either 0.625 mg CEE and 2.5 mg MPA or placebo each day during 5.6 years of follow-up. The participants were women aged 50–79 and all had an intact uterus. Diabetes incidence was ascertained by self-report of treatment with insulin or oral hypoglycaemic medication. Fasting glucose, insulin and lipoproteins were measured in a random sample at baseline and at 1 and 3 years.

The cumulative incidence of treated diabetes was 3.5% in the EPT group and 4.2% in the placebo group (hazard ratio 0.79; 95% CI; range 0.67–0.93) (Table 5.2). There was little change in the hazard ratio after adjustment for changes in BMI and waist circumference. During the first year of follow-up, changes in fasting glucose and insulin indicated a significant fall in insulin resistance in actively treated women compared to the control subjects. The interpretations of the data suggest that CCHRT reduces the incidence of type 2 diabetes. Thus the study confirms the observations made in the HERS in women with established CHD,

The menopause

Table 5.2 Self reported diabetes incidence by treatment assignment in the WHI trial. Adapted from (34).

Treatment	CEE + MPA (n = 7352)	Placebo (n = 7016)	Hazard ratio	95% CI	P
Number of cases	277	324	0.79	0.67–0.93	0.004

CEE, conjugated equine oestrogen; CI, confidence interval; MPA, medroxyprogesterone acetate. Adapted with permission from reference 24.

as a subset of the participants also had blood samples taken for fasting glucose and insulin at baseline and during follow-up. This randomly selected cohort represented 8.6% of the population and was stratified by age, clinical centre and ethnicity. At 1 year of follow-up, the HOMA of insulin resistance was calculated from fasting levels of glucose and insulin and was found to be significantly lower in women on HRT. By year 3, this difference in HOMA had disappeared, probably because of lower numbers and poorer adherence to the HRT regimen, but the observations provide evidence that reduced insulin resistance may be the mechanism by which HRT reduced the incidence of diabetes in this group, possibly mediated by a decrease in insulin resistance unrelated to body size.

As in the HERS only one combination of HRT with continuous administration of CEE + MPA was investigated. Further differentiated information on the oestrogen and progestogen effect will only be obtained when all data from the ET arm of the WHI are analysed. Meanwhile, the HERS and WHI have shown that women on HRT are less likely to progress to type 2 diabetes. Whether the results should also favour the prescription of HRT to diabetic women remains to be answered. A search for the optimal and probably 'low-dose' HRT is needed. The reported increased risk of stroke and 'early harm' CHD effect is of concern and points to the importance of adjusting underlying risk factors such as hypertension, hyperlipidaemia and elevated plasma glucose. In particular, women at risk of diabetes should be advised on lifestyle changes including eating restrictions and exercise. In diabetic women there are, however, some reports giving substantial information on better glycaemic and clinical CHD outcome during HRT administration although an increased CHD risk may exist in diabetic women with manifest atherosclerotic lesions, e.g. earlier MI.[3,8]

CONCLUSION

The association between the deterioration of glucose metabolism and CHD has been observed in numerous studies. During recent decades, research has demonstrated that the commonly used term 'insulin resistance syndrome' promotes atherothrombosis and includes insulin resistance with or without glucose intolerance, abdominal obesity, atherogenic dyslipidaemia, raised blood pressure, a proinflammatory state and a prothrombotic state. In the vessel wall, insulin stimulates the proliferation and migration of smooth muscle cells, the binding of LDL to receptors in monocytes and the activity of major enzymes in lipogenesis. In any individual, insulin resistance is genetically determined, and the clinical expression is linked to age and is more frequently found in middle-aged women as compared with men. Endogenous and exogenous sex steroids have a modulating effect. In postmenopausal women exogenous oestrogens may decrease insulin resistance although the effect may be weakened by the increased synthesis of growth factors and decreased hepatic insulin clearance following the first-pass effect of orally administered hormones. Moreover, the administration of progestogens with oestrogens may counteract the oestrogen effects on insulin resistance. At present, the results from the HERS and WHI are encouraging for preventing type 2 diabetes with postmenopausal use of HRT, although more information is needed before clinical recommendations or guidelines can be defined. In diabetic women, HRT may have a bimodal effect preventing the development of CHD in women without pre-existing manifestation of CHD but accelerating the thrombotic process in those with established disease.

References

1. Barret-Connor E, Laakso M 1990 Ischemic heart disease risk in postmenopausal women. Effects of estrogen use on glucose and insulin levels. Arteriosclerosis 10:531–534

2. Cagnacci A, Soldani R, Carriero P L et al 1992 Effects of low doses of transdermal 17-beta estradiol on carbohydrate metabolism in postmenopausal women. The Journal of Clinical Endocrinology and Metabolism 74:1396–1400

3. Crespo C J, Smit E, Snelling A et al 2002 Hormone replacement therapy and its relationship to lipid and glucose metabolism in diabetic and nondiabetic postmenopausal women: results from the Third National Health and Nutrition Examination Survey (NHANES III). Diabetes Care 25:1675–1680

4. Cucinelli F, Paparella P, Soranna L et al 1999 Differential effect of transdermal estrogen plus progestagen replacement therapy on insulin metabolism in postmenopausal women: relation to their insulinemic secretion. European Journal of Endocrinology 140:215–223

5. DeFronzo R A, Ferrannini E 1991 Insulin resistance. A multifaceted syndrome responsible for NIDDM, obesity, hypertension, dyslipidemia, and atherosclerotic cardiovascular disease. Diabetes Care 14:173–194

6. Duncan A C, Lyall H, Roberts R N et al 1999 The effect of estradiol and a combined estradiol/progestagen preparation on insulin sensitivity in healthy postmenopausal women. The Journal of Clinical Endocrinology and Metabolism 84:2402–2407

7. Espeland M A, Hogan P E, Fineberg S E et al 1998 Effect of postmenopausal hormone therapy on glucose and insulin concentrations. PEPI Investigators. Postmenopausal Estrogen/Progestin. Interventions. Diabetes Care 21:1589–1595

8. Ferrara A, Quesenberry C P, Karter A J et al 2003 Current use of unopposed estrogen and estrogen plus progestin and the risk of acute myocardial infarction among women with diabetes: the Northern California Kaiser Permanente Diabetes Registry, 1995–1998. Circulation 107:43–48

9. Ford E S, Giles W H, Dietz W H 2002 Prevalence of the metabolic syndrome among US adults: findings from the third National Health and Nutrition Examination Survey. The Journal of the American Medical Association 287:356–359

10. Gaspard U J, Wery O J, Scheen A J et al 1999 Long-term effects of oral estradiol and dydrogesterone on carbohydrate metabolism in postmenopausal women. Climacteric 2:93–100

11. Godsland I F, Gangar K, Walton C et al 1993 Insulin resistance, secretion, and elimination in postmenopausal women receiving oral or transdermal hormone replacement therapy. Metabolism 42:846–853

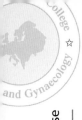

12. Godsland I F, Manassiev N A, Felton C V et al 2004 Effects of low- and high-dose oestradiol and dydrogesterone therapy on insulin and lipoprotein metabolism in healthy postmenopausal women. Clinical Endocrinology 60:541–549

13. Goodman-Gruen D, Barrett-Connor E 1997 Sex hormone-binding globulin and glucose tolerance in postmenopausal women. The Rancho Bernardo Study. Diabetes Care 20:645–649

14. Grundy S M, Hansen B, Smith S C, Jr et al 2004 Clinical management of metabolic syndrome: report of the American Heart Association/National Heart, Lung, and Blood Institute/American Diabetes Association conference on scientific issues related to management. Circulation 109:551–556

15. Hanson R L, Imperatore G, Bennett P H et al 2002 Components of the 'metabolic syndrome' and incidence of type 2 diabetes. Diabetes 51:3120–3127

16. Isomaa B, Almgren P, Tuomi T et al 2001 Cardiovascular morbidity and mortality associated with the metabolic syndrome. Diabetes Care 24:683–689

17. Kanaya A M, Herrington D, Vittinghoff E et al 2003 Glycemic effects of postmenopausal hormone therapy: The Heart and Estrogen/progestin Replacement Study. A randomized, double-blind, placebo-controlled trial. Annals of Internal Medicine 138:1–9

18. King H, Rewers M 1993 Global estimates for prevalence of diabetes mellitus and impaired glucose tolerance in adults. WHO Ad Hoc Diabetes Reporting Group. Diabetes Care 16:157–177

19. King H, Aubert R E, Herman W H 1998 Global burden of diabetes, 1995–2025: prevalence, numerical estimates, and projections. Diabetes Care 21:1414–1431

20. Kurmagai S, Hokmang A, Bjorntorp P 1993 The effects of oestrogen and progestogen on insulin sensitivity in female rats. Acta Physiologica Scandinavica 49:91–97

21. Lindheim S R, Buchanan T A, Duffy D M et al 1994 Comparison of estimates of insulin sensitivity in pre- and postmenopausal women using the insulin tolerance test and the frequently sampled intravenous glucose tolerance test. Journal of the Society for Gynecologic Investigation 1:150–154

22. Lindheim S R, Duffy D M, Kojima T et al 1994 The route of administration influences the effect of estrogen on insulin sensitivity in postmenopausal women. Fertility and Sterility 62:1176–1180

23. Manson J E, Rimm E B, Colditz G A et al 1992 A prospective study of postmenopausal estrogen therapy and subsequent incidence of non-insulin-dependent diabetes mellitus. Annals of Epidemiology 2:665–673

24. Margolis K L, Bonds D E, Rodabough R J et al 2004 Women's Health Initiative Investigators. Effect of oestrogen plus progestin on the incidence of diabetes in postmenopausal women: results from the Women's Health Initiative Hormone Trial. Diabetologia 47:1175–1187

25. Matthews D R, Hosker J P, Rudenski A S et al 1985 Homeostasis model assessment: insulin resistance and beta-cell function from fasting plasma glucose and insulin concentrations in man. Diabetologia 28:412–419

26. Morin-Papunen L C, Vauhkonen I, Ruokonen A et al 2004 Effects of tibolone and cyclic hormone replacement therapy on glucose metabolism in non-diabetic obese postmenopausal women: a randomized study. European Journal of Endocrinology 150:705–714

27. Nawrocki A R, Scherer P E 2004 The delicate balance between fat and muscle: adipokines in metabolic disease and musculoskeletal inflammation. Current Opinions in Pharmacology 4:281–289

28. Reaven M 1988 Banting Lecture 1988. Role of insulin resistance in human disease. Diabetes 37:1595–1607

29. Sitruk-Ware R 2004 Pharmacological profile of progestins. Maturitas 47:277–283

30. Skouby SO 1988 Oral contraceptives: effect on glucose and lipid metabolism in insulin-dependent diabetic women and women with previous gestational diabetes. A clinical and biochemical assessment. Danish Medical Bulletin 35:157–167

31. Sutherland J, McKinnley B, Eckel R H 2004 The Metabolic Syndrome and Inflammation. Metabolic Syndrome and Related Disorders 2:82–104

32. Trayhurn P, Wood I S 2004 Adipokines: inflammation and the pleiotropic role of white adipose tissue. The British Journal of Nutrition 92:347–355

33. Walton C, Godsland I, Proudler A et al 1993 The effects of the menopause on insulin sensitivity, secretion and elimination in non-obese, healthy women. European Journal of Clinical Investigation 23:466–473

34. Wiegratz, I, Starflinger F, Tetzoff W et al 2002 Effect of tibolone compared with sequential hormone replacement therapy on carbohydrate metabolism in postmenopausal women. Maturitas 41:133–141

35. Wu S I, Chou P, Tsai S T 2001 The impact of years since menopause on the development of impaired glucose tolerance. Journal of Clinical Epidemiology 54:117–120

6

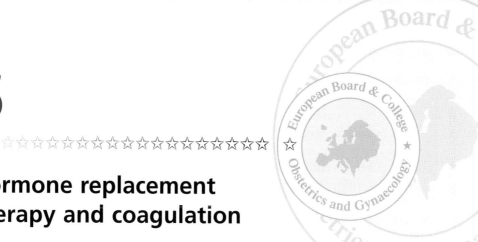

Hormone replacement therapy and coagulation

Per Morten Sandset   Else Høibraaten   Anette Løken Eilertsen

ABSTRACT

In recent years, large observational studies and randomized clinical trials have shown that oral fixed-dose hormone replacement therapy (HRT) increases the risk of arterial and venous thromboembolism. This review concerns the use of coagulation markers as surrogate end-points to detect the increased risk of thrombosis on HRT. There is compelling evidence that oral HRT containing conventional doses of conjugated equine oestrogen (CEE) or oestradiol is associated with increased levels of markers of activated coagulation, which can be attributed to reduced levels of coagulation inhibitors and acquired resistance to activated protein C. Lower doses of oral HRT as well as transdermal HRT are associated with marginal or no activation of coagulation, which is consistent with the lower risk of thrombosis on transdermal therapy. Effects on coagulation markers should therefore be used as surrogate markers in early pharmacodynamic studies to evaluate the risk associated with different doses and new formulations of oestrogens.

KEYWORDS

Activated protein C resistance, coagulation factors, coagulation inhibitors, hormone replacement therapy (HRT)

INTRODUCTION

Before the mid 1990s, numerous epidemiological studies suggested that HRT was associated with a protective effect on coronary atherothrombosis[3] and with no excess risk of venous thromboembolism (VTE),[15] and HRT was therefore widely prescribed by many physicians to protect women against thrombosis.

However, in retrospects many of these studies were biased and could not rule out clinically relevant effects on the risk of thrombosis. Over the last decade, several new epidemiological studies,[13,14,22,23,28] as well as randomized clinical trials in healthy women[11] and in women at risk of thrombosis,[20,27] have provided compelling evidence that HRT is associated with an increased risk of VTE. There is also strong evidence that HRT is associated with an early increased risk of coronary heart disease[19,39] and an increased risk of thromboembolic stroke.[8,63] This chapter will mainly review the effects of HRT on blood coagulation, which may, to a large extent, account for the prothrombotic effects of HRT.

A BRIEF OVERVIEW OF BLOOD COAGULATION AND MARKERS OF ACTIVATED COAGULATION

Blood coagulation is normally initiated by tissue factor, which is constitutively produced in extravascular tissue, and which is especially abundant in the placenta and in the brain (for a review, see reference 39). In healthy individuals, the vascular endothelium, along with circulating anticoagulants, provides an anticoagulant barrier that keeps blood flowing. However, by vascular damage, e.g. rupture of the vessel wall in trauma and surgery or rupture of atherosclerotic plaques, tissue factor may gain access to the circulating blood. Tissue factor may also be produced in circulating blood monocytes after cytokine stimulation, which is thought to be the mechanism leading to disseminated intravascular coagulation in cancer and sepsis.

Tissue factor exposed to circulating blood immediately binds to coagulation factor VII, and the tissue factor–factor VII complex then initiates a series of reactions in which native coagulation factors are sequentially activated by enzymatic cleavage, one by the other, and which converge on thrombin generation (Fig. 6.1). Thrombin is responsible for fibrin formation but also a number of other reactions including feedback activation of the cofactors V and VIII, platelet activation, inhibition of fibrinolysis and activation of the protein C anticoagulant pathway. Elevated levels of coagulation factors VII,[59] VIII[49,59] and IX[62] have been shown to be risk factors for venous thrombosis, whereas increased levels of fibrinogen and factor VII have been associated with the risk of arterial thrombosis.[21]

The activation of coagulation is dampened and sequentially downregulated by coagulation inhibitors; tissue factor pathway inhibitor (TFPI) inhibiting tissue factor–factor VIIa (see Fig. 6.1); the protein C–protein S anticoagulant pathway degrading activated cofactors V and VIII, and antithrombin inhibiting activated coagulation proteases (see Fig. 6.1). Familial deficiency of antithrombin (AT), protein C and protein S caused by numerous mutations in their respective genes is often associated with an increased risk of venous thrombosis.[49] Although familial deficiency of TFPI has not yet been detected, low levels of TFPI have recently proven to be a risk factor for VTE.[12]

The factor V Leiden mutation is a specific point mutation in the coagulation factor V gene, which causes an arginine to glutamine shift at position 506 and

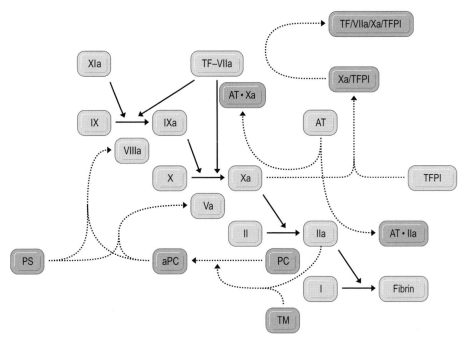

Fig 6.1 A simplified overview of the blood coagulation system. Native coagulation factors are denoted by roman numerals, activate factors by the suffix `a'. AT, antithrombin; PC, protein C; PS, protein S; TF, tissue factor; TFPI, tissue factor pathway inhibitor; TM, thrombomodulin.

thereby prevents cleavage and inactivation of activated factor V by activated protein C.[4] This results in sustained coagulation activation in the presence of activated protein C and is therefore called activated protein C (APC) resistance. In 5–10% of cases, APC resistance is also found in the absence of the factor V Leiden mutation, e.g. during pregnancy and on oral contraceptives. APC resistance, both in the presence or absence of the factor V Leiden mutation, has proven to be a weak risk factor for VTE.[49]

The net activity of blood coagulation can be assessed by markers of the final stages of coagulation (Fig. 6.2). Prothrombin fragments 1+2 (F_{1+2}) is formed by the cleavage of prothrombin and is a marker of thrombin generation. Fibrinopeptide A is formed by the cleavage of fibrinogen and is a marker of fibrin formation. The thrombin–antithrombin (TAT) complex is a marker of thrombin and its inactivation by AT. D-Dimer is a specific fibrin split product which is a marker of fibrin formation and consequent degradation of fibrin by plasmin. D-Dimer is thereby both a marker of activated coagulation and ongoing fibrinolysis. Normally, all these markers are found at low concentrations in plasma, but by the activation of coagulation the concentrations can be dramatically increased. Another marker of coagulation activation is the endogenous thrombin potential, which is the time integral of thrombin generation in plasma triggered by a low concentration of tissue factor.

Recent studies have shown that minor disturbances, e.g. a marginal increase of clotting factors with or without a marginal decrease of inhibitors, may induce

Hormone replacement therapy and coagulation

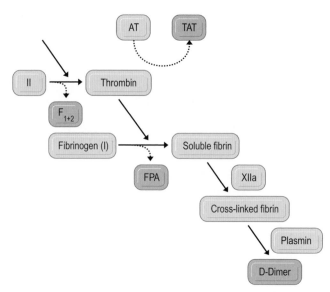

Fig 6.2 Overview of markers of activated coagulation. F_{1+2}, prothrombin fragments 1+2; FPA, fibrinopeptide A; TAT, thrombin–antithrombin complex.

thrombin generation and thereby potentially trigger thrombosis.[38] It is therefore possible that marginal changes in coagulation factors – even within their normal reference ranges, e.g. induced by HRT and other agents – can be of importance for the risk of thrombosis. It may therefore be time for a critical reappraisal of the use of coagulation factors as surrogate markers to assess the risk of thrombosis on HRT.

PHYSIOLOGICAL CHANGES IN COAGULATION AFTER MENOPAUSE

The menopause induces minor changes in the levels of coagulation factors. These changes involve minor increases in the levels of clotting factors including levels of fibrinogen,[18,33,41–43] factor VII[42,53] and factor VIII,[2] but also minor increases in the levels of the coagulation inhibitors AT,[43] PC[56] and TFPI.[12] So far, there is no evidence that these changes are associated with the net activation of coagulation as judged by the levels of F_{1+2} and TAT,[47,50] which suggests overall balanced physiological changes of coagulation during and after menopause.

THE EFFECTS OF HORMONE REPLACEMENT THERAPY ON MARKERS OF ACTIVATED COAGULATION

There is now consistent evidence that *oral HRT*, either oestrogen alone or combined HRT, increases the levels of F_{1+2}.[7,9,26,31,45,51,54,57,60] The effects of oral HRT on TAT[26,31,60] and D-dimer[10,26,29,35,51,57,60,61] have shown conflicting results although more recent studies suggest that oral HRT also increases these parameters.[26,57] In a randomized placebo-controlled study of women with a history of

VTE, we found that oral combined 17β-oestradiol (2 mg) and norethisterone acetate (1 mg) significantly increased the levels of F_{1+2}, TAT and D-dimer. Interestingly, the increase in F_{1+2} was higher in those women who subsequently developed recurrent VTE.[26]

In clinical practice and in most randomized clinical trials, the same dose of oestrogen has been prescribed, but proper testing of the dose–response effects on relevant clinical end-points and biochemical markers including coagulation has not yet been performed. However, one very small study did report that 0.625 mg conjugated oestrogen induced half-activation of coagulation as compared with 1.25 mg as judged by changes in the levels of F_{1+2} and fibrinopeptide A.[7] It is therefore a possibility that lower oestrogen doses may induce less (or no) activation of coagulation and thereby be associated with less risk of thrombosis.

Most studies suggest that *transdermal oestrogen* is not associated with activation of coagulation,[9,25,29,45,48,51,55,61,64] which may be attributed to a lack of 'first-pass' hepatic effects oestrogen after transdermal administration. These findings are consistent with recent clinical findings suggesting that transdermal oestrogen does not increase the risk of VTE.[52]

There is, so far, no evidence that conjugated oestrogens and oestradiol exert differential effects on coagulation and the risk of thrombosis. There is also no evidence that additional progestins or different progestins significantly alter the effects of oestrogens on coagulation.

THE EFFECTS OF HORMONE REPLACEMENT THERAPY ON PROCOAGULANTS

Several epidemiological studies initially reported lower levels of fibrinogen on HRT, which at the time was taken as further evidence for cardioprotective effects of HRT.[33,40,44] Theoretically, low fibrinogen will lower the substrate concentration for fibrin formation and plasma viscosity. Later controlled trials have found inconsistent results.[1,10,17,25,26,32,58]

The effects of HRT on factor VII are confusing. Most studies using oral oestrogen alone have reported increases in factor VII activity.[18,31,34,60,61] Since this activity is associated with triglyceride levels (see Ch. 4), the increase in factor VII activity can partly be explained by an adverse increase in triglyceride levels on oestrogen alone. Progestins counteract this increase in triglycerides, and may therefore explain why oral combined HRT is not associated with increased factor VII activity[51] or even reductions in factor VII activity.[6,26,46]

In contrast to combined oral contraceptives there are few reports on the effects of HRT and other coagulation factors. One study has reported that HRT may increase factor IX levels and the risk of VTE,[36,37] whereas other studies have found no effect on factor VIII levels.[26,37,44] A recent finding that oral HRT is associated with an increase in tissue factor activity[30] is of theoretical interest as an underlying mechanism for a prothrombotic effect, but this needs confirmation in further studies.

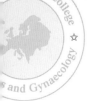
THE EFFECTS OF HORMONE REPLACEMENT THERAPY ON ANTICOAGULANTS AND ACTIVATED PROTEIN C RESISTANCE

Numerous studies have found that oral HRT significantly impairs natural antico-agulant pathways. AT is lowered by 5–10%,[7,25,26,29,44,51,60] protein C by 5–15%,[25,26,54] protein S by 0–5%[7,18,25,26,45,54,60] and TFPI[5,24–26,30,45,46] by 10–30%. The strong reductions on TFPI levels are comparable to the effects observed with combined oral contraceptives.[12] In our study of women with a history of VTE, we found that the reduction in TFPI levels on oral combined HRT (in women with a history of VTE) was a significant predictor for the increase in prothrom-botic markers[26] and for acquired APC resistance.[24] There is also evidence that reduced levels of TFPI can increase tissue factor activity.[30] These data strongly support the hypothesis that changes in TFPI levels during HRT play an impor-tant role for the increased risk of thrombosis.

An important effect of oral HRT may be the induction of acquired APC resist-ance, which can be detected using the sensitive thrombin generation assay.[24,45] We found that high-dose oral HRT in women with a history of VTE induced an APC-resistant phenotype similar to that observed in heterozygous carriers of the factor V Leiden mutation, whereas heterozygous carriers displayed a phenotype more like homozygous individuals. Changes in TFPI and protein S, but not factor VIII, were important predictors for the APC-resistant phenotype.[24] Oger et al observed a sim-ilar but much less pronounced effect of low-dose oral HRT containing half-dose oestradiol on APC resistance.[45] The reduction of TFPI was less pronounced. They also found that transdermal oestradiol did not induce an APC-resistant phenotype.

CONCLUSION

The compiled literature on the effects of HRT on coagulation now strongly sug-gests that conventional doses of oral oestrogen (2 mg 17β-oestradiol or 0.625 mg CEE) either alone or in combination with progestins induce a prothrombotic phenotype with increased levels of markers of activated coagulation, reduced lev-els of natural anticoagulants and an acquired APC-resistant phenotype. Except for one small study, direct comparisons of different doses of oestrogens on coag-ulation are lacking, but studies using lower oestrogen doses have detected markedly smaller effects on markers of activated coagulation. These findings raise the hypothesis of a threshold by which oestrogens may induce activation of coag-ulation and trigger thrombosis. So far, clinical data on adverse effects of oral HRT on the risk of thrombosis have almost exclusively been generated from studies using high doses of oestrogens, and there is a possibility that lower oestrogen doses can be associated with much lower or no excess risk of thrombosis. Over-all, transdermal oestrogen has proven to be associated with only minimal or no adverse effects on coagulation, which is consistent with clinical data suggesting a very low excess risk of thrombosis.

An important question is whether the effects of HRT on blood coagulation markers can be used as surrogate markers to predict the risk of arterial and venous thrombosis at an early stage. This overview provides evidence that markers of activated coagulation, such as F_{1+2} and D-dimer, can most probably be used to predict adverse prothrombotic effects of oestrogens. Well-designed pharmacodynamic studies in a limited number of subjects using blood coagulation surrogate end-points could therefore be an important tool for the selection of new oestrogen formulations and doses in the future. Maybe there is time for a reappraisal of use of coagulation markers as surrogate end-points for the assessment of thrombotic risk associated with oestrogens?

References

1. Andersen L F, Gram J, Skouby S O et al 1999 Effects of hormone replacement therapy on hemostatic cardiovascular risk factors. American Journal of Obstetrics and Gynecology 180:283–289

2. Balleisen L, Bailey J, Epping P H et al 1985 Epidemiological study on factor VII, factor VIII and fibrinogen in an industrial population. I. Baseline data on the relation to age, gender, body-weight, smoking, alcohol, pill-using, and menopause. Thrombosis and Haemostasis 54:475–479

3. Barrett-Connor E, Bush T L 1991 Estrogen and coronary heart disease in women. The Journal of the American Medical Association 265:1861–1867

4. Bertina R M, Koeleman B P, Koster T et al 1994 Mutation in blood coagulation factor V associated with resistance to activated protein C. Nature (5 May) 369:64–67

5. Bladbjerg E M, Skouby S O, Andersen L F et al 2002 Effects of different progestin regimens in hormone replacement therapy on blood coagulation factor VII and tissue factor pathway inhibitor. Human Reproduction 17:3235–3241

6. Borgfeldt C, Li C, Samsioe G 2004 Low-dose oral combination of 17beta-estradiol and norethisterone acetate in postmenopausal women decreases factor VII, fibrinogen, antithrombin and plasminogen activator inhibitor-1. Climacteric 7:78–85

7. Caine Y G, Bauer K A, Barzegar S et al 1992 Coagulation activation following estrogen administration to postmenopausal women. Thrombosis and Haemostasis 68:392–395

8. Cherry N 2002 Oestrogen therapy for prevention of reinfarction in postmenopausal women: a randomised placebo-controlled trial. The Lancet 360:2001–2008

9. Cieplluch R, Czestochowska E 1996 Influence of hormone replacement therapy (17 beta-OH estradiol and medroxyprogesterone acetate) on plasma concentration of prothrombin fragment F1+2 and thrombin-antithrombin III complex in postmenopausal women. Acta Haematologica Polonica 27:21–25

10. Conard J, Gompel A, Pelissier C et al 1997 Fibrinogen and plasminogen modifications during oral estradiol replacement therapy. Fertility and Sterility 68:449–453

11. Cushman M, Kuller L H, Prentice R et al 2004 Estrogen plus progestin and risk of venous thrombosis. The Journal of the American Medical Association 292:1573–1580

12. Dahm A, van Hylckama Vlieg A, Bendz B et al 2003 Low levels of tissue factor pathway inhibitor (TFPI) increase the risk of venous thrombosis. Blood 101:4387–4392

13. Daly E, Vessey M P, Hawkins M M et al 1996 Risk of venous thromboembolism in users of hormone replacement therapy. The Lancet 348:977–980

14. Daly E, Vessey M P, Painter R et al 1996 Case-control study of venous thromboembolism risk in users of hormone replacement therapy. The Lancet 348:1027

15. Devor M, Barrett-Connor E, Renvall M et al 1992 Estrogen replacement therapy and the risk of venous thrombosis. The American Journal of Medicine 92:275–282

16. Folsom A R, Wu K K, Davis C E et al 1991 Population correlates of plasma fibrinogen and factor VII, putative cardiovascular risk factors. Atherosclerosis 91:191–205

17. Frohlich M, Schunkert H, Hense H W et al 1998 Effects of hormone replacement therapies on fibrinogen and plasma viscosity in postmenopausal women. British Journal of Haematology 100:577–581

18. Gottsater A, Rendell M, Hulthen U L et al 2001 Hormone replacement therapy in

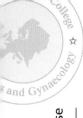

healthy postmenopausal women: a randomized, placebo-controlled study of effects on coagulation and fibrinolytic factors. The Journal of Internal Medicine 249:237–246

19. Grady D, Herrington D, Bittner V et al 2002 Cardiovascular disease outcomes during 6.8 years of hormone therapy. Heart and Estrogen/progestin Replacement Study follow-up (HERS II). The Journal of the American Medical Association 288:49–57

20. Grady D, Wenger N K, Herrington D et al 2000 Postmenopausal hormone therapy increases risk for venous thromboembolic disease. The Heart and Estrogen/progestin Replacement Study. Annals of Internal Medicine 132:689–696

21. Grant P J 2003 The genetics of atherothrombotic disorders: a clinician's view. Journal of Thrombosis and Haemostasis 1:1381–1390

22. Grodstein F, Stampfer M J, Goldhaber S Z et al 1996 Prospective study of exogenous hormones and risk of pulmonary embolism in women. The Lancet 348:983–987

23. Høibraaten E, Abdelnoor M, Sandset P M 1999 Hormone replacement therapy with estradiol and risk of venous thromboembolism – a population-based case-control study. Thrombosis and Haemostasis 82:1218–1221

24. Høibraaten E, Mowinckel M C, de Ronde H et al 2001 Hormone replacement therapy and acquired resistance to activated protein C: results of a randomized, double-blind, placebo-controlled trial. British Journal of Haematology 115:415–420

25. Høibraaten E, Os I, Seljeflot I et al 2000 The effects of hormone replacement therapy on hemostatic variables in women with angiographically verified coronary artery disease. Results from the Estrogen in Women with Atherosclerosis study. Thrombosis Research 98:19–27

26. Høibraaten E, Qvigstad E, Andersen T O et al 2001 The effects of hormone replacement therapy (HT) on hemostatic variables in women with previous venous thromboembolism – results from a randomized, double-blind, clinical trial. Thrombosis and Haemostasis 85:775–781

27. Høibraaten E, Qvigstad E, Arnesen H et al 2000 Increased risk of recurrent venous thromboembolism during hormone replacement therapy – results of the randomized, double-blind, placebo-controlled Estrogen in Venous Thromboembolism Trial. Thrombosis and Haemostasis 84:961–967

28. Jick H, Derby L E, Myers M W et al 1996 Risk of hospital admission for idiopathic

venous thromboembolism among users of postmenopausal oestrogens. The Lancet 348:981–983

29. Koh K K, Horne M K, III, Cannon R O, III 1999 Effects of hormone replacement therapy on coagulation, fibrinolysis, and thrombosis risk in postmenopausal women. Thrombosis and Haemostasis 82:626–633

30. Koh K K, Ahn J Y, Kim D S et al 2003 Effect of hormone replacement therapy on tissue factor activity, C-reactive protein, and the tissue factor pathway inhibitor. The American Journal of Cardiology 91:371–373

31. Kroon U B, Silfverstolpe G, Tengborn L 1994 The effects of transdermal estradiol and oral conjugated estrogens on haemostasis variables. Thrombosis and Haemostasis 71:420–423

32. Kroon U B, Tengborn L, Rita H et al 1997 The effects of transdermal oestradiol and oral progestogens on haemostasis variables. British Journal of Obstetrics and Gynaecology 104 (Suppl 16):32–37

33. Lee A J, Lowe G D, Smith W C et al 1993 Plasma fibrinogen in women: relationships with oral contraception, the menopause and hormone replacement therapy. British Journal of Haematology 83:616–621

34. Lindberg U B, Crona N, Stigendal L et al 1989 A comparison between effects of estradiol valerate and low-dose ethinyl estradiol on haemostasis parameters. Thrombosis and Haemostasis 61:65–69

35. Lip G Y, Blann A D, Jones A F et al 1997 Effects of hormone replacement therapy on hemostatic factors, lipid factors, and endothelial function in women undergoing surgical menopause: implications for prevention of atherosclerosis. American Heart Journal 134:764–771

36. Lowe G, Woodward M, Vessey M et al 2000 Thrombotic variables and risk of idiopathic venous thromboembolism in women aged 45–64 years. Relationships to hormone replacement therapy. Thrombosis and Haemostasis 83:530–535

37. Lowe G D, Upton M N, Rumley A et al 2001 Different effects of oral and transdermal hormone replacement therapies on factor IX, APC resistance, t-PA, PAI and C-reactive protein – a cross-sectional population survey. Thrombosis and Haemostasis 86:550–556

38. Mann K G 1999 Biochemistry and physiology of blood coagulation. Thrombosis and Haemostasis 82:165–174

39. Manson J E, Hsia J, Johnson K C et al 2003 Estrogen plus progestin and the risk of

coronary heart disease. The New England Journal of Medicine 349:523–534

40. Meade T W 1997 Hormone replacement therapy and haemostatic function. Thrombosis and Haemostasis 78:765–769

41. Meade T W, Dyer S, Howarth D J et al 1990 Antithrombin III and procoagulant activity: sex differences and effects of the menopause. British Journal of Haematology 74:77–81

42. Meade T W, Imeson J D, Haines A P et al 1983 Menopausal status and haemostatic variables. The Lancet 321:22–24

43. Meilahn E N, Kuller L H, Matthews K A et al 1992 Hemostatic factors according to menopausal status and use of hormone replacement therapy. Annals of Epidemiology 2:445–455

44. Nabulsi A A, Folsom A R, White A et al 1993 Association of hormone-replacement therapy with various cardiovascular risk factors in postmenopausal women. The New England Journal of Medicine 328:1069–1075

45. Oger E, Alhenc-Gelas M, Lacut K et al 2003 Differential effects of oral and transdermal estrogen/progesterone regimens on sensitivity to activated protein C among postmenopausal women: a randomized trial. Arteriosclerosis, Thrombosis, and Vascular Biology 23:1671–1676

46. Peverill R E, Teede H J, Smolich J J et al 2001 Effects of combined oral hormone replacement therapy on tissue factor pathway inhibitor and factor VII. Clinical Science (London) 101:93–99

47. Pinto S, Rostagno C, Coppo M et al 1990 No signs of increased thrombin generation in menopause. Thrombosis Research 58:645–651

48. Post M S, van der Mooren M J, van Baal W M et al 2003 Effects of low-dose oral and transdermal estrogen replacement therapy on hemostatic factors in healthy postmenopausal women: a randomized placebo-controlled study. American Journal of Obstetrics and Gynecology 189:1221–1227

49. Rosendaal F R 1999 Venous thrombosis: a multicausal disease. The Lancet 353:1167–1173

50. Saleh A A, Dorey L G, Dombrowski M P et al 1993 Thrombosis and hormone replacement therapy in postmenopausal women. American Journal of Obstetrics and Gynecology 169:1554–1557

51. Scarabin P Y, Alhenc-Gelas M, Plu-Bureau G et al 1997 Effects of oral and transdermal estrogen/progesterone regimens on blood coagulation and fibrinolysis in postmenopausal women. A randomized controlled trial. Arteriosclerosis, Thrombosis, and Vascular Biology 17:3071–3078

52. Scarabin P Y, Oger E, Plu-Bureau G 2003 Differential association of oral and transdermal oestrogen-replacement therapy with venous thromboembolism risk. The Lancet 362:428–432

53. Scarabin P Y, Vissac A M, Kirzin J M et al 1996 Population correlates of coagulation factor VII. Importance of age, sex, and menopausal status as determinants of activated factor VII. Arteriosclerosis, Thrombosis, and Vascular Biology 16:1170–1176

54. Sidelmann J J, Jespersen J, Andersen L F et al 2003 Hormone replacement therapy and hypercoagulability. Results from the Prospective Collaborative Danish Climacteric Study. British Journal of Obstetrics and Gynaecology 110:541–547

55. Stevenson J C, Oladipo A, Manassiev N et al 2004 Randomized trial of effect of transdermal continuous combined hormone replacement therapy on cardiovascular risk markers. British Journal of Haematology 124:802–808

56. Tait R C, Walker I D, Islam S I et al 1993 Protein C activity in healthy volunteers – influence of age, sex, smoking and oral contraceptives. Thrombosis and Haemostasis 70:281–285

57. Teede H J, McGrath B P, Smolich J J et al 2000 Postmenopausal hormone replacement therapy increases coagulation activity and fibrinolysis. Arteriosclerosis, Thrombosis, and Vascular Biology 20:1404–1409

58. The Writing Group for the PEPI trial 1995 Effects of estrogen or estrogen/progestin regimens on heart disease risk factors in postmenopausal women. The Postmenopausal Estrogen/Progestin Interventions (PEPI) trial. The Journal of the American Medical Association 273:199–208

59. Tsai A W, Cushman M, Rosamond W D et al 2002 Coagulation factors, inflammation markers, and venous thromboembolism. The Longitudinal Investigation of Thromboembolism Etiology (LITE). The American Journal of Medicine 113:636–642

60. Van Baal W M, Emeis J J, van der Mooren M J et al 2000 Impaired procoagulant-anticoagulant balance during hormone replacement therapy? A randomised, placebo-controlled 12-week study. Thrombosis and Haemostasis 83:29–34

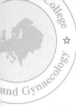

The menopause

61. Vehkavaara S, Silveira A, Hakala-Ala-Pietila T et al 2001 Effects of oral and transdermal estrogen replacement therapy on markers of coagulation, fibrinolysis, inflammation and serum lipids and lipoproteins in post-menopausal women. Thrombosis and Haemostasis 85:619–625

62. Vlieg A v H, van der Linden I K, Bertina R M et al 2000 High levels of factor IX increase the risk of venous thrombosis. Blood 95:3678–3682

63. Wassertheil-Smoller S, Hendrix S, Limacher M et al 2003 Effect of estrogen plus pro-gestin on stroke in postmenopausal women. The Women's Health Initiative. A randomi-zed trial. The Journal of the American Medical Association 289:2673–2684

64. Zegura B, Keber I, Sebestjen M et al 2003 Double-blind, randomized study of estradiol replacement therapy on markers of inflammation, coagulation and fibrinolysis. Atherosclerosis 168:123–129

7

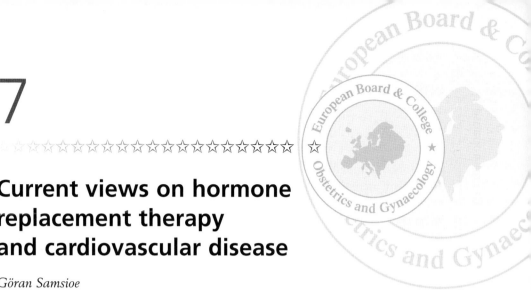

Current views on hormone replacement therapy and cardiovascular disease

Göran Samsioe

ABSTRACT

Coronary heart disease (CHD) remains the most common cause of mortality for both genders. A 50-year-old woman has a 46% risk of developing CHD and a 31% risk of dying from it. However, female CHD is specific in several ways. Firstly, risk factors comprise not only cholesterol but also high triglycerides. Depression is another prudent female risk factor. Women have instable angina more often than men and mortality rates after acute myocardial infarction (MI) are higher in women, particularly in diabetics. The frequency of CHD also increases by age in women but there is no abrupt jump at the time of the menopause. Accumulating and compelling evidence from mechanistic and experimental studies suggests that oestrogens are cardioprotective. This includes laboratory and event data from non-primates as well as primates. A huge number of observational studies strongly concur to the notion that oestrogen reduces CHD. It was astonishing when randomized controlled trials (RCTs) such as the HERS and WHI studies failed to confirm this rationale. Even if RCTs are considered pivotal in the hierarchy of evidence, they are not problem free. Apart from several technicalities they can only study one preparation at a time. Subjects in these trials do not constitute the clinical target group as they are generally older and without climacteric symptoms. Neither risks nor benefits by hormone replacement therapy (HRT) in published clinical trials should therefore readily be transferred to the major target population. Indeed, a synthesis of results from all types of studies probably constitutes the best platform for the clinicians' and patients' choices.

KEYWORDS

Heart disease, hormone replacement therapy (HRT), oestrogen, venous thromboembolism (VTE)

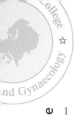
The menopause

INTRODUCTION

The use of oestrogen to mitigate classic climacteric symptoms such as hot flushes and sweats dates back to the 1950s, and by the mid-1970s around 40% of women in the USA were using oestrogens for the alleviation of climacteric symptoms. Compelling evidence then suggested that there were time- and dose-dependent increases of endometrial cancer by oestrogen monotherapy, which led to the introduction of combined oestrogen–progestogen remedies, particularly the continuous combined oestrogen–progestogen therapy (CCHRT), which, in addition to protection against endometrial cancer, also provided a bleed-free regimen much appreciated by the consumer. An increase of the use of hormone replacement therapy (HRT) was noted again, which, by 1997, had reached figures around 40% both in Europe and in the USA.

During the 1990s, evidence-based medicine developed, emphasizing the double-blind randomized control trial (RCT) as the gold standard for the basis of clinical recommendations. However, RCTs are not problem free. It goes without saying that breast cancer development could not be the primary end-point in such studies. Another very important point is that RCTs could not be made double-blind as placebo has an insufficient effect on climacteric symptoms. Therefore, participants in RCTs on HRT are void of symptoms and about 10 years older than the clinical target population.

Prior to the publication of the HERS trial in 1998 primary and especially secondary prevention of heart disease by HRT was regarded as almost established medicine.[10] Admittedly, cardiac prevention was never an established official indication but more or less all available data pointed to this possibility. Apart from beneficial effects on several surrogate markers for cardiovascular disease (CVD) observational and experimental data came together. Several observational studies on hard end-points, as well as angiographic data on the extent of coronary arteriosclerosis, strongly suggested a cardioprotective effect. These data were also backed up by animal experiments – the results on the *Cynomolgus* monkey were considered pivotal. These concepts formed the rationale for the HERS, which, to our surprise, could not verify the hypothesis. Despite well-founded criticism of the HERS, an era of negativism regarding CVD and HRT has prevailed ever since. Nonetheless oestrogens and oestrogen–progestin combinations have repeatedly and positively been shown to influence several factors of pivotal importance for the subsequent development of CVD.

FEMALE CORONARY HEART DISEASE

Coronary heart disease (CHD) is the most common cause of morbidity and mortality in both women and men. At the younger ages men are at a significantly greater risk of developing CHD, but as women age, their risk for CHD approaches that of men. The prevalence of CHD in women aged between 45 and 64 years is 1 in 7; over the age of 65 years, the prevalence is 1 in 3. A significant number of women have atherosclerotic lesions even if they have no clinical signs of CHD. Mortality rises by age in both genders. The male:female ratio is 5:1 for those aged 35–44 years, but only 1.5:1 for those over 75 years old. One in four women aged 60 and over will eventually die of CHD. A 50-year-old woman has a 46% risk of developing CHD and a 31% risk of dying from it.

Women hospitalized with MI have a mortality rate twice that of men. The high risk of death emphasizes the need for a better understanding of heart disease in women. Only 50% of cases are related to predictable risk factors, suggesting the need for a different approach to risk factors in women. Despite the fact that CHD incidence increases at the time of the menopause, the change is gradual rather than abrupt. Deaths from CHD and cancer are approximately equal in younger women but, over 65 years of age, CHD is the major cause of death. Although CHD overall represents a greater risk of morbidity and mortality, cancer remains a woman's greatest fear even among university graduates who are normally better informed of CHD risks.

Women have a different clinical presentation of an acute ischaemic event as compared to men. Indeed, women have unstable angina more frequently than men, while men have acute ischaemic syndromes more frequently. Women have a worse outcome after acute MI, in part because they receive slower medical attention, with a greater delay in receiving care and later and less thrombolysis. In addition, they present more risk factors and higher rates of complications, due to their different pathophysiology or other as-yet-unknown reasons.

Over the last few years data have accumulated to suggest that a high risk of several diseases inclusive of CVD is closely linked to fetal development. Infants born after intrauterine growth retardation tend to grow old at a quicker pace. Risk results in an overall increased risk of CVD but also induces an earlier menopause.

The development of atherosclerosis is delayed in women compared to men, and normal ovarian hormone production seems to counteract the development of atherosclerosis, while oestrogen deficiency is associated with the development of atherosclerosis and CHD. However, one should remember that several other mechanisms may also contribute.

The highest mortality rates from ischaemic heart disease in Europe are found in northern European countries, while central and eastern Europe have intermediate rates. The risk differs in different countries in different parts of the world, in relation to ethnic group, diet and lifestyle. Populations characterized by different patterns of mortality may have different HRT risk/benefit balances with regard to mortality. These epidemiological differences should be considered in the evaluation of the HRT risk/benefit profile as they may well differ by country and ethnic group.

CARDIOVASCULAR DISEASE RISK FACTORS IN WOMEN

Women share several CVD risk factors with men, such as family history, diet, obesity, smoking, unfavourable lipid profile, high homocysteine levels, high fibrinogen, low physical activity, diabetes mellitus and hypertension. In addition, women have the unique risk factor of the menopause. Women have a greater relative risk than men if they are diabetic, have raised triglyceride levels, low levels of high-density lipoprotein (HDL) or if they are smokers. CHD is more common in countries with high saturated fat diets and high cholesterol levels. In addition, hypercholesterolaemic patients are prone to early CHD, while cholesterol lowering reduces CHD. For CHD in middle-aged women, high triglyceride levels are more important than high LDL cholesterol levels. We do not yet know whether the HDL level or the triglyceride level is the more important factor in women. Nevertheless, CHD prevention trials using statins have demonstrated that women benefit from LDL cholesterol reduction as much as men. Recent studies have revealed that intensive multiple interventions such as lifestyle modifications, including diet, weight reduction, smoking cessation and exercise, may reduce the risk of CHD and can result in fewer cases of heart disease in a very cost-effective manner. Aspirin, beta-blockers and cholesterol-lowering drugs are beneficial also for women with documented CVD.

MENOPAUSE AND CARDIOVASCULAR DISEASE

Women tend to develop CHD about 10 years later than men. Being male and above 45 years of age is a risk factor for CHD, whereas females are not considered at risk until they reach 55 years of age. This '10-year advantage' can be lost, however, if a woman starts menopause prematurely or if she has other risk factors, such as smoking or diabetes mellitus.

Large cross-sectional studies indicate that, in addition to the effect of ageing, menopause *per se* is associated with lipid modifications, such as an increase in total cholesterol, low-density lipoprotein cholesterol (LDL-C) and triglycerides that can cause an increased risk of developing CVD. This increase in total cholesterol results from increases in levels of LDL-C, and increases in very-low-density lipoprotein (VLDL) and lipoprotein (a); the oxidation of LDL-C is also enhanced. High-density lipoprotein cholesterol (HDL-C) levels may decrease over time but these changes are small and insignificant relative to the increases in LDL-C. The coagulation balance is not altered significantly with menopause because a counterbalance of changes occurs – some procoagulation factors increase (e.g. factor VII and fibrinogen) but so do certain fibrinolytic factors, such as antithrombin III and plasminogen. In addition, at the time of menopause, changes in vascular reactivity take place: prostacyclin production decreases, endothelin levels increase and the endothelium-dependent vasodilation is impaired. At the same time, increases in blood pressure and body weight, and changes in body fat distribution, plus alterations in insulin sensitivity and glucose metabolism have been reported. In healthy, non-obese, postmenopausal women, carbohydrate tolerance decreases as a result of an increase in insulin resistance.[13]

HORMONE REPLACEMENT THERAPY AND THE LIPID PROFILE

Oestrogen replacement can improve the lipid profile in postmenopausal women. The various oestrogen formulations, and the route of administration, seem to have different effects on lipid profile over time, although the exact weight of these differences and their clinical significance for CVD risk are still open to discussion. No conclusive evidence suggests that the addition of progestogens, at the doses needed to exert endometrial protection, accentuates in a clinically significant way the effects of oestrogen on lipid profiles, although the effect may vary depending on the type and the dose of different progestogens. Besides the negative effect on HDL-C, data are available on some beneficial effects of tibolone on the lipid profile but to date there is no information on cardiovascular events.

HORMONE REPLACEMENT THERAPY AND CARBOHYDRATE METABOLISM

Menopausal women exhibit features of the metabolic syndrome X. Postmenopausal women have greater insulin resistance than premenopausal, and menopause is followed by a progressive fall in insulin sensitivity. Oestrogen replacement increases insulin sensitivity in postmenopausal women, while oestrogen–progestin regimens may decrease insulin sensitivity. However, the data are very limited. Thus, progestins may accentuate the beneficial actions of oestrogen on glucose tolerance: this effect is related to the type, the route of administration and the dose of progestin. In women with type 2 diabetes, oestrogen therapy (ET) and some forms of HRT have recently been shown to improve glucose control, HDL and LDL cholesterol, with minimal or no increase in blood triglycerides. However, all of the existing studies in diabetic women have a small number of participants and are short-term studies. There was clear agreement by the expert panel that more research is needed to determine the effects of ET/HRT on glucose metabolism and cardiovascular risk in diabetic women.

HORMONE REPLACEMENT THERAPY AND BLOOD PRESSURE

In addition to the age-related increase in blood pressure levels, women show a more evident increase in both diastolic and, chiefly, systolic blood pressure during the climacteric transition. This phenomenon seems not to be related principally to the menopause-related increase in body weight and central, android body fat distribution. HRT has a neutral effect on blood pressure in normotensive women. However, limited data are available concerning the effects of HRT on blood pressure in borderline and hypertensive postmenopausal women.

HORMONE REPLACEMENT THERAPY AND BODY WEIGHT

Overweight and obesity are associated with an increase in morbidity and mortality. In particular, the central distribution of body fat may be considered as an independent predictor of CVD in women. Evidence for an increase in body weight, and a shift to a more central, android fat distribution in normal women throughout the climacteric period has been reported. Perimenopausal hormonal changes (rather than the ageing process) seem to be relevant for the accelerated increase in body weight and body fat, and these can be counteracted, at least in part, by HRT. Most interventional studies indicate that HRT can also accentuate the accumulation of central body fat in postmenopausal women compared with control or placebo-treated women.

HORMONE REPLACEMENT THERAPY AND VASCULATURE

In recent years, exciting new scientific information has emerged regarding how oestrogens are able to influence blood vessel function and structure directly and indirectly. Recent studies have shown that the cells of the blood vessels and heart also contain oestrogen receptors (ERS). Furthermore, in a number of studies it has become clear that oestrogen binds to ERs in the cardiovascular system and causes important changes in how these tissues work. At the molecular level, oestrogen works by binding to ERs, but other non-genomic mechanisms may play a role in inducing the oestrogenic effects. Experimental data show that oestrogens in animal models can improve endothelial function, inhibit LDL oxidation, intimal thickening, vascular smooth muscle cell migration and proliferation and, thus, can prevent or inhibit atherogenesis. In women, oestrogens can exert an antiatherogenic effect through their actions on lipid and glucose metabolism. Also, oestrogen administration can cause coronary vasodilation, and can preserve endothelial function. Premenopausal normotensive women are protected against the effect of ageing on endothelial function. Oestrogen administration restores the endothelium-dependent vasodilation and/or nitric oxide availability. The role of oestrogen administration in elderly postmenopausal women with various risk factors is still controversial. However, HRT can effectively reduce the vascular wall intima and media thickness in hypercholesterolaemic, postmenopausal women. Further studies (taking into account co-medication with drugs with an impact on CVD such as statins) are needed to assess the effect of HRT upon the progression from its early stages of coronary atherosclerosis in women.

All available data support a role for ERs in preventing vascular injury. Thus these studies provide hope that new tissue-selective oestrogens can act selectively on the heart and blood vessels, avoiding the possible side-effects associated with existing hormonal replacement therapies. In postmenopausal women, the selective ER modulator raloxifene reduces some risk factors of coronary artery disease such as total cholesterol, LDL-C, homocysteine and fibrinogen, while it does not induce any significant change in triglycerides, HDL-C, plasminogen activation inhibitor 1 (PAI-1) and C-reactive protein (CRP). In addition, raloxifene exerts effects similar to those of oestradiol at the endothelial level. Ongoing randomized clinical trials are evaluating the effect of raloxifene on the incidence of coronary events.

HORMONE REPLACEMENT THERAPY AND CARDIOVASCULAR EVENTS

DEEP VEIN THROMBOSIS

Current, but not past, use of HRT in early postmenopausal women is associated with a two- to threefold increase of venous thromboembolism (VTE). Consistently, the results for all studies indicate that, among healthy postmenopausal women, an excess risk of one to two cases of idiopathic VTE per 10 000 women per year can be attributed to current use of HRT (estimated incidence of idiopathic VTE per 10 000 women per year of one among non-users and of two or three among oestrogen users). Thus, the absolute risk is small and the mechanism largely unclear. The risk is more prominent in the first year of therapy and appears to be dose-dependent. However, caution in high-risk situations must be advised, such as low pretreatment PAI-1 values, which may negate any cardiovascular benefit and result in a substantial increase of the thromboembolic risk. Despite an increase in VTE events, no increase in mortality from pulmonary embolism has been reported. The use of raloxifene or tamoxifen is associated with an excess risk of VTE events similar to that associated with HRT. Transdermal oestradiol seems to be associated with a lower risk of VTE but it is still higher than in untreated postmenopausal women.

THE HERS AND WHI DATA

The *post-hoc* analyses of the HERS data showed a statistically significant time trend, with more CHD events in the hormone group than in the placebo group during the first year of treatment, and fewer in years 3 to 5.

The HERS II study[6] was a follow-up to women enrolled in HERS. In HERS II, treatment assignment was unblinded in 1998. Subsequent use of HRT was based on decisions made by women and their physicians. Of the 2763 women enrolled in HERS, 2510 were alive at the time of enrolment in HERS II (1260 in the placebo group and 1250 in the hormone group). Of these, 2321 (92%) agreed to enrol in HERS II (1165 in the placebo group and 1156 in the hormone group). At the end of HERS II, close-out telephone contacts were completed for 99% of surviving women in both the placebo and hormone groups. The results of the study were published after an average additional follow-up of 2.7 years; the non-CVD outcomes were also published in the same issue.[9] Among women randomly assigned to HRT in HERS, the proportion reporting 80% or higher adherence to hormones was 81% during the first year and declined to 45% during the sixth year of follow-up in HERS II. The results showed no differences between women originally assigned to the hormone or placebo groups in regard to the rates of CHD events during HERS.[6]

Less than one week after the publication of the HERS II results, the US National Heart, Lung and Blood Institute announced that it had stopped the trial of the CCHRT arm versus placebo in healthy postmenopausal women because of increased numbers of breast cancer and an overall measure suggesting that the harms outweighed the benefits. The trial was one component of the large WHI. Participants were randomized to a continuous combined combination of 0.625 mg daily of conjugated equine oestrogens (CEE) and 2.5 mg daily of medroxyprogesterone acetate (MPA) or placebo (the same commercial preparation that was used in the HERS I and II studies).

The WHI was the first randomized trial to address directly whether continuous combined oestrogen plus progestin had a favourable or unfavourable effect on CHD incidence and on overall risks and benefits in predominantly healthy women, since only 7.7% of participating women reported having prior CVD. The trial was stopped early due to health risks that exceeded health benefits over an average follow-up of 5.2 years.

The WHI extends these findings to include younger women and those without clinically apparent CHD. The findings in the WHI for stroke are consistent with HERS, whereas the pattern in the WHI related to the occurrence of VTE is an expected complication of the postmenopausal hormones, and also consistent with the findings from HERS.[15]

In the WHI report the magnitude of the relative risks is impressive. However, absolute risks are small per 10 000 woman-years, an abstract figure of extrapolation that does not reflect the actual results – at the end of 5.2 years there were 7968 women in the treated group and 7608 in the placebo group. Therefore, if the absolute risks are plotted as percentages, instead of the additional eight strokes, seven heart attacks and eight breast cancers per 10 000 woman-years, one would have, respectively, 0.8, 0.7 and 0.8 cases per 1000 woman years, a figure that is easier to interpret. It would suggest that if 1000 women were treated during one year there would be less than one woman with an adverse effect.

Combining all the monitored outcomes, women taking oestrogen plus progestin might expect 19 more events per year per 10 000 women than women taking placebo. These figures underline the need to present the absolute risk and not relative figures in order to prevent public scares and confusion among users. Moreover, the differences in relative risks were small, and applying the adjusted CI relatively weak and few statistical differences were found. One obvious limitation of the WHI study is mentioned by the authors – the trial tested only one specific drug regimen: CEE, 0.625 mg daily plus 2.5 mg MPA. The results do not necessarily apply to lower dosages, to other formulations of oral oestrogens and progestins, or to their administration via non-oral routes.

In 2003, the final results from the WHI combined arm were presented.[6] It was now evident that there was no statistically significant increase of CHD, and, similar to HERS there was a statistically significant trend towards a protection with time (Fig. 7.1).

Apart from a lack of primary CVD prevention not much new information was added to our existing knowledge although the balance between harmful and beneficial outcomes seems not to favour long-term HRT in symptom-free postmenopausal women.[19]

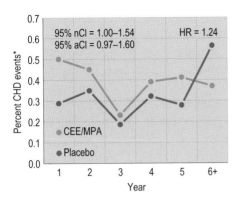

Year	Hazard ratio	95% CI
1	1.81	(1.09–3.01)
2	1.34	(0.82–2.18)
3	1.27	(0.64–2.50)
4	1.25	(0.74–2.12)
5	1.45	(0.81–2.59)
6+	0.70	(0.42–1.14)

Manson JE, et al. N Engl J Med. 2003;523–34.

Fig 7.1 An updated analysis of the annual risk of a CHD event through the termination of the WHI trial on 7 July 2002. In this analysis, the investigators used centrally adjudicated end-points for the primary coronary outcome of nonfatal MI or death due to CHD to enhance the uniformity of the documentation of outcomes. Previous analyses were based on local adjudication.

   This illustration compares yearly rates (annualized percent) of CHD events in the CEE/MPA and placebo groups. Annualized percent represents the percent of women experiencing CHD events in the patient group during that particular year. For example, an annualized percent of 0.29 represents 0.29% of women in that treatment group who had a CHD event during that year. The annualized percent of CHD events in the CEE/MPA and placebo groups were variable.

   The boxed figures are the hazard ratios (HR) and confidence intervals (CI) for CHD events with CEE/MPA use on a year-to-year basis. Statistical tests for linear trends detected a significant decrease (z score = –2.36; P = 0.02) in the risk associated with CEE/MPA over time. For the entire follow-up period examined, overall HR for CHD was 1.24, with a 95% nCI of 1.00–1.54 and a 95% aCI of 0.97–1.60.[16,24]
* Includes nine silent MIs.

The WHI finding (that CEE plus continuous administration of MPA does not confer benefit for preventing CHD among women with a uterus) concurs with the HERS study.

BENEFICIAL EFFECTS OF OESTROGEN

In conjunction with the cohort studies showing benefit, there are many mechanisms of oestrogen's cardioprotective effects, which lend credibility to the positive effects of oestrogen on cardiovascular risk. Beneficial effects on lipids and lipoproteins, endothelial function and inflammation have been documented. A controversy developed recently when it was found that an inflammatory marker CRP was increased with CEE use.[20] However, this appears to be a first-pass effect of oral ingestion in that transdermal oestrogen has been shown not to increase, but rather lower, CRP levels. The WHI trial has shed extra light on the important issue of mechanisms of action. What was apparent in both arms was the striking age dependence. There was no increased risk of CVD for women aged 50–59 in the combined arm and a 44% reduction, which almost reached statistical significance in the oestrogen-only arm.[1]

These findings suggest that the stage of atherosclerosis, which is a function of age, may play a pivotal role in the understanding of oestrogen effects. Losordo et al[14] demonstrated a loss of detectable ERs in atherosclerotic arteries yielding a lesser possibility for oestrogen-mediated vasodilatation. Koh et al[12] reported that CEE did not affect the flow-mediated dilatory response to hyperaemia in postmenopausal women with type 2 diabetes.

Inflammation plays a key role in the pathogenesis of CHD in the late stages of atherosclerosis. The role of CRP in plaque vulnerability is uncertain. While naturally occurring plasma levels of this marker appear associated with a risk of CHD, the pharmacological increase by oral oestrogens does not seem to influence risk.[20]

Acute coronary events are not necessarily associated with the degree of coronary artery atherosclerosis but more often result from a rupture of instable small to medium-sized plaques, which in turn are heavily infiltrated by macrophages. These macrophages readily produce matrix metalloproteinases (MMPs). The MMPs 9 and 7 seem particularly sensitive to oestrogens' influence whereby their activity is increased. This leads to a weakening of the fibrous cap and eventually to plaque rupture with subsequent mural thrombosis and arterial occlusion. The gene that controls production of MMP 9 is downregulated by statins and upregulated by oestrogens. In the combined arm of WHI the hazard ratio for women using statins was 0.99 and for those without statins 1.27. Also, in the HERS study there was no increased risk of CVD events in women on concomitant statin medication.

THE ROLE OF PROGESTOGEN

Although there have been many concerns about the attenuating effects of progestogens on the cardiovascular benefits of oestrogen, observational trials have not demonstrated any difference between ET and HRT regimens. While the null effects of the CCHRT regimen compared to placebo in HERS was criticized on the basis of continuous progestogen use, there was no difference between this regimen and oestrogen alone in an angiographic trial.[8] Nevertheless, because several clinical studies have shown attenuating effects of progestogen on certain parameters (HDL-C, blood flow, carbohydrate tolerance) on a theoretical basis, there should still be some caution exercised over the excessive use of progestogens.

Stroke is a cardiovascular end-point, which is more difficult to assess in terms of risks and benefits. Although some observational data have suggested a benefit of oestrogen in its incidence and changes in mortality, one of the studies that did find an increase in risk has suggested that this risk is dependent on the dose.[7] Here the statistical increase in risk was only confirmed in women using larger doses of CEE (≥0.625 mg). The dose of 0.3 mg (which showed a similar coronary benefit as with 0.625 mg) was shown not to increase the incidence of stroke. The lower dose having been beneficial for CHD suggests that lower doses of oestrogen should be considered for long-term use.

CLINICAL IMPLICATIONS

It is not an easy task to opt between results of observational and clinical trials. High-quality observational studies may extend evidence over a wider population and a wider time span. The incidence of harmful effects in the WHI study was really very small in terms of individual health. There is no reason to avoid post-menopausal hormone medication in women with climacteric symptoms.

It should be stressed that the main goal for all healthcare should be the improvement of women's health and not just hormonal therapies. The Nurses' Health Study[23] showed that between 1980 and 1994 there was a 31% reduction in CHD. Better nutrition, smoking cessation and HRTs in the menopause were responsible for the 18%, 13% and 9% of the reduction, respectively.

Our main goal should remain the maintenance of health as well as the primary and secondary prevention of disabling diseases, in particular those that are more prevalent after age 50.

Over the years several meta-analyses have been performed and published. However, it is questionable if they add anything to our knowledge except for providing a summary of the existing data. The problem with meta-analysis is that if a bias or confounder exists in observational studies, this cannot be corrected for. The plain meta-analysis does not control for size duration or quality of the studies included in such an analysis. A grading by quality is often made by the authors prior to performing the statistics leading to the results of the meta-analysis. This procedure is subjective and hence subject to bias.

One meta-analysis[11] attempted to minimize such bias by using established criteria on study quality issued by an independent body, in this case the US Preventive Services Task Force criteria. From the literature comprising 3035 papers evaluating primary prevention and published between 1966 and 2000, only 24 cohort studies, 18 case-control studies and one RCT were found to meet the criteria of the US Task Force. Whether it is justifiable to disregard 99.5% of the literature is another question. This meta-analysis by Humphrey et al[11] also differs from previous work by evaluating potential explanatory variables of the relationship between HRT and CVD. The results revealed a reduction of incidence and mortality in CHD in current users and a decreased mortality among current users of HRT in total CVD. There were no statistically significant effects in past ever or any users of HRT (Table 7.1). Still, the WHI is an important study even though it does not necessarily introduce new rules into good clinical practice.

In most western countries women suffer more cardiovascular events than men, and female mortality is higher, particularly when occurring in women with coexisting diabetes. A MI occurs as a result of a preceding CVD usually in the form of arteriosclerosis, which, in turn, develops over decades.

Several studies have also produced compelling evidence that CVD increases after oophorectomy. At premenopausal ages CVD is more common in women with premature menopause. In premenopausal women, who were struck by CVD events, oestradiol levels were almost half of the values in matched controls

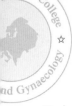
Table 7.1 A meta-analysis of 18 case-control studies, 24 cohort studies and one randomized controlled study of risk ratio of mortality or incidence of coronary heart disease with regard to use of HRT as compared with placebo[11]

	Mortality	Incidence
Current users	0.62[a]	0.80[a]
Past users	0.76	0.89
Ever users	0.81	0.91
Any users	0.74	0.88

without CVD. Furthermore, the attacks of instable angina seem to occur most frequently just prior to menses when oestrogen levels are particularly low. In conclusion, nature suggests that the premature loss of ovarian function is associated with a higher incidence of CVD.

Numerous attempts have been made to mimic the natural hormonal situation in women by producing a huge variety of HRTs. As CVD is also the main killer for women, the effect of HRT on cardiovascular morbidity and mortality has been meticulously studied. Given the enormous variation among various HRT regimens only a few have been studied to produce results as to the treatment or prevention of CVD. Concerning hard end-points we have limited data on oestrogens and doses other than CEE of 0.625 or 1.25 mg per day.

There are almost no data on transdermal administration but in a recent UK publication,[3] involving a fairly small number of patients, no benefit but no harm either was encountered after use of a transdermal patch. As in many other recent studies on HRT and CVD, doses used were high, in this case 80 µg per day compared to the standard dose of 25–50 µg per day, which is commonly used to treat menopausal symptoms.

In the limited number of studies on combined HRT, only oral MPA at doses 2.5–10 mg per day have produced data. In other words, when using the term 'HRT' this must be interpreted with care as it refers to a very limited number from the huge family of HRT preparations. In addition, the majority of data on CVD events is from the USA with only few European studies and no data from Asia, Africa or Latin America. A generalization of conclusions is therefore not justifiable.

Cardiovascular disease is multifactorial and the risk of a cardiovascular event depends largely on the occurrence of one or several risk factors. Some of these, such as male gender, age and family history, are not possible to change whereas others, such as perturbations of lipid and carbohydrate metabolism, obesity, hypertension and (oxidative) stress, are clearly modifiable. Also, a healthy diet, smoking cessation and increased physical activity impact heavily on future risk.

The WHI also has an observational arm, which recently produced data on exercise and cardiovascular events in postmenopausal women belonging to the

WHI population. This study[16] compared, prospectively, walking with vigorous exercise for the prevention of cardiovascular events among 73 743 post-menopausal women aged 50–79. Increasing physical activity had a strong inverse association with the risk of both coronary events and total CVD. Walking and vigorous exercise were associated with similar risk reductions provided they produced similar energy expenditure. Expressed in quintiles from lowest to highest energy expenditure, the relative risks were 1.00, 0.73, 0.69, 0.68 and 0.47, the trend being highly statistically significant (Box 7.1). Again, compelling evidence suggests that the reduction of one or several established risk factors by pharmacological or non-pharmacological means reduces subsequent events.

Several studies on various HRT regimens and CVD have been undertaken. These range from animal experiments and the lowering of metabolic risk factors to observational studies on actual events in humans. A few RCTs also exist but are limited in size and time of observation.

In line with nature's own experiments as outlined above almost all experimental data on animals, as well as humans, suggest a reduction of surrogate markers for atherosclerosis as well as of the extent of atherosclerotic plaques by oestrogens, and commonly also by combinations of oestrogens and progestogens.

Recently, long-term studies, which included tens of thousands, leading up to over 100 000 woman-years, have been pushed aside because of shorter-term and smaller-scale studies designed with a superior methodology by being double-blind, placebo-controlled and randomized.

A prospective cohort study by Fioretti et al[4] assessed the role of menopause on the risk of nonfatal MI and could not demonstrate an effect when data were controlled for age, BMI, education and the use of HRT. Furthermore, the substantial decrease (31%) in CVD reported by the Nurses' Health Study investigators[23] between 1980 and 1994 was mainly attributed to lifestyle changes such as smoking cessation and improved diet rather than to the use of HRT.

While shortcomings and interpretation problems with surrogate end-point studies and observational data are well recognized, the magnitude and diversity of these studies are such that the overall results should carry considerable weight in our understanding of the relationship between HRT and CVD. RCTs are not problem free and are subject to bias[17,21] as exemplified by the following.

Box 7.1 Walking or vigorous exercise leading to a reduction of coronary events[16]

- 73 743 postmenopausal women aged 50–79 years
- 345 CHD and 1551 CVD events in 5.9 years
- walking or vigorous exercise
- both reduce CVDs by 30–40%
- reduction increases with increasing energy expenditure.

1. RCTs have inclusion and exclusion criteria that are much more rigid than observational studies, many of which have implications for CVD, such as hypertension, high BMI, lipid abnormalities and impaired hepatic or renal function, leading to the recruitment of a lower than average risk population. Hence results are only valid for those who meet those inclusion and exclusion criteria.

2. According to the Helsinki Declaration, information to RCT participants must be such that they understand the current scientific knowledge on which the hypothesis of the RCT is based, recognizing that there is a 50% chance of being on placebo for a long time. This is likely to recruit a population at lower than average risk into RCTs, which seems to be the case for both HERS and WHI.

3. Subjects are new starters, but whether they had never used HRT, or used HRT for a considerable time prior to the trial, is not without importance for the development of CVD. Of particular relevance for primary prevention is the possibility that women void of climacteric symptoms, and with previously higher endogenous oestrogens, are recruited into RCTs.

4. RCTs use one preparation at one given dose and mode of administration. Interpretation of the results should be limited to this and to the target group of the RCT, and not generalized to include all populations and all HRT preparations regardless of their composition, dose and mode of administration. In addition, the composition of the target population regarding age and concomitant medication must be considered, as this may impact on steroid pharmacology.

5. RCTs are usually short-term and are at present limited to some 5 years' observation time.

In summary, both RCTs as well as observational studies are subject to bias but such biases are likely to be different between the two study types. Another important difference is the fact that an RCT will bear weight for the initial phase of a chronic treatment whereas cohort studies are poor captures of this phase. RCTs are extremely poor at giving us data on effects beyond 5 years of treatment, whereas observational data readily supply this. Time seems to be crucial in several studies, and in many observational studies a clear reduction cannot be seen until after 4 or 5 years of HRT. However, this time effect could well be influenced by drop-outs.

CVDs are multifactorial and can be influenced by lifestyle. For both primary and secondary prevention of CVD, much could be gained by modifying lifestyle factors, i.e. stopping smoking, using a well-balanced low-fat diet and exercising regularly. There is no controversy over adjusting these very important risk factors; lifestyle modifications should be emphasized to all women as well as men.

Incidence and mortality can also be modified by use of pharmacological agents other than HRT. There is evidence that antifibrinolytic medications, beta-blockers, ACE inhibitors and statins all may lower risk, both in primary but especially secondary prevention settings. Despite their proven benefits, it should be remembered that all these agents are not natural compounds to humans. Widespread long-term use of such compounds may lead to other untoward effects, as exemplified by the recent withdrawal of a marketed statin due to side-effects.

A recent publication from the MORE trial[2] indicates that raloxifene does not impose an increased risk of CVD. In the subset of 1035 women with risk factors for CVD, this even induced protection with a relative risk of 0.60 (95% CI; range 0.38–0.95). This occurred despite the fact that raloxifene in earlier reports was shown to induce a similar increased risk of VTE as oestrogens. One way of explaining this finding is that raloxifene may lack an induction of an inflammatory response. The increase by oral oestrogens of CRP could be indicative of such an induction by oral oestrogens, which in turn may promote instable atherosclerotic plaques to rupture and thereby initially induce CVD events.

Data based almost exclusively on CEEs suggest that HRT in doses used to treat climacteric symptoms increases the incidence of VTE, but only during the first 1–3 years of usage.[18] The reason for this remains obscure. Our current insufficient understanding of HRT administration and surveillance should encourage further research, especially on the effects of lower doses and non-oral approaches. This was further highlighted by a French case-control study showing an increased hazards ratio with oral (hazard ratio 3.5) but not with patches (hazard ratio 0.9).[22] Findings on VTE should not impact on the overall concept, which is that oestrogens may well be beneficial for the heart.

FUTURE DEVELOPMENTS

Hence, in the aftermath of HERS and WHI, it is essential to revisit the current situation and provide ideas for the future role of HRT regarding its effects on CVD. As mentioned above, the use of a healthy diet should be encouraged. Such a diet should be low in saturated fat but should have a high content of polyunsaturated fatty acids (PUFAs) especially from the so-called omega-3 series, i.e. n-3 fatty acids. Such a diet should also be rich in fibres and contain appropriate amounts of vitamins, antioxidants and trace elements.

The antioxidant properties of vitamins C end E are well documented as is the same property by several oestrogens, and antioxidation is believed to be cardio-protective. Port and red wine contain antioxidants and so could be included in the diet but not more than one or two glasses per day.

Seafood is a rich source of PUFA, particularly in salmon and other fish with a high fat content. It is also well known that the Inuit have a low risk of thromboembolism and longer bleeding time than, for example, Caucasians. This phenomenon is ascribed to the high content of PUFA in their diet. In addition, it is possible to reduce blood coagulability by the ingestion of cod liver oil. Another important quality of PUFA is to reduce triglycerides and particularly to stabilize the heart rate. The latter was demonstrated clearly in GISSI 3,[5] an Italian study on secondary prevention. The administration of PUFA from the n-3 series was associated with an increased survival rate after MI, which was ascribed to the antiarrhythmic effect (Box 7.2).

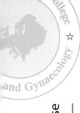

Box 7.2 GISSI-3 trials[5]

- 11 324 MI survivors
- randomized to (n-3) fatty acids or vitamin E, or both, controls
- 3–5 years of follow-up
- (n-3) fatty acids but not vitamin E alone decreased CVD recurrence by 10 15%; $P < 0.05$
- risk of arrhythmia markedly reduced.

Given the results of HERS and the later HERS II, as well as the WHI study, it is intriguing to suggest a combination of oestrogens and a healthy diet. This could also be complemented by the low-dose administration of acetylsalicylic acid to reduce the risk of early thrombosis, which is particularly prudent in secondary preventive trials.

CONCLUSION

A reasonable view to conclude at present is that there are multiple protective mechanisms afforded by oestrogen on the cardiovascular system and therefore this would be expected to translate into beneficial effects on CVD in women. Accordingly, it is still envisioned that oestrogen has a significant role in the primary prevention of CVD. However, this does not appear to be the case in older women with established disease, who may or may not have had a cardiovascular event, such as MI. In this setting, unless a woman is already on oestrogen and benefiting from this therapy for other indications when she experiences an event, there is no reason to prescribe oestrogen for the first time for the purpose of cardioprotection. On the other hand, women who have been taking oestrogen and happen to experience an event may be better protected from death. Recent data have suggested the efficacy of using lower doses of oestrogen for a variety of disorders including CVD. Along these lines, it appears to be prudent to consider using lower doses of oestrogen in all women for long-term use, and particularly for older women.

Until we have further evidence, it seems wise not to include CVD prevention as a sole indication for HRT. There is also no good evidence to deny HRT to women with increased CVD risk, including those with established CVD. So far, most studies have been performed with CEE on its own or combined with MPA. Indeed, one randomized trial[8] using oestradiol showed less progression of vascular wall intima and media thickness as compared to controls, suggesting that it may well be the composition of the HRT that is the overall culprit. However, it must be pointed out that due to the low number of participants, this study badly warrants confirmation. Therefore we cannot make firm recommendations until further studies on a variety of HRT preparations and regimens inclusive of different delivery systems, doses and construction have been performed, and these are obviously urgently required.

References

1. Anderson G L, Limacher M, Assaf A R et al 2004 Effects of conjugated equine estrogens in postmenopausal women with hysterectomy: The Women's Health Initiative randomized controlled trial. The Journal of the American Medical Association 291:1701–1712

2. Barrett-Connor E, Grady D, Sashegyi A et al 2002 Raloxifene and cardiovascular events in osteoporotic postmenopausal women. The Journal of the American Medical Association 287:847–857

3. Clarke S C, Kelleher J, Lloyd-Jones H et al 2002 A study of hormone replacement therapy in postmenopausal women with ischaemic heart disease. The Papworth HRT Atherosclerosis Study. British Journal of Obstetrics and Gynaecology 109:1056–1062

4. Fioretti F, Tavani A, Gallus S et al 2000 Menopause and risk of non-fatal acute myocardial infarction. An Italian case-control study and a review of the literature. Human Reproduction (review) 15:599–603

5. GISSI Investigators 1999 Dietary supplementation with n-3 polyunsaturated fatty acids and vitamin E after myocardial infarction. Results of the GISSI-Prevenzione trial. Gruppo Italiano per lo Studio della sopraavvivenza nell'infarto miocardico. The Lancet 354:447–455

6. Grady D, Herrington D, Bitner V et al 2002 Cardiovascular disease outcomes during 6.8 years of hormone therapy. Heart and Estrogen/progestin Replacement Study follow-up (HERS II). The Journal of the American Medical Association 288:49–57

7. Grodstein F, Manson J E, Colditz G A et al 2000 A prospective, observational study of postmenopausal hormone therapy and primary prevention of cardiovascular disease. Annals of Internal Medicine 133:933–941

8. Hodis H N, Mack W J, Lobo R A et al 2001 Estrogen in the prevention of atherosclerosis. A randomised double-blind, placebo-controlled trial. Annals of Internal Medicine 135:939–953

9. Hulley S, Furberg C, Barret-Connor E et al 2002 Noncardiovascular disease outcomes during 6.8 years of hormone therapy. Heart and Estrogen/progestin Replacement Study follow-up (HERS II). The Journal of the American Medical Association 288:58–66

10. Hulley S, Grady D, Bush T et al 1998 Randomized trial of estrogen plus progestin for secondary prevention of coronary artery disease in post menopausal women. The Journal of the American Medical Association 280:605–613

11. Humphrey L, Chan B, Sox H 2002 Postmenopausal hormone replacement therapy and the primary prevention of cardiovascular disease. Annals of Internal Medicine 137:273–284

12. Koh K K, Kang M H, Jin D K et al 2001 Vascular effects of estrogens in type II diabetic postmenopausal women. Journal of the American College of Cardiology 38:1409–1415

13. Lidfeldt J, Nerbrand C, Samsioe G et al 2001 A screening procedure detecting high yield candidates for OGTT. The Women's Health in the Lund Area (WHILA) study. A population-based study of middle-aged women. European Journal of Epidemiology 17:943–951

14. Losordo D W, Kearny M, Kim E A et al 1994 Variable expression of the estrogen receptor in normal and atherosclerotic coronary arteries of postmenopausal women. Circulation 89:1501–1510

15. Manson J, Hsia J, Johnson K et al 2003 Estrogen plus progestins and the risk of coronary heart disease The New England Journal of Medicine 349:523–534

16. Manson J E, Greenland P, Lacroix A Z et al 2002 Walking compared with vigorous exercise for the prevention of cardiovascular events in women. The New England Journal of Medicine 347:755–756

17. Neves-e-Castro M, Doren M, Samsioe G et al 2002 Results from WHI and HERS-II. Implications for women and the prescriber of HRT. Maturitas 9:255

18. Perez-Gutthann S P, Rodríguez L G, Castellsague J et al 1997 Hormone replacement therapy and risk of venous thromboembolism: population based case-control study. British Medical Journal 314:796–800

19. Petitti D B 2002 Hormone replacement therapy for prevention. More evidence, more pessimism (Editorial). The Journal of the American Medical Association 288(1):99–101

20. Ridker P M, Hennekens C H, Rifai N et al 1999 Hormone replacement therapy and increased plasma concentration of C-reactive protein. Circulation 100:713–716

21. Samsioe G, Neves-e-Castro M, Pines A et al 2001 Critical comments. Maturitas 40:5–15

Current views on hormone replacement therapy and cardiovascular disease

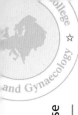

22. Scarabin P Y, Oger E, Plu-Bureau G 2003 Differential association of oral and transdermal oestrogen-replacement therapy with venous thromboembolism risk. The Lancet 362:428–432

23. Stampfer M J, Hu F B, Manson J E et al 2000 Primary prevention of coronary heart disease in women through diet and lifestyle. The New England Journal of Medicine 343:16–22

24. Writing Group for the Women's Health Initiative Investigators 2002 Risks and benefits of estrogen plus progestin in healthy postmenopausal women. The Journal of the American Medical Association 288:321–333

8

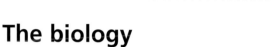

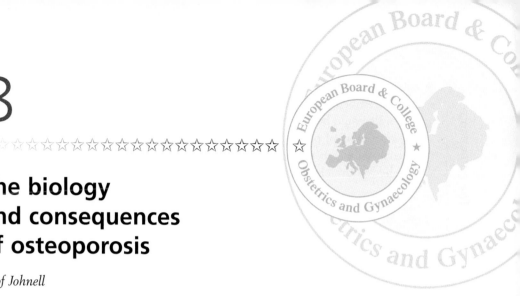

The biology and consequences of osteoporosis

Olof Johnell

ABSTRACT

Bone is a living tissue, constantly remodeling, with a sequence of initial resorption by osteoclasts and then new bone is formed by osteoblasts. An imbalance in this process can cause osteoporosis. The diagnosis of osteoporosis is based on a measurement of bone mineral density (BMD). The clinical consequences of osteoporosis are osteoporotic fractures; several fractures can be regarded as osteoporotic fractures, not only hip, vertebrae, shoulder and wrist fractures. Several of the osteoporotic fractures have a high mortality and morbidity.

KEYWORDS

Fractures, morbidity, mortality, osteoblasts, osteoclasts, osteoporosis, remodelling

INTRODUCTION

Bone is a living tissue – it is always remodelling. Bone can be divided into cortical or compact bone (approximately 80% of the total skeleton) while the rest is cancellous trabecular bone.[5] Around 65% of the bone is mineral, mainly hydroxyapatite, and 35% is matrix. Of the dry weight, 90% of the matrix is collagen. The residual 10% comprises proteins, lipids and peptides, which are important for the function of bone and can also be detected in bioassays. The bone consists mainly of three different cells:

- osteoblasts, which are derived from mesenchymal progenitor cells and can synthesize the bone matrix; when osteoblasts are not forming bone they are flat and called resting osteoblasts;

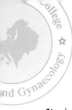
☆☆☆☆☆☆☆☆☆☆☆☆☆☆☆☆☆☆☆☆☆☆

- osteocytes, which are osteoblasts that have stopped synthesizing the matrix and are embedded in the bone. They have a connection with the osteoblasts. One role could be responding to mechanical stress and might play a role in the regulation of plasma minerals;
- osteoclasts, which are cells that originate from haematopoetic cells and are usually multinuclear cells; their role is to resorb bone.

The osteoblasts and osteoclasts are involved in bone turnover, which occurs at a rate of 5–10% per year: bone is a living tissue. The turnover starts with a signal to the osteoblasts, which give a signal to the osteclasts to start resorbing bone. They resorb a pit on the surface of cancellous bone and thereafter the osteoblasts start to fill the pit with matrix, which is later mineralized. This process is called remodelling and goes on throughout life to replace old bone with new. This bone turnover is in balance in young adulthood but after the menopause an imbalance occurs in that relatively more resorption to formation occurs and thus bone is lost. The imbalance can either be that resorption is increased, as in the menopause, or formation is decreased in relation to resorption, which mostly occurs in the very elderly.

To regulate this turnover, there are three main hormones: the parathyroid hormone; calcitriol (vitamin D); and calcitonin. Other hormones are also involved, and several cytokines are involved in bone resorption. Recently, a factor for osteoclast differentiation has been found, called a rank ligand. It has a decoy receptor called osteoprotegrin.

Apart from losing mineral, bone also changes size after the menopause in that there is a medullary expansion and periosteal apposition, probably to counteract the lower bone mineral content.

THE CONSEQUENCES OF OSTEOPOROSIS

The diagnosis of osteoporosis is based on BMD measurement.[17] However, the currently accepted definition of osteoporosis is 'a systematic skeletal disease characterized by low bone mass and micro-architectural deterioration of bone tissue, with a consequent increase in bone fragility and susceptibility to fracture risk.' This shows that it is important to prevent fracture risk. Furthermore, clinical consequences depend on the fracture that occurs; low BMD by itself gives no major symptoms. The description of consequences of osteoporosis is to describe the consequences of the fracture that arises due to osteoporosis.

Which fractures are osteoporotic? The answer is that most fractures can occur due to low bone mass. Kanis et al have a stricter definition as the fracture was selected based on whether it was associated with low BMD and increasing incidence by age after the age of 50.[9,10] The fractures considered to be due to osteoporosis were vertebral, rib, pelvis, humerus, forearm, hip, other femoral fractures, clavicle, scapula and sternum. This was in men and women, and in women there were also tibia and fibula fractures. Kanis et al describe the relationship in morbidity between all these fractures.[9,10]

HIP FRACTURES

A hip fracture is the one that causes the greatest reduction in quality of life, an increase in mortality for the patient and the largest cost to society. Hip fractures often occur when falling sideways onto the trochanter. They can be divided into cervical and trochanteric hip fractures, which have different healing patterns and require different surgical treatments. Since most studies have lumped them together, the description is for both types.

Morbidity

The hip fracture creates a huge increase in morbidity and a decrease in quality of life for the patient. Several studies have confirmed this. Sernbo and Johnell studied, prospectively, 1500 consecutive fracture patients and found that after a year only 50% regained their pre-fracture status concerning function and 50% needed help from society for tasks such as shopping.[15] Virtually all hip fractures are operated on, the cervical by nailing or hip replacement and the trochanteric by sliding nail and screw or intramedullar nail. The quality of life is very low just after the fracture and thereafter partly regained. Even after a year most of the lost quality of life has not been regained. Zethraeus et al included 95 hip fractures in a prospective study by using the quality of life instruments EQ5D and SR-36.[18] Several of the patients died during the first year and 42 were available for follow-up over 1 year. The social tariff values from EQ5D were 0.42 after 2 weeks, 0.64 after 6 months, 0.60 after 9 months and 0.58 after 12 months. This is far below the values in quality of life of the average population. This indicates that the effect is long-standing and affects the patient after more than 1 year. Before the hip fracture this patient is already frailer than the general population.

Mortality

Several studies have shown increased mortality after hip fractures with around 20–30% of hip fracture patients dying during the first year.[8] A part of this increased mortality is due to comorbidity, i.e. these patients have many other diseases that increase mortality. In a study we have used the national databases and compared these with the general population. We found that the relative risk was increased three- to fourfold even after adjusting for other diseases; this was more pronounced in men than women.[9,10] Center et al studied mortality after fractures in Australia and found a more than doubled risk of dying after a hip fracture as compared with those in the same cohort without hip fractures.[2] Even higher figures were found by Cauley et al.[1] In an attempt to study comorbidity, Kanis et al used the Swedish National Database and found that the main mortality occurred a short time after the fracture, and after roughly a year the increased mortality leveled off and was in line with the general population.[9,10] The authors assumed that when it was in line it was due to comorbidity but that the excess during the first year was due to the fracture. Approximately 30% of the increased mortality after a hip fracture was due to the hip fracture itself.

The cost of hip fractures

Several studies have tried to evaluate the cost of hip fractures. The problem is that the cost in hospital is usually one-third of the total cost in the first year and very few studies have followed the patients for more than a year. The cost has been estimated in a review paper by Johnell and shows that the total cost over the first year was US$20 000 and roughly one-third of that cost was the initial cost in hospital.[8] The rest was due to increased rehabilitation and nursing home costs. A detailed study by Zethraeus et al showed that this cost is age-dependent and also depends on where the patient comes from.[18] If the patient comes from a geriatric hospital the increased cost (as compared with the cost before the fracture) is much less compared with patients coming from their homes and is referred to a nursing home. Thus the cost is very high for society: an estimate of the total cost of hip fracture worldwide is US$131.5 billion.

VERTEBRAL FRACTURES

The problem with vertebral fractures is that they can be divided in clinical and radiological/morphometric fractures and that they are difficult to treat. The next step is that the doctor does not take an X-ray and if he does, it is important that the radiologist will find the fractures. Therefore, radiological/morphometric fractures are probably more accurate to describe. However, most data are from clinical vertebral fractures. Radiological/morphometric fractures are defined from population studies where X-rays are taken of a population and a dedicated radiologist either measures the height of the vertebrae or studies the spine X-ray for fractures.

Morbidity

There are few studies on reduction in quality of life after clinical vertebrae/spine fractures. Zethraeus et al followed fractures prospectively over a year.[18] However, the number of fractures in the study was low and the reduction in quality of life measured by EQ5D expressed as utilities was 0.21 after 2 weeks, 0.49 after 6 months, 0.51 after 9 months and 0.57 and 12 months. This indicates that in this small sample the spine fracture had a similar loss in quality of life as hip fractures (see above from the same study). A few other studies have shown similar results in a more pronounced quality of life loss than most had expected.

Mortality

In an Australian study, the relative risk of death of a woman after a clinical vertebral fracture was 1.66 (95% CI; range 1.51–1.80).[2] In a study performed in the Fracture Intervention Trial, the relative risk for a patient with a clinical spine fracture for mortality was 8.6, thus indicating a very high mortality, only slightly lower than for hip fractures.[12]

Morphometric fractures

Morphometric fractures were studied by Hasserius et al who found a relative risk of 2 of death, for men and women, if they had a baseline morphometric vertebral fracture.[7] Silverman et al also found that morphometric fractures were associated with a reduction in quality of life.[16] A similar effect has been shown by Oleksik et al.[14] Nevitt et al have shown, regarding severe back pain, that morphometric fractures had an only slightly lower number of bed days compared with the symptom-giving clinical vertebral fracture, indicating that there is a gradient and that a large number of vertebral fractures must be undetected.[13]

Costs

Costs can be divided among hospitalized vertebral fractures.[4] Gehlbach et al studied hospitalized patients and found that the total charges averaged US$8000–10 000 per hospitalization and were higher in men.[6] More than 50% of the discharged patients needed some form of continuing care. The authors also found that the cost of hospitalization was about half of that of hip fractures. In a European study it was estimated that the cost of hospitalization due to vertebral fracture was 377 million euro per year and that the fracture costs were, on average, 63% of that of hip fractures.[15]

A pilot study was carried out in Sweden by Zethraeus et al with a low number of fractures. The direct cost of all vertebral fractures, both for outpatients and hospitalized patients, was 3300 euro; the indirect cost was 3400 euro.[5] A large study is underway to calculate the correct cost of clinical vertebral fractures. In a recent study from the Mayo Clinic, Melton et al studied the cost in a case-control series and it was found to be almost US$2000 per year for 283 vertebral fractures that were investigated.[12]

For morphometric fractures, the most cited investigation is the Rotterdam study where they have analysed the additional cost of medical care, i.e. the incremental cost, and it was averaged to US$500 per year.[3] The study was over 3 years.

WRIST FRACTURES

Wrist fractures seem to have a lower morbidity than hip and vertebral fractures.

Morbidity

In previous studies, wrist fractures have been shown to have a 6–10% poor outcome. In the study by Zethraeus et al, wrist fractures were followed prospectively and the reduction in the quality of life expressed as utilities were 0.54 after 2 weeks, 0.76 after 6 months, 0.81 after 9 months and 0.82 after 12 months.[18] Thus there was an initial decrease in quality of life but after 6 months these patients had almost regained the quality of life of the general population.

Mortality

Mortality after wrist fractures has, in several studies, been similar to that of the general population.[8] However, in the DUBBO study[2] there was also a tendency of increased mortality after a wrist fracture.

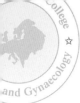
The menopause

Costs

There are few studies on wrist fractures and estimates of costs have been from US$800 upwards. Zethraeus et al found the direct cost after a wrist fracture was 2000 euro and the indirect cost 350 euro, a much lower cost than of the vertebral and hip fractures.[18]

SHOULDER FRACTURES

Morbidity

A study by Zethraeus et al showed that shoulder fractures created a loss of quality of life expressed as utilities somewhere between hip and wrist fractures, i.e. generally a loss in quality of life.[18]

Mortality

It has been shown that the mortality rate is increased in patients with a shoulder fracture.

Costs

Zethraeus et al showed that the direct cost was 3400 euro and the indirect cost was 450 euro.[18] The direct cost was fairly similar to that for spine fractures.

REPEATED FRACTURES

Another important aspect of the consequences of a fracture is that after the individual has sustained the fracture there is a very high probability of acquiring a new fracture. Klotzbuecher et al found that in pre- and postmenopausal women the relative risk for having a new fracture after a previous one is 2.0 (95% CI; range 1.8–2.1).[11]

CONCLUSION

The consequences of osteoporosis, and therefore osteoporotic fractures, are high. Hip and vertebral fractures seem to have a similar morbidity as several other major healthcare problems, indicating that osteoporotic fractures are as difficult to treat as these other problems. Mortality is also high. The question is how much of this is due to comorbidity and how much to the fracture. A part is definitely due to the fracture, which also shows the importance of preventive strategies. Another aspect is the societal aspect, and the cost of fractures, especially of hip fractures but also vertebral fractures, is high and is also very similar to major diseases.

References

1. Cauley J A, Thompson D E, Ensrud K C et al 2000 Risk of mortality following clinical fractures. Osteoporosis International 11:556–561
2. Center J R, Nguyen T V, Schneider D et al 1999 Mortality after all major types of osteoporotic fracture in men and women: an observational study. The Lancet 353:878–882
3. De Laet C E, van Hout B A, Burger H et al 1999 Incremental cost of medical care after hip fracture and first vertebral fracture. The Rotterdam study. Osteoporosis Internatio- nal 10:66–72

4. Finnern H W, Sykes D 2003. The hospital cost of vertebral fractures in the EU. Estimates using national datasets. Osteoporosis International 14:429–436

5. Fleisch H 1997 Bisphosphonates in bone disease: from the laboratory to the patient, 3rd edn. Parthenon Publishing, New York

6. Gehlbach S H, Burge R T, Puleo E et al 2003 Hospital care of osteoporosis-related vertebral fractures. Osteoporosis International 14:53–60

7. Hasserius R, Karlsson M K, Nilsson B E et al for the European Vertebral Osteoporosis Study 2003 Prevalent vertebral deformities predict increased mortality and increased fracture rate in both men and women. A 10-year population-based study of 598 individuals from the Swedish cohort in the European Vertebral Osteoporosis Study. Osteoporosis International 14:61–68

8. Johnell O 1997 The socioeconomic burden of fractures: today and in the 21st century. The American Journal of Medicine 103:20S–6S

9. Kanis J A, Odén A, Johnell O et al 2001 The burden of osteoporotic fractures. A method for setting intervention thresholds. Osteoporosis International 12:417–427

10. Kanis J A, Odén A, Johnell O et al 2003 The components of excess mortality after hip fracture. Bone 32:468–473

11. Klotzbuecher C M, Ross P D, Landsman P B et al 2000 Patients with prior fractures have an increased risk of future fractures. A summary of the literature and statistical synthesis. Journal of Bone and Mineral Research 15:721–739

12. Melton L J, III, Gabriel S E, Crowson D X et al 2003 Cost-equivalence of different osteoporotic fractures. Osteoporosis International 14:383–388

13. Nevitt M C, Thompson D E, Black D M et al 2000 Effect of alendronate on limited-activity days and bed-disability days caused by back pain in postmenopausal women with existing vertebral fractures. Fracture Intervention Trial Research Group. Archives of Internal Medicine 160:77–85

14. Oleksik A, Lips P, Dawson A et al 2000 Health-related quality of life in postmenopausal women with low BMD with or without prevalent vertebral fractures. Journal of Bone and Mineral Research 15:1384–1392

15. Sernbo I, Johnell O 1993 Consequences of a hip fracture. A prospective study over 1 year. Osteoporosis International 3:148–153

16. Silverman S L, Minshall M E, Shen W et al 2001 The relationship of health-related quality of life to prevalent and incident vertebral fractures in postmenopausal women with osteoporosis. Results from the Multiple Outcomes of Raloxifene Evaluation Study. Arthritis and Rheumatism 44:2611–2619

17. WHO Study Group report 1994 Assessment of fracture risk and its application to screening for postmenopausal osteoporosis. World Health Organization Technical Report Series 843:1–129

18. Zethraeus N, Borgström F, Johnell O et al 2002 Costs and quality of life associated with osteoporosis-related fractures. Results from a Swedish survey. SSE/EFI Working Paper Series in Economics and Finance, No 512

9

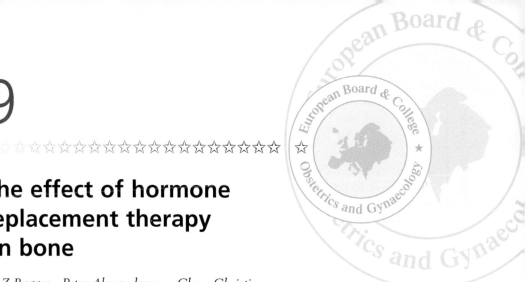

The effect of hormone replacement therapy on bone

Yu Z Bagger   Peter Alexandersen   Claus Christiansen

ABSTRACT

Hormone replacement therapy (HRT) is given mainly to suppress menopausal symptoms. Epidemiological as well as clinical studies have demonstrated the protective effects of HRT against postmenopausal osteoporosis. HRT inhibits bone resorption, reduces postmenopausal bone loss and decreases the incidence of osteoporotic fractures by about 50%. The recent Women's Health Initiative (WHI) study has confirmed the antifracture efficacy of HRT, yet demonstrated an increased risk for cardiovascular diseases (CVDs) and breast cancer, which apparently outweighed the overall benefits. Accordingly, the use of HRT for long-term prevention is no longer recommended. Since HRT remains the only therapy for suppression of menopausal symptoms and is usually prescribed to women for a few years, results from longitudinal studies assessing the long-term antifracture effect of short-term HRT (2–3 years) are awaited.

KEYWORDS

Bone mass, hormone replacement therapy (HRT), fractures

INTRODUCTION

Hormone replacement therapy (HRT) is given mainly to suppress menopausal symptoms but it has also been a common therapy for the prevention of post-menopausal osteoporosis. Despite irrefutable data that demonstrate the efficacy of postmenopausal oestrogen administration in preventing bone loss and osteoporotic fractures, the majority of women will stop taking HRT after 2–5 years. An important reason why women stop taking HRT after a relatively short time is the fear of adverse events and an increased risk of breast cancer. The recent WHI study

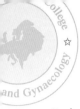
☆☆☆☆☆☆☆☆☆☆☆☆☆☆☆☆☆☆☆☆☆

using conjugated equine oestrogen (CEE) combined with medroxyprogesterone did not find any benefits in terms of prevention of CVD, and actually showed harm, which was evident 5.2 years after treatment initiation.[31] In spite of these results, the WHI study actually signified the strong protective effect of HRT against fractures. Over the last two decades, new oestrogen-like substances (analogues) have been developed to prevent and treat postmenopausal osteoporosis as alternatives to conventional HRT. These compounds elicit tissue-specific rather than systemic effects due to mixed oestrogen agonist/antagonist actions.

In this chapter, the most important clinical studies published on conventional HRT on postmenopausal bone loss, fracture prevention and the withdrawal effect, and of oestrogen-like substances on fracture risk are outlined. Since the structural and functional entity for the action on bone of all these agents is turnover or remodelling of bone, a description of the cellular events involved in this process is useful.

BONE REMODELLING AND COUPLING

BONE REMODELLING

The skeleton undergoes constant dynamic changes throughout its life via two continuous but opposite actions, namely bone resorption and bone formation, also collectively called bone remodelling. This temporally and spatially coordinated process of bone cell function is characterized by discrete foci of metabolic activity, orchestrated primarily by cellular and humoral mechanisms.[23] The cells involved in this process consist of bone resorptive cells, osteoclasts and bone forming cells (osteoblasts) mediating their respective effects through coupled mechanisms.

Bone remodelling is increased in several pathological conditions, for instance in primary hyperparathyroidism, Paget's disease and osteolytic bone diseases due to malignancy (e.g. myeloma); it also occurs at an increased rate after the menopause.

The initial step of bone remodelling is osteoclast activation, the stimulus of which is still unknown but may in part be linked to oestrogen deficiency. Osteoclast activation in turn leads to bone resorption. Due to coupling, bone resorption does not continue indefinitely but seems to be tightly regulated and lasts for approximately 10 days. The resorptive phase is followed by the migration of osteoblast precursors to the resorptive site, presumably mediated through chemotaxis by the osteoclasts. Osteoblast precursors proliferate and mature into osteoblasts and they start repairing the defect left by the osteoclasts, which eventually disappear. A matrix (osteoid) is thus produced by the osteoblasts and subsequently mineralizes, forming new bone. The entire process takes approximately three months.[12]

Bone resorption and bone formation may be evaluated by biochemical markers in the urine, and more recently in the serum. New markers have been found to be specific and sensitive, depending on the markers used.

COUPLING

Bone coupling mechanisms remain unclear but several theories have been proposed to explain this phenomenon. Most likely is the involvement of humoral factors (cytokines) that are released from the degradation of osteoclastically mediated bone resorption and which attract osteoblast precursors to the site of bone resorption.[16] Candidates for this crucial role in bone coupling are insulin-like growth factor (IGF-) I and transforming growth factor (TGF-) β but several, partly unidentified, cytokines may modulate this complex process. This widely held notion of humoral factors being responsible for bone coupling has been challenged by some authors,[19] suggesting that the cytokine responsible for activating the osteoclasts, and thereby bone resorption, although at a much slower rate, is responsible for the subsequent bone formation. Still others have speculated that preosteoclasts may recognize the resorptive site through receptors located at the surface of the cells, stimulating them to proliferate and differentiate into mature osteoblasts.

In premenopausal women with an intact production of female sex steroids, the resorption of bone is followed by the complete replacement of new bone, thus bone balance is maintained through a dynamic equilibrium of bone mass.

BONE MASS, BONE TURNOVER AND MENOPAUSE

Menopause is the time when oestrogen production declines in women and bone loss starts to accelerate from the existing peak bone mass, i.e. the maximum bone mass obtained at skeletal maturity. Bone loss occurs in postmenopausal women as a result of an increase in the rate of bone remodelling and an imbalance between the activity of osteoclasts and osteoblasts. When the processes of bone resorption and bone formation are not matched, the result is a remodelling imbalance that leads to bone loss. It is likely that if the imbalance is caused by increased osteoclast activity (as occurs in the immediate postmenopausal period) this is more damaging to the bone structure than if it is caused by decreased osteoblast activity, as during the slow phase of bone loss with ageing. Therefore excessive osteoclast activity may result in the perforation and loss of entire bone trabeculae and thus the subsequent bone formation phase is eliminated. In contrast, decreased osteoblast activity leads chiefly to thinning of the trabeculae.[24] The increased bone turnover is maintained throughout life.

Bone loss in postmenopausal women occurs in two phases: rapid and slow.[27] The rapid initiating phase (approximately 3% per year in the spine) lasts approximately 5 years and is mainly attributed to oestrogen deficiency. Bone loss during these years accounts for 50% of all bone loss occurring over the female lifespan. In support of the role of oestrogen, oestrogen receptors have been demonstrated on both osteoblasts and osteoclasts. However, the regulation and action mechanisms are only partly understood. The slow phase of bone loss in women starts at about the age of 55 and may be largely attributed to an increase in parathyroid hormone (PTH) levels and osteoblast senescence. The

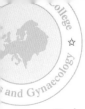
☆ ☆☆☆☆☆☆☆☆☆☆☆☆☆☆☆☆☆☆☆☆☆☆

increase in PTH is a result of decreased renal calcium resorption and decreased intestinal absorption. The latter is accompanied by reduced circulating concentrations of total 1,25-dihydroxyvitamin D and decreased 1α-hydroxylase activity in the kidney. Moreover, there is evidence that declining serum levels of vitamin D stimulate PTH release, leading to an increased bone turnover. It was recently shown that more than 50% of postmenopausal women with hip fractures were vitamin D deficient.[17] Although other factors may be very important, there is evidence that calcium and vitamin D deficiency plays a role in bone loss in the elderly population.[26]

Figure 9.1 shows the changes in bone resorption, formation and bone mass in response to oestrogen deficiency after menopause.

THE EFFECT OF OESTROGEN THERAPY OR COMBINED OESTROGEN–PROGESTOGEN THERAPY ON BONE

DEFINITION OF OESTROGEN AND PROGESTOGEN

Oestrogen (oestradiol, 17β-oestradiol) can be defined as compounds that are able to produce vaginal cornification or uterotrophic effects in oophorectomized rats or mice.[15] Oestrogen can be divided into four main groups:

1. Synthetic oestrogen-like substances without a steroid skeleton (often stilbestrol derivatives).
2. Synthetic oestrogen-like substances with a steroid skeleton.
3. Nonhuman oestrogen, produced from an equine source (conjugated oestrogens).
4. Native human oestrogens or compounds that are transformed into native oestrogen in the body.

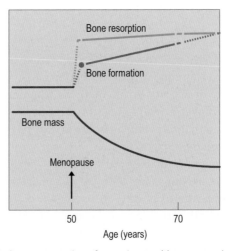

Fig 9.1 The changes in bone resorption, formation and bone mass in response to oestrogen deficiency after menopause.

For postmenopausal therapy, CEEs are most commonly prescribed in the USA, whereas in Europe there has been a tradition for using native human oestrogen (i.e. 17β-oestradiol) or oestradiol valerate.

Progestogens differ greatly in their additional properties but they have at least one property in common: they are all able to cause secretory transformation of an oestrogen-primed endometrium.[22] The classes of progestogen can be divided into three subgroups:

1. 19-norethisterone (norethindrone) derivatives, with a relatively strong androgenic effect.
2. 17-hydroxyprogesterone derivatives, with less androgenic activity.
3. Natural human progesterone, which is available in a micronized form for oral therapy.

The progestogens may be given in either a cyclical regimen (CSEPT) or in a continuous combined regimen (CCEPT). The CSEPT mimics the natural premenopausal cycle and thus provokes monthly menstrual-like bleeding. In the CC-EPT, the endometrium is kept atrophic continuously and bleeding is avoided in many but not all users.

THE EFFECT OF HORMONE REPLACEMENT THERAPY ON BONE MASS AND FRACTURES

Hormone replacement therapy is a well-established mode of prevention and treatment for osteoporosis. It results not only in arresting bone loss but also in an improvement in bone density and a reduction in the risk of osteoporotic fractures. Epidemiological as well as clinical data consistently support this finding. Oestrogen therapy primarily decreases bone resorption and only secondarily decreases bone formation, resulting in a temporary positive bone balance. In this period, as the resorption lacunae are filled up, bone density increases. After some time, when the rate of formation has made up this difference, the increase in bone density levels off. Hormone replacement therapy will result in a stabilization of bone density without a further increase; HRT can be administered orally, subcutaneously, transdermally and nasally. Several clinical trials have shown that the oral, transdermal and nasal routes appear to be equally effective in conserving bone.[1,6,21,30,32] Bone mineral density (BMD) has been shown to increase by up to 6–10% in postmenopausal women treated with HRT.

HRT induces a dose-dependent decrease in bone markers, which reaches a plateau maintained for the duration of treatment. Under adequate doses of either oral, percutaneous, transdermal or nasal oestrogen, the mean decrease is 40–70% for urinary carboxyl-terminal crosslinking (CTX) and N-terminal crosslinking telopeptide of type I collagen (NTX), slightly less for serum CTX, and is reached within a few months of treatment.[2,6,10,20,29] The delayed decrease in bone formation markers is reached after 6–12 months of HRT. Once the plateau is reached, the mean decrease in serum osteocalcin ranges from 10–45% with transdermal 17β-oestradiol, from 22% to 27% with nasal 17β-oestradiol, and from 25% to 50% with oral oestrogen.[2,6,10,20,29] The decrease in bone formation markers is even less pronounced when oestrogen is combined with norethisterone acetate.[8,28] The combination of 17β-oestrdiol and norethisterone acetate may even induce uncoupling, leading to considerable increases in bone mass, which probably reflects the unique stimulating activity of this progestogen on osteoblast activity.

Although HRTs have been widely accepted as the agents of choice for osteoporosis management, data from clinical trials investigating the effect of HRT on fracture risk in postmenopausal women with osteoporosis are sparse. The WHI study has shown strong protective effects of HRT against osteoporotic fractures. The risk of hip and vertebral fractures was reduced by 34% after 5.2 years of HRT.[31] However, the Heart and Estrogen/progestin Replacement Study (HERS) with clinical fractures as a secondary outcome did not show significant benefit of HRT for osteoporotic fractures.[4] Most observational studies suggest that postmenopausal women who used HRT have reduced fracture risk by 50% if HRT is taken for more than 5 years.[5,34]

WITHDRAWAL EFFECT OF HORMONE REPLACEMENT THERAPY

When HRT is discontinued, bone loss recurs although the withdrawal effect of HRT on bone mass remains controversial. Some authors have shown that the rate of bone loss after stopping HRT was accelerated compared to average postmenopausal bone loss.[18,33] Trémollières et al observed that the rate of bone loss in the spine accelerated within the first 2 years after HRT withdrawal, which was identical to untreated women within the first 2 years after menopause. Then, the annual rate of bone loss was decreased as observed following the menopause in the untreated women.[33] Others have shown that the rate of bone loss after cessation of HRT is similar to average bone loss.[7,14], indicating the residual effect of HRT on bone mass maintained many years after withdrawal of HRT. However, long-term prospective studies are still lacking.

EFFECT OF OESTROGEN-LIKE SUBSTANCES ON BONE

Raloxifene

Raloxifene is a nonsteroidal benzothiophene compound with tissue-specific oestrogen agonist and antagonist actions. It is also the only selective oestrogen receptor modulator (SERM) currently approved by the US Food and Drug Administration (FDA) for osteoporosis prevention;[25] raloxifene is now avaiable in several countries, including the USA and many parts of Europe. This substance is known to exert its skeletal effects through binding to the oestrogen receptors and produces oestrogen agonist effects on bone.[9] The effect of raloxifene (60 mg per day) on BMD has been demonstrated – a significant 2.4% increase in the BMD of the lumbar spine and of total hip, 2.5% in BMD of the femoral neck and 2.0% in BMD of the total body over 2 years.

Also, raloxifene lowered urinary CTX by approximately 25%, as well as serum osteocalcin by approximately 20%,[9] although this inhibitory effect is somewhat less than that observed by HRT. Furthermore, a fracture study has shown a significant reduction (30%) of vertebral fractures in elderly women treated with raloxifene compared to women treated with calcium only.[13]

In contrast, the influence on the endometrium and breast is oestrogen antagonistic, indeed the risk of breast cancer may be decreased in postmenopausal women treated with raloxifene for osteoporosis prevention.[11]

Tibolone

Tibolone is an interesting compound that possesses oestrogenic, progestogenic and even androgenic effects. It is primarily used in early postmenopausal women to alleviate climacteric symptoms, particularly hot flushes, and is well tolerated.

The effect of tibolone on bone has been evaluated in clinical osteoporosis prevention studies.[3] In late postmenopausal women (>10 years after menopause), tibolone results, like HRT, in a steady and equal increase in BMD by approximately 5–6%. This increase in BMD is mirrored by decreases in biochemical markers of bone resorption (urinary CTX and hydroxyproline) and bone formation (serum osteocalcin), respectively. Therefore tibolone prevents bone loss in the forearm in late postmenopausal women. A large ongoing fracture study (LIFT) will determine whether tibolone can also prevent incidental fractures in elderly women with low bone mass.

CONCLUSION

HRT is essential for a large proportion of women around the menopause in order to alleviate menopausal symptoms such as hot flushes. However, HRT is not an ideal solution for all postmenopausal women: individual needs are incredibly different. In spite of the benefits of HRT for an improvement in quality of life and the prevention of bone loss in postmenopausal women, a short-term use of HRT is recommended in order to avoid the adverse effects of HRT. Nowadays, HRT is no longer recommended for the sole purpose of preventing chronic disease, such as CVD or osteoporosis, as other alternatives are becoming available.

The only oestrogen-like substance so far approved by the FDA for prevention of postmenopausal bone loss is raloxifene. A number of SERMs are also currently in phase II or III clinical studies for prevention of osteoporosis and may become available in the future as alternatives to raloxifene, provided that all efficacy and safety issues are met. Well-designed and well-conducted clinical trials (and preferably also head-to-head comparisons with new versus approved drugs in clinically meaningful doses) will continue to be the scientific basis of future drugs in the prevention and treatment of postmenopausal osteoporosis.

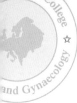

References

1. Bjarnason N H, Byrjalsen I, Hassager C et al 2000 Low doses of estradiol in combination with gestodene to prevent early postmenopausal bone loss. American Journal of Obstetrics Gynecology 183:550–560

2. Bjarnason N H, Christiansen C 2000 An early response in biochemical markers predicts long-term response in bone mass during HRT in early postmenopausal women. Bone 26:551–552

3. Bjarnason N H, Bjarnason K, Haarbo J et al 1996 Tibolone: prevention of bone loss in late postmenopausal women. Journal of Clinical Endocrinology and Metabolism 81:2419–2422

4. Cauley J A, Black D M, Barrett-Connor E et al 2001 Effects of hormone replacement therapy on clinical fractures and height loss. The Heart and Estrogen/progestin Replacement Study (HERS). The American Journal of Medicine 110:442–450

5. Cauley J A, Seeley D G, Ensrud K et al 1995 Estrogen replacement therapy and fractures in old women. Study of Osteoporotic Fractures Research Groups. Annals of Internal Medicine 122:9–16

6. Christiansen C, Bagger Y, Chetaille E et al 2002 Pulsed estrogen therapy prevents postmenopausal bone loss. A 2-year randomised placebo-controlled study. Climacteric 5:87

7. Christiansen C, Christensen M S, Transbol I 1981 Bone mass after withdrawal of oestrogen replacement. The Lancet 1:1053–1054

8. Christiansen C, Riis B J 1990 17 Beta-estradiol and continuous norethisterone: a unique treatment for established osteoporosis in elderly women. The Journal of Clinical Endocrinology and Metabolism 71:836–841

9. Delmas P D, Bjarnason N H, Mitlak B H et al 1997 Effects of raloxifene on bone mineral density, serum cholesterol concentrations, and uterine endometrium in postmenopausal women. The New England Journal of Medicine 337:1641–1647

10. Delmas P D, Pornel B, Felsenberg D 1999 A dose-ranging trial of a matrix transdermal 17β-estradiol for the prevention of bone loss in early postmenopausal women. Bone 24:517–523

11. Dunn B K, Ford L G 2001 From adjuvant therapy to breast cancer prevention: BCPT and STAR. The Breast Journal 7:144–157

12. Eriksen E F, Langdahl B, Vesterby A et al 1999 Hormone replacement therapy prevents osteoclastic hyperactivity. A histomorphometric study in early postmenopausal women. Journal of Bone and Mineral Research 14:1217–1221

13. Ettinger B, Black D M, Mitlak B H et al 1999 Reduction of vertebral fracture risk in postmenopausal women with osteoporosis treated with raloxifene. Results from a 3-year randomized clinical trial. Multiple Outcomes of Raloxifene Evaluation (MORE) Investigators. The Journal of the American Medical Association 282:637–645

14. Greendale G A, Espeland M, Slone S et al 2002 Bone mass response to discontinuation of long-term hormone replacement therapy. Results from the Postmenopausal Estrogen/Progestin Interventions (PEPI) Safety Follow-up Study. Archives of Internal Medicine 162:665–672

15. Hammond C B, Maxson W S 1982 Current status of estrogen therapy for the menopause. Fertility and Sterility 37:5–25

16. Howard G A, Bottemiller B L, Turner R T et al 1981 Parathyroid hormone stimulates bone formation and resorption in organ culture: evidence for a coupling mechanism. Proceedings of the National Academy of Sciences of the USA 78:3204–3208

17. LeBoff M S, Kohlmeier L, Hurwitz S 1992 Occult vitamin D deficiency in postmenopause US women with acute hip fracture. The Journal of the American Medical Association 281:505–511

18. Lindsay R, Hart DM, MacLean A et al 1978 Bone response to termination of oestrogen treatment. The Lancet 1:1325–1327

19. Manolagas S C, Jilka R L 1995 Bone marrow, cytokines, and bone remodeling. Emerging insights into the pathophysiology of osteoporosis. The New England Journal of Medicine 332:305–311

20. Marcus R, Holloway L, Well B 1999 The relationship of biochemical markers of bone turnover to bone density changes in postmenopausal women. Results from the Postmenopausal Estrogen/Progestin Interventions (PEPI) trial. Journal of Bone and Mineral Research 14:1583–1595

21. Marslew U, Overgaard K, Riis B J et al 1992 Two new combinations of estrogen and progestogen for prevention of postmenopausal bone loss. Long-term effects on bone, calcium and lipid metabolism, climacteric symptoms, and bleeding. Obstetrics and Gynecology 79:202–210

22. Neumann F 1978 The physiological action of progesterone and the pharmacological effects of progesterone. A short review. Postgraduate Medicine 54:11–24

23. Parfitt A M 1994 Osteonal and hemi-osteonal remodeling: the spatial and temporal framework for signal traffic in adult human bone. Journal of Cellular Biochemistry 55:273–286

24. Parfitt A M, Mathews C H, Villanueva A 1983 Relationships between surface, volume, and thickness of iliac trabecular bone in aging and in osteoporosis. Implications for the microanatomic and cellular mechanisms of bone loss. The Journal of Clinical Investigation 72:1396–1409

25. Raloxifene for postmenopausal osteoporosis. The Medical Letter on Drugs and Therapeutics 1998, 40:29–30. Erratum in The Medical Letter on Drugs and Therapeutics 1998, 40:54

26. Reid IR, Ames RW, Evans MC et al 1993 Effect of calcium supplementation on bone loss in postmenopausal women. The New England Journal of Medicine 328:460–464. Erratum in The New England Journal of Medicine 329:1281

27. Riggs B L, Khosla S, Melton L J, III 1998 A unitary model for involutional osteoporosis: estrogen deficiency causes both type I and type II osteoporosis in postmenopausal women and contributes to bone loss in aging men. Journal of Bone and Mineral Research 13:763–773

28. Riis B J, Lehmann H J, Christiansen C 2002 Norethisterone acetate in combination with estrogen: effects on the skeleton and other organs. A review. American Journal of Obstetrics and Gynecology 187:1101–1116

29. Riis B J, Overgaard K, Christiansen C 1995 Biochemical markers of bone turnover to monitor the bone mass response to post-menopausal hormone replacement therapy. Osteoporosis International 5:276–280

30. Riis B J, Thomsen K, Strom V et al 1987 The effect of percutaneous estradiol and natural progesterone on postmenopausal bone loss. American Journal of Obstetrics and Gynecology 156:61–65

31. Rossouw J E, Anderson G L, Prentice R L et al; Writing Group for the Women's Health Initiative Investigators 2002 Risks and benefits of estrogen plus progestin in healthy postmenopausal women. Principal results from the Women's Health Initiative randomized controlled trial. The Journal of the American Medical Association 288:321–333

32. Stevenson J C, Cust M P, Ganger K F 1990 Effects of transdermal versus oral hormone replacement therapy on bone density in spine and proximal femur in postmenopausal women. The Lancet 335:265–269

33. Trémollières F A, Pouilles J M, Ribot C 2001 Withdrawal of hormone replacement therapy is associated with significant vertebral bone loss in postmenopausal women. Osteoporosis International 12:385–390

34. Weiss NS, Ure CL, Ballard JH et al 1980 Decreased risk of fractures of the hip and lower forearm with postmenopausal use of estrogen. The New England Journal of Medicine 303:1195–1198

10

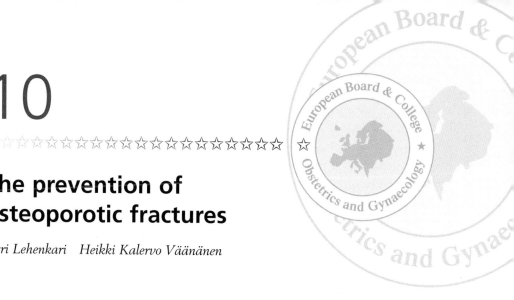

The prevention of osteoporotic fractures

Petri Lehenkari   Heikki Kalervo Väänänen

ABSTRACT

Osteoporotic fractures are the combined expression of a trauma and low bone strength. Strategies for their prevention should therefore focus on the prevention of trauma and the pathogenesis behind the weakness of bone. For this to work, several different sectors of society must be included in the process; healthcare personnel have a central role in initiating these activities in their local communities. These may include innovative building solutions of homes and the living environment of the elderly as well as the good maintenance of the pavements and roads. At an individual level, special attention should be given to carefully checking on any inappropriate medication, which may contribute to falls.

The use of personal protectors, such as hip protectors, must also be considered if the patient has either a history of falls or an increased probability of falling. Carefully planned exercise programmes and diet instructions may be of value in improving coordination and muscle strength.

Finally, there are several ways of using pharmacological therapy to increase bone mass and strength as a primary prevention, or after the first fracture, to prevent any further skeletal decay.

KEYWORDS

Fracture, osteoporosis, prevention

INTRODUCTION: OSTEOPOROTIC FRACTURES

Osteoporotic fractures can occur at any skeletal site. Typical sites include the hip, spine, wrist, pelvis, ribs, proximal humerus, distal femur and proximal tibia, ankle and in general the metaphyseal areas of long bones.[35,36,41,46,51] In particular, the proximal metaphyses of the longest bones in the body seem to be susceptible to fractures, possibly due to bone geometry and biomechanical properties, hence the collum of the femur and humerus are often referred as the fragility sites.

The metaphyses of long bones consist of trabecular bone, which is more susceptible to excess bone resorption and which is commonly recognized as a main pathophysiological process of the disease.[64,65] This imbalance in bone remodelling, bone resorption exceeding bone formation, does, however, eventually also lead to a loss of cortical bone mass. Thus even diaphyseal fractures of long bones can be caused by osteoporosis. Hence, an osteoporotic fracture can be defined as any fracture that occurs with a force of trauma that is lower than expected for a healthy adult skeleton.

Osteoporotic fractures often, though not always, are caused by a fall or injury that is not tolerated by the weakened skeleton.[1,56] Risk factors for falls include increased age, muscle weakness, functional limitations (e.g. paralysis), environmental risk factors, use of psychoactive medications and a previous history of falls.[8] If these are compared to the known risk factors for hip fractures, which include decreased physical activity, low body mass index, a previous low energy fracture, osteoporosis, and age,[41,53] a pattern of age-related frailty can easily be recognized. Women aged above 85 years are nearly eight times more likely to be hospitalized for hip fractures than women aged 65–74 years. Skeletal health and susceptibility to falling are indistinguishable entities that have synergistic manifestation in the incidence and prevalence of osteoporotic fractures.

In terms of osteoporotic fracture prevention, the most studied and best known subjects are the disabling fractures of the hip and spine. According to Johnell and Kanis in 1990 there were 1.31 million new hip fractures worldwide.[34] The prevalence of hip fractures with marked disability was 4.48 million; 740 000 deaths were estimated to be associated with hip fracture. The 1.75 million disability-adjusted life-years lost are, however, distributed unevenly. Osteoporotic fractures are concentrated in the established market economies, representing 1.4% of the disease burden among these women whereas the global burden is markedly smaller, only 0.1% of the global burden of disease in females. It is a known fact that white aged women are at a higher risk for hip fracture than black aged women.[21]

Hip fracture data are generally considered a very reliable indicator of osteoporotic fracture.[3] This can be explained by the critical need to treat these immobilizing fractures. Osteoporotic fractures of the spine often occur without any clinically detectable end-points, such as hospital records, operations, etc.[51] In some cases the traumatic force is small or even unrecognizable; osteoporotic fractures of the spine are commonly misdiagnosed.[12,32] However, it is generally accepted that the incidence of such fractures is rapidly, even exponentially, increasing.[36,47] Whether this is caused by a change in the demographics of western industries and elsewhere is not known. However, at present one in two women and one in eight men over 50 will have an osteoporosis-related fracture.[47]

Approximately 33% of women over 65 will experience a fracture of the spine. Both hip and vertebral fractures are also associated with excess mortality.[6,7,30,62] Also, 20% of hip fracture patients die within 6 months from conditions caused by lack of activity, such as embolism and pneumonia.[18,19] A 50-year-old woman has a 2.8% risk of death related to a hip fracture during her remaining lifetime. This risk is equivalent to the risk of death from breast cancer and four times higher than that from endometrial cancer.[19] The mortality rates are unquestionably higher in older patients. However, deaths in younger patients (i.e. aged <70 years) contribute substantially to the excess mortality and short survival associated with osteoporotic fractures.[7]

Osteoporosis is an asymptomatic disease and too often its first symptom – osteoporotic fracture – is devastating for the patient. Thus there is an urgent need to develop and implement primary and secondary fracture prevention strategies. In this chapter we summarize the current knowledge on the prevention of such fractures.

NUTRITIONAL MEASURES IN FRACTURE PREVENTION

A decreased level of physical activity has a direct effect on bone biology as the bone becomes adjusted to the lower strain. Physical activity also has another role in the preservation of skeletal health: not only does it decrease the probability of injury from a severe fall but it also increases the consumption of nutrients accompanied by energy sources, adding nutrition to the needs of skeletal health. Several studies have shown that older individuals with low protein intakes lose more bone and have an increased risk of fractures.[23,27,44] Amongst all nutrients, dairy products are the most valuable from the perspective of skeletal nutrient demand in that they supply both protein and calcium. Indeed, it is commonly accepted that calcium and vitamin D intake are the key factors in the maintenance of skeletal health as well as the prevention of osteoporotic fractures.

CALCIUM AND VITAMIN D SUPPLEMENTATION

Besides pharmaceutical interventions against osteoporotic fractures, the strongest evidence for fracture prevention is from calcium and vitamin D supplementation. Combined treatment in the elderly institutionalized is shown to reduce the risk of nonvertebral fractures.[10,11,48] In a randomized, placebo-controlled study (n = 3270) over 36 months, the intention-to-treat analysis showed that supplementation reduced the incidence of hip fractures by 29% and of all nonvertebral fractures by 24%.[10] The benefit of supplementation emerged within 12 months and the number needed to treat (NNT) to prevent any vertebral or nonvertebral fracture was 41. The reduction in hip fracture risk with supplementation was consistent with the changes in bone mineral density (BMD). Similar studies and subsequent meta-analyses have confirmed these observations.[20,49,52,60]

In the clinical and scientific community there is a general agreement on the beneficial effects of calcium. However, recent studies have suggested that the beneficial effect of vitamin D might also require an accompanying calcium supplementation.[43,49] Even more strikingly, as well as bone effects, vitamin D might have an important influence on muscular capacity and hence explain the reduced risk of fractures by a decreased risk of falls. In a study by Bischoff et al, this hypothesis was tested and it was shown that a group of 122 elderly institution- alized women had a significant improvement after 3 months of therapy with cal- cium and vitamin D; there was no significant improvement in women treated with calcium alone over the same period.[5] It is not surprising that the Cochrane meta-analysis fails to combine all this to some extent contradictory data.[24,42] The inconsistencies between the studies are probably due to differences in the type of supplement used, the addition of a calcium supplement, the characteristics of the patients (such as degree of vitamin D deficiency at baseline), study design and/or the study end-points.

There is strong evidence that calcium and vitamin D supplementation is a beneficial and cost-effective treatment in the prevention of osteoporotic frac- tures in elderly individuals with calcium and/or vitamin D deficiency.[40] Calcium and vitamin D should therefore be considered an essential component of an inte- grated management strategy for the prevention and treatment of osteoporosis, although maximal benefit will generally be derived from combination therapy with an antiresorptive agent.[13]

OTHER VITAMINS AND DIETARY FACTORS

In addition to calcium, other nutrients also deserve attention. In terms of effects of other vitamins there are two well-documented Swedish studies of retinol intake and risk for hip fracture.[45,50] Both studies confirmed the same result: an increased dietary intake of retinol is linked to an increase in the odds for hip frac- ture (at least twofold).

Vitamin K is involved in the γ-carboxylation of osteocalcin and it has been suggested that deficient intake may increase the risk of proximal femoral frac- tures. The administration of vitamin K_2 may reduce bone loss in postmenopausal women.[22,31,67] It is interesting that the ratio of total serum osteocalcin to decar- boxylated osteocalcin was found to be a better predictor of fractures in a cohort of old women than total osteocalcin.[43]

The role of phosphorus in the treatment of osteoporosis has risen in impor- tance through the literature. There is, however, increasing evidence of the ambivalent effect of phosphorus on the skeleton: it does increase BMD but, par- adoxically, it does not prevent but rather increases the likelihood of fractures.[26] This observation has strengthened the concept of bone quality as the main deter- minant of the skeleton in the persistence of fractures.

Besides the factors named above, there are several observations of other nutri- tional factors and skeletal health. The most popular of these 'initiatives' include caffeine and phyto-oestrogens. To date there is no convincing proof that caffeine adversely affects bone mass, particularly in patients with an adequate calcium intake. Although some studies might suggest otherwise, these studies commonly fail to eradicate the effect of the major constituents, i.e. calcium and vitamin D, from the study set up, and hence no definite conclusions can be made.[28,29] The same applies to studies concerning phyto-oestrogens.

Phyto-oestrogens comprise a family of plant derivatives whose chemical structure has some similarities to that of 17β-oestradiol and hence they are said to have oestrogen-like effects on bone. Isoflavones, most notably genisteine and daidzeine, are by far the most extensively studied phyto-oestrogens. So far, the studies provide no conclusive data although some phyto-oestrogens might have some beneficial effect on BMD, similarly with hormone replacement therapy (HRT).[2,55]

Because of complex dietary behaviour, we might never be able to analyse perfectly all factors influencing osteoporotic fractures. Although compelling evidence of the beneficial effects on bone of a specific diet is not always available, a physician's common sense should lead to the recommendation of a balanced and varied diet, together with stopping smoking and only a modest intake of alcohol.

NON-PHARMACEUTICAL FRACTURE PREVENTION

The epidemiological data suggest a strong correlation for repeated osteoporotic fractures – if an individual has a first fracture then they are more susceptible to later fractures.[9,19,37,61] Hence most effective fracture prevention should be aimed at those patients who are likely to have their first osteoporotic fracture. This would then naturally require efficient screening for the entire ageing population. Since there are no validated screening methods that would recognize the susceptibility for a fall and weak bone, the non-pharmaceutical prevention is usually secondary prevention and aimed at those individuals who are at obvious risk of a fall. However, it is also important that special exercise is recommended for all elderly individuals not only to prevent osteoporosis and fractures but also for other obvious reasons.

A SAFE PHYSICAL ENVIRONMENT

The first priority for non-pharmaceutical fracture prevention consists of the reorganization of the physical environment, i.e. the removal of obstacles, unattached carpeting, etc.[25] Mechanical supports should be mounted along critical walking pathways and areas at home and in public places. Specific attention should also be focused on the maintenance of pavements and roads, especially during icy weather. Those individuals who are not able to control their risk should be predisposed to appropriate monitoring and help if possible.

Personal protectors
Second, individuals with a high fracture risk should be advised to use appropriate protectors, such as hip protection suits and wrist supports. Hip protection has been shown to be an efficient way of preventing hip fractures.[39,54] The problem in their use is related to compliance.

Physical exercise
Third, a very well-documented non-pharmaceutical fracture prevention is physical exercise,[33,59] which can have a beneficial effect in two different ways. First,

exercise improves the physical strength and coordination that are prerequisites in the preparation for unpredictable events, such as falls. Second, exercise directly improves BMD and skeletal strength and may also improve the nutritional status of the elderly. It is important that exercise programmes and instructions are such that they provide sufficient loading on critical parts of the skeleton. Suitable exercise regimens are, for example, balance and strength exercises. However, these programmes should not be too demanding and, of course, should not themselves contain features that increase the risk of a fall. The unquestionable proof that exercise really does reduce fragility fractures is still lacking and must come from well-designed and well-executed, prospective, randomized, controlled trials. These studies are still urgently needed.

PHARMACEUTICAL FRACTURE PREVENTION

Every physician taking care of elderly patients, and especially those who have an elevated number of risk factors for fractures, should carefully review the current medication of their patients bearing in mind that a high risk for falls means a high risk for fractures. In particular, the need for medication with a potential influence on balance and coordination should be carefully evaluated in elderly patients.[70] It should also be kept in mind that several drugs, especially corticosteroids and immunosuppressants, can rapidly damage the microstructure of bone.[57,66]

CURRENT PHARMACOLOGICAL TREATMENT OPTIONS

Several different drugs have been shown to maintain or increase BMD. These include, for example, several forms of bisphosphonates,[13,14] HRT,[68] selective oestrogen receptor modulators,[15] calcitonin,[14] and as the newest options, parathyroid hormone and strontium ranelate. However, only a proportion of these have been shown to reduce the risk of fractures.[13] Each treatment option must be weighed with the experience of the clinician and available data from various fracture prevention studies. Currently there are many options for any pharmaceutical intervention in osteoporosis, for which a clinician should take enough time to review the positive effects as well as the side-effects that are mentioned in the literature. It might be demanding for a clinician to make the final choice from a number of treatment options, although the number of options also give the possibility to 'personalize' the treatment for each individual patient.

Vertebral fractures seem to be easier to prevent with various anti-osteoporotic drugs than nonvertebral fractures. The explanation is in the high amount of trabecular bone in the vertebrae, which responds more readily to antiresorptive treatment than cortical bone. Several bisphosphonates, namely alendronate, etidronate and risedronate, have been shown to reduce the risk of vertebral fractures.[16,17] It is likely that some other bisphosphonates will do the same but those data do not exist yet. In addition to bisphosphonates, calcitonin, vitamin D and raloxifene significantly reduce the number of vertebral fractures.[13–15] Calcitonin also appears to be effective in the management of acute pain, which is often associated with osteoporotic vertebral compression fracture. It may therefore be beneficial to shorten the time to effective mobilization.[38] As mentioned above, vitamin D may also have other beneficial effects which should be considered when a decision for treatment is evaluated.[52] The role of HRT in the prevention and treatment of osteoporosis is discussed elsewhere in this book. However, it is important to note here that according to recent meta-analysis HRT,[69] calcium[58] and fluoride treatments[26] have a tendency to reduce vertebral fractures.

In contrast, published data on vertebral fracture analysis suggest that only two aminobisphosphonates (namely alendronate and risedronate) have the ability to significantly reduce the relative risk for nonvertebral fractures. This was also confirmed in a recent meta-analysis where NNT values of nonvertebral fractures for aledronate and risedronate were calculated to be 24 and 43, respectively.[16,17]

FUTURE TRENDS OF PHARMACEUTICAL INTERVENTIONS IN OSTEOPOROSIS

Several new pharmaceutical treatment options for osteoporosis have been launched in recent years and some of them also seem to be effective in fracture prevention. However, we are still looking for new therapeutic possibilities to prevent and treat osteoporosis. Fortunately, several new therapies are developing and may, in the near future, challenge current therapy regimens. The anabolic effect of parathyroid hormone and analogues and strontium ranelate, for instance, are interesting new compounds that seem to have the capacity to rebuild the damaged microarchitecture of trabecular bone. It remains to be conclusively seen how well this property will be reflected in fracture prevention.

Since pharmaceutical intervention for osteoporosis should be planned to last several years, it is of special interest to see whether the bisphosphonate treatment could be applied by dosing a drug only very infrequently, even once a year. Considering the pharmacokinetics of these compounds, it may well be the case, and it has already been shown that this mode of treatment does increase bone density.[13]

References

1. Albrand G, Munoz F, Sornay-Rendu E et al 2003 Independent predictors of all osteoporosis-related fractures in healthy postmenopausal women: the OFELY Study. Bone 32:78–85
2. Alekel D L, St Germain A, Peterson C T et al 2000 Isoflavone-rich soy protein isolate attenuates bone loss in the lumbar spine of perimenopausal women. The American Journal of Clinical Nutrition 72:844–852
3. Baron J A, Karagas M, Barrett J et al 1996 Basic epidemiology of fractures of the upper and lower limb among Americans over 65 years of age. Epidemiology 7:612–618
4. Bischoff H A, Stahelin H B, Dick W et al 2003 Effects of vitamin D and calcium supplementation on falls: a randomized controlled trial. Journal of Bone and Mineral Research 18:343–351
5. Black D M, Cummings S R, Karpf D B et al 1996 Randomised trial of effect of alendronate on risk of fracture in women with existing vertebral fracture. The Lancet 348:1535–1541
6. Cauley J A, Thompson D E, Ensrud K C et al 2000 Risk of mortality following clinical fractures. Osteoporosis International 11:556–561
7. Center J R, Nguyen T V, Schneider D et al 1999 Mortality after all major types of

osteoporotic fracture in men and women: an observational study. The Lancet 353:878–882

8. Chang J T, Morton S C, Rubenstein L Z et al 2004 Interventions for the prevention of falls in older adults: systematic review and meta-analysis of randomised clinical trials. British Medical Journal 328(7441):80.

9. Chapurlat R D, Bauer D C, Nevitt M et al 2003 Incidence and risk factors for a second hip fracture in elderly women. The Study of Osteoporotic Fractures. Osteoporosis International 14:130–136

10. Chapuy M C, Arlot M E, Delmas P D et al 1994 Effect of calcium and cholecalciferol treatment for three years on hip fractures in elderly women. British Medical Journal 308:1081–1082

11. Chapuy M C, Arlot M E, Duboeuf F et al 1992 Vitamin D_3 and calcium to prevent hip fractures in elderly women. The New England Journal of Medicine 327:1637–1642

12. Cooper C, Atkinson E J, O'Fallon W M et al 1992 Incidence of clinically diagnosed vertebral fractures: a population-based study in Rochester, Minnesota, 1985–1989. Journal of Bone and Mineral Research 7:221–227

13. Cranney A, Guyatt G, Griffith L et al, the Osteoporosis Methodology Group and the Osteoporosis Research Advisory Group 2002 Meta-analyses of therapies for post-menopausal osteoporosis. IX. Summary of meta-analyses of therapies for postmeno-pausal osteoporosis. Endocrine Reviews 23:570–578

14. Cranney A, Tugwell P, Zytaruk N et al 2002 Meta-analyses of therapies for postmenopausal osteoporosis. VI. Meta-analysis of calcitonin for the treatment of postmenopausal osteoporosis. Endocrine Reviews 4:540–541

15. Cranney A, Tugwell P, Zytaruk N et al 2002 Meta-analyses of therapies for post-menopausal osteoporosis. IV. Meta-analysis of raloxifene for the prevention and treat-ment of postmenopausal osteoporosis. Endocrine Reviews 4:524–528

16. Cranney A, Tugwell P, Adachi J et al 2002 Meta-analyses of therapies for postmeno-pausal osteoporosis. III. Meta-analysis of risedronate for the treatment of postmeno-pausal osteoporosis. Endocrine Reviews 4:517–523

17. Cranney A, Wells G, Willan A et al 2002 Meta-analyses of therapies for postmenopausal osteoporosis. II. Meta-analysis of alendronate for the treatment of postmenopausal women. Endocrine Reviews 4:508–516

18. Cummings S R, Black D M, Rubin S M 1989 Lifetime risks of hip, Colles, or vertebral fracture and coronary heart disease among white postmenopausal women. Archives of Internal Medicine 149:2445–2448

19. Cummings S R, Nevitt M C, Browner W S et al 1995 Risk factors for hip fracture in white women. The New England Journal of Medicine 332:767–773

20. Dawson-Hughes B, Harris S S, Krall E A et al 1997 Effect of calcium and vitamin D supplementation on bone density in men and women 65 years of age or older. The New England Journal of Medicine 337:670–676

21. Fang J, Freeman R, Jeganathan R et al 2004 Variations in hip fracture hospitalization rates among different race/ethnicity groups in New York City. Ethnicity & Disease 14:280–284

22. Feskanich D, Weber P, Willet W C et al 1999 Vitamin K intake and hip fractures in women: a prospective study. The American Journal of Clinical Nutrition 69:74–79

23. Geinoz G, Rapin C H, Rizzoli R et al 1993 Relationship between bone mineral density and dietary intakes in the elderly. Osteoporosis International 3:242–248

24. Gillespie W J, Avenell A, Henry D A et al 2001 Vitamin D and vitamin D analogues for preventing fractures associated with involutional and post-menopausal osteoporosis. Cochrane Database of Systematic Reviews 1:CD000227

25. Greenspan S L, Myers E R, Maitland L A et al 1994 Fall severity and bone mineral density as risk factors for hip fractures in ambulatory elderly. The Journal of the American Medical Association 271:128–133

26. Gutteridge D H, Stewart G O, Prince R L et al 2002 A randomized trial of sodium fluoride (60 mg) +/– estrogen in postmenopausal osteoporotic vertebral fractures: increased vertebral fractures and peripheral bone loss with sodium fluoride. Concurrent estrogen prevents peripheral loss, but not vertebral fractures. Osteoporosis International 13:158–170

27. Hannan M T, Tucker K L, Dawson-Hughes B et al 2000 Effect of dietary protein on bone loss in elderly men and women: the Framingham Osteoporosis Study. Journal

of Bone and Mineral Research 15:2504–2512

28. Hansen A., Folsom A R, Kushi L H et al 2000 Association of fractures with caffeine and alcohol in postmenopausal women: the Iowa Women's Health Study. Public Health Nutrition 3:253–261

29. Heaney R P 2002 Effects of caffeine on bone and calcium economy. Food and Chemical Toxicology 40:1263–1270

30. Ismail A A, O'Neill T W, Cooper C et al 1998 Mortality associated with vertebral deformity in men and women: results from the European Prospective Osteoporosis Study (EPOS). Osteoporosis International 8:291–297

31. Iwamoto J, Takeda T, Ichimura S 2000 Effect of combined administration of vitamin D_3 and vitamin K_2 on bone mineral density of the lumbar spine in postmenopausal women with osteoporosis. Journal of Orthopaedic Science 5:546–551

32. Jackson S A, Tenenhouse A, Robertson L and the CaMos Study Group 2000 Vertebral fractures definition from population-based data: preliminary results from the Canadian Multicentre Osteoporosis Study (CaMos). Osteoporosis International 11:680–687

33. Joakimsen R M, Ronnebo V, Magnus J H et al 1998 The Tromso study: physical activity and the incident of fractures in a middle-age population. Journal of Bone and Mineral Research 13:1149–1157

34. Johnell O, Kanis J A 2004 An estimate of worldwide prevalence, mortality and disability associated with hip fracture. Osteoporosis International 15:897–902

35. Kanis J A, Oden A, Johnell O et al 2001 The burden of osteoporotic fractures: a method for setting intervention thresholds. Osteoporosis International 12:417–427

36. Kannus P, Niemi S, Parkkari J et al 1993 Hip fractures in Finland between 1970 and 1997 and predictions for the future. The Lancet 353:802–805

37. Klotzbuecher C M, Ross P D, Landsman P B et al 2000 Patients with prior fractures have an increased risk of future fractures: a summary of the literature and statistical synthesis. Journal of Bone and Mineral Research 15:721–739

38. Knopp J A, Diner B M, Blitz M et al 2004 Calcitonin for treating acute pain of osteoporotic vertebral compression fractures: a systematic review of randomized, controlled trials. Osteoporosis International 22 December (epub ahead of print)

39. Lee S H, Dargent-Molina P, Breart G 2002 Risk factors for fractures of the proximal humerus: results from the EPIDOS prospective study. Journal of Bone and Mineral Research 17:817–825

40. Lilliu H, Pamphile R, Chapuy M-C et al 2003 Calcium–vitamin D_3 supplementation is cost-effective in hip fractures prevention. Maturitas 44:299–305

41. Lips P 1997 Epidemiology and predictors of fractures associated with osteoporosis. The American Journal of Medicine 103:3S–11S

42. Lips P, Graafmans W C, Ooms M E et al 1996 Vitamin D supplementation and fracture incidence in elderly persons: a randomized, placebo-controlled clinical trial. Annals of Internal Medicine 124:400–406

43. Luukinen H, Käkönen S M, Pettersson K et al 2000 Strong prediction of fractures among older adults by the ratio of carboxylated to total osteocalcin. Journal of Bone and Mineral Research 15: 2473–2478

44. Matkowic V, Kostial K, Simonivic I et al 1979 Bone status and fracture rates in two regions of Yugoslavia. The American Journal of Clinical Nutrition 32:540–549

45. Melhus H, Michaelsson K, Kindmark A et al 1998 Excessive dietary intake of vitamin A is associated with reduced bone mineral density and increased risk of hip fracture. Annals of Internal Medicine 129:770–778

46. Melton L J 1998 Evidence-based assessment of pharmaceutical interventions. Osteoporosis International 8:S17–S20

47. Melton L J, III, Chrischilles E A, Cooper C et al 1992 Perspective. How many women have osteoporosis? Journal of Bone and Mineral Research 7:1005–1010

48. Meunier P J, Chapuy M C, Arlot M E et al 1994 Can we stop bone loss and prevent hip fractures in the elderly? Osteoporosis International 4 (Suppl 1):S71–S76

49. Meyer H E, Smedshaug G B, Kvaavik E et al 2002 Can vitamin D supplementation reduce the risk of fractures in the elderly? A randomized controlled trial. Journal of Bone and Mineral Research 17:709–715

50. Michaelsson M D, Lithell H, Vessby B et al 2003 Serum retinol levels and risk of fracture. The New England Journal of Medicine 348:287–294

51. Nguyen T V, Center J R, Sambrook P H et al 2001 Risk factors for proximal humerus, forearm, and wrist fractures in elderly men and women. The Dubbo Osteoporosis

Epidemiology Study. American Journal of Epidemiology 153:587–595

52. Papadimitropoulos E, Wells G, Shea B et al 2002 Meta-analyses of therapies for post-menopausal osteoporosis. VIII. Meta-analysis of the efficacy of vitamin D treatment in preventing osteoporosis in postmenopausal women. Endocrine Reviews 4:560–569

53. Perry B C 1982 Falls among the elderly: a review of the methods and conclusions of epidemiologic studies. Journal of the American Geriatrics Society 30:367–371

54. Pfeifer M, Begerow B, Minne HW et al 2000 Effects of a short-term vitamin D and calcium supplementation on body sway and secondary hyperparathyroidism in elderly women. Journal of Bone and Mineral Research 15:1113–1118

55. Potter S M, Baum J A, Teng H et al 1998 Soy protein and isoflavones: their effects on blood lipids and bone density in post-menopausal women. The American Journal of Clinical Nutrition 68:1375S–1379S

56. Prudham D, Evans J G 1981 Factors associated with falls in the elderly: a community study. Age and Ageing 10:141–146

57. Reid I 1998 Glucocorticoid-induced osteoporosis: assessment and treatment. Journal of Clinical Densitometry 1:65–73

58. Shea B, Wells G, Cranney A et al 2002 Meta-analyses of therapies for postmenopausal osteoporosis. VII. Meta-analysis of calcium supplementation for the prevention of postmenopausal osteoporosis. Endocrine Reviews 23:552–559

59. Sorock G S, Bush T L, Golder A L et al 1988 Physical activity and fracture risk in a free-living elderly cohort. The Journals of Gerontology 43:M134–M139

60. Trivedi D P, Doll R, Khaw K T 2003 Effect of four-monthly oral vitamin D_3 (cholecalciferol) supplementation on fractures and mortality in men and women living in the community: randomised double-blind controlled trial. British Medical Journal 326:469–472

61. Trombetti A, Herrmann F, Hoffmeyer P et al 2002 Survival and potential years of life lost after hip fracture in men and age-matched women. Osteoporosis International 13:731–737

62. Tromp A M, Ooms M E, Popp-Snijders C et al 2000 Predictors of fractures in elderly women. Osteoporosis International 11:134–140

63. Ushiroyama T, Ikeda A, Veki M 2002 Effect of continuous combined therapy with vitamin K_2 and vitamin D_3 on bone mineral density and coagulofibrinolysis function in postmenopausal women. Maturitas 41:211–221

64. Väänänen H K 1991 Pathogenesis of osteoporosis. Calcified Tissue International (Suppl) 49:S11–S14

65. Väänänen H K 1993 Mechanism of bone turnover. Annals of Medicine 25:353–360

66. Väänänen HK, Härkönen P L 2002 Bone effects of glucocorticoid therapy. Ernst Schering Research Found Workshop. Review. In: Cato A B C, Schäcke H, Asadullah K (eds) Recent Advances in Glucocorticoid Receptor Action, Volume 40. Berlin, Springer-Verlag, p 55–64

67. Van der Voort D J M, Geusens P P, Dinant G J 2001 Risk factors for osteoporosis related to their outcome: fractures. Osteoporosis International 12:630–638

68. Wells E G, Shea B et al 2002 Meta-analysis of the efficacy of vitamin D treatment in preventing osteoporosis in postmenopausal women. Endocrine Reviews 23:560–569

69. Wells G, Tugwell P, Shea B et al 2002 Meta-analyses of therapies for post-menopausal osteoporosis. V. Meta-analysis of the efficacy of hormone replacement therapy in treating and preventing osteoporosis in postmenopausal women. Endocrine Reviews 4:529–539

70. Whooley M A, Kip K E, Cauley J A et al 1999 Depression, falls and risk of fracture in older women. Study of Osteoporotic Fractures Research Group. Archives of Internal Medicine 159: 484–500

11

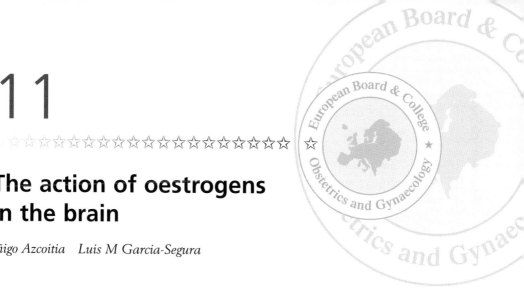

The action of oestrogens in the brain

Iñigo Azcoitia   Luis M Garcia-Segura

ABSTRACT

Oestrogens have a wide range of actions in the brain, regulating the physiological and pathological responses of neurones and glial cells. Oestradiol (E_2) affects the survival and differentiation of brain cells and regulates synaptic communication. Furthermore, the hormone has neuroprotective properties, preventing neuronal loss in several animal models of neurodegenerative disease. New advances in the knowledge of the molecular mechanisms and cellular targets involved in the action of E_2 in the central nervous system (CNS) are reviewed. The roles of oestrogen receptors (ERs), intracellular signalling and neurotransmitter receptors in hormonal actions are analysed, as well as the cellular targets involved.

KEYWORDS

Aromatase, cell signalling, glia, insulin-like growth factor I (IGF-I), neurones, neuroprotection, neurotrophins, oestradiol (E_2), oestrogen receptors (ERs), synapses

INTRODUCTION

In 1849, Adolf Berthold published the results of the first experiments relating behaviour, and therefore the brain, to gonadal secretions. Later, after the identification of the molecular structure of gonadal hormones, specific neural events that were affected by sex steroids were recognized. These included the sexual differentiation of the brain and spinal cord, and the regulation of neuroendocrine events and sex behaviours. However, in the past fifteen years, it has become evident that sex steroids, including E_2, exert an additional broad

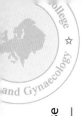
spectrum of actions in the nervous system which are similar to those exerted by trophic factors and neuromodulators, and which are not directly involved in the control of reproduction.

E_2 regulates gene expression, neuronal survival, neuronal and glial differentiation, and synaptic transmission in many CNS areas.[15] It is also well established that E_2 has neuroprotective and reparative properties.[2,10,11] The hormone prevents cognitive and neuronal loss in several experimental animal models of neurodegeneration. However, there has not been an unambiguous translation of the data from animal models to human studies and the results from hormone replacement therapy (HRT, oestrogens and progestins) or oestrogen-only therapy (ET), on neurological and cognitive functions in women, are not yet conclusive.[20]

Most studies suggest that ET increases memory and cognitive functions in healthy women. In addition, it has been reported that ET may reduce the motor disability associated with Parkinson's disease, decrease the risk of stroke in postmenopausal women, prevent or delay the onset of Alzheimer's disease and improve cognition for women with Alzheimer's disease. However, other studies indicate that ET or HRT have no effect on Parkinson's disease, do not reduce mortality or the recurrence of stroke in postmenopausal women with cerebrovascular disease and do not improve cognition of women with Alzheimer's disease.[4,6–9,14,17,18] The Women's Health Initiative (WHI) randomized trial, where participants received 1 daily tablet of 0.625 mg of conjugated equine oestrogen plus 2.5 mg of medroxyprogesterone acetate (MPA), or a matching placebo, suggests an increased risk of dementia and stroke as a result of long-lasting hormonal treatment several years after the menopause.

Several explanations for the discrepancies among different studies – such as differences in dose, formulation, route of administration, length of treatment, sample size and age of the women receiving the treatment – have been proposed. In particular, MPA may have several undesirable effects. It cannot be excluded that natural progesterone – as it can be transformed into the neuroprotective metabolites dihydroprogesterone and tetrahydroprogesterone by neural tissue – may have better cognitive effects. However, the oestrogen-alone arm of the WHI study has not provided any support for the expected beneficial effects of E_2 in the brain.

It should be noted that the WHI data are relevant for long-term HRT started in women aged 65 or over. The risks and benefits of either short-term or long-term HRT or ET on younger women are not yet known. The focus of the WHI study on women who are already many years beyond the onset of the menopause is a serious limitation. There are reasons to think that the perimenopause may be a critical period for the highest efficacy of HRT on the prevention of brain disorders. During this period, the brain may be adapting local steroid synthesis to the new situation created by the loss of ovarian function; steroid receptor machinery is probably still not affected by the new situation. In any case, the results of the WHI study emphasize the need for a better understanding of the effects of E_2 in the brain.

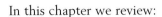

In this chapter we review:

1. The current knowledge of the molecular mechanisms of the action of E_2 in the brain.
2. The cell types that are affected by the hormone.
3. A better understanding of these molecular and cellular targets of E_2 in the brain as well as of the regulation of its local synthesis, which is indispensable for predicting the potential outcome of HRTs on brain function.

E_2 ACTS IN THE BRAIN BY MULTIPLE MECHANISMS

As in other tissues, the effects of E_2 in the nervous system may be exerted by the activation of classical nuclear ERs (Fig. 11.1). These receptors are ligand-dependent transcription factors that mediate multiple effects in different tissues. The two mammalian ERs cloned to date, α and β, are expressed in the human brain. ERs belong to the steroid/thyroid nuclear receptor superfamily and, once activated, homo- or heterodimerize, interact with DNA and recruit a cohort of transcriptional cofactors to the regulatory regions of target genes (see Fig. 11.1). Also, E_2 may elicit rapid actions in the nervous system by the interaction with the cytoplasmic and membrane compartments of neurones and glial cells.[3,5,13,15]

E_2 may also act in the nervous system through non-specific receptors, such as neurotransmitter ion channels (see Fig. 11.1), and through non-receptor-mediated mechanisms, for example as an antioxidant.[1,2] The actions of E_2 at the membrane and the nuclear receptors are inextricably linked: the gene products generated by the E_2-dependent activation of nuclear receptors and transcription can be post-transcriptionaly modified by cell signals activated by membrane ERs. Transcription itself can be augmented or reduced by coactivators and co-repressors previously modified through membrane-associated oestrogen actions (see Fig. 11.1). Finally, E_2 not only drives the transcription of genes whose promoters bind to nuclear ERs, but also of genes that are transactivated by other transcription factors modified after membrane E_2 signalling.[1]

OESTROGEN RECEPTORS IN THE BRAIN

Oestrogen binding in the brain was first described in the late 1960s. The presence of ERs in the brain has been confirmed by radioligand binding, steroid hormone autoradiography, immunocytochemistry, *in-situ* hybridization and polymerase chain reaction. In addition, *in-vivo* imaging techniques have recently been used to demonstrate the transcription of ER-dependent genes in the brain of both mature and immature rodents. Immunocytochemical analyses and *in-situ* hybridization studies revealed the presence of abundant ERα expression in neurones in many brain areas.[11] The predominant localization of ERs in neurones is in the cell nucleus. However, ultrastructural analyses have demonstrated that ERα

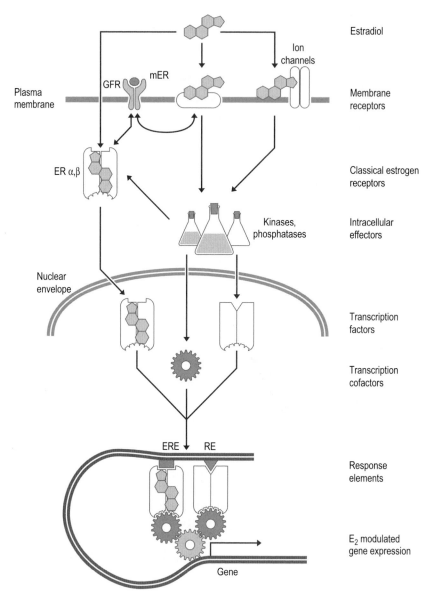

Fig 11.1 Membrane and cytoplasmic actions of E_2 in the brain. E_2 signalling includes classic oestrogen receptors (ERs) α and β and putative membrane ERs (*mR*). In addition, E_2 can alter the membrane conductance of ion channels and ERs can interact and modulate growth factor receptors. After cytoplasmic crosstalk, transcription factors, including ERα and β, are activated and translocated to the cell nucleus where they bind to cognate response elements, recruit transcriptional cofactors and drive gene expression.

immunoreactivity is also present in neuronal processes: dendritic spines, axons and axon terminals.[15] ERβ is also expressed in several neuronal subtypes and in some brain areas, such as the cerebellum, it is the predominant form of ER.

Glial cells also express ERs, although the constitutive expression of ERs in glia is low. However, there is a marked increase in expression of both ERα and ERβ in reactive astrocytes after brain injury. Endothelial cells in the brain are also affected by E_2, and immunoreactivity for ERα has been described in these cells in the guinea-pig brain by electron microscopy.

The expression of ERs in the brain is developmentally regulated, and developmental sex differences in the expression of ERs may participate in the generation of sex differences in adult brain functions. The distribution and level of expression of ERs is regulated by E_2. In most brain areas, ERs are upregulated when E_2 levels are low and downregulated by ET.

MEMBRANE AND CYTOPLASMIC ACTIONS OF E_2 IN THE BRAIN

As in other organs, E_2 acts in the brain not only through ERs but also through putative non-nuclear ERs.[1] As mentioned above, ERs have been detected in neuronal and glial cell processes, in a position that could favour non-nuclear signalling.[15] To date, the molecular identity of non-nuclear ERs in the brain has not been characterized and the extranuclear functions of E_2 may be mediated by receptors identical to the nuclear ERs, but in some way modified (for instance palmitoylated) in order to prevent, at least temporarily, their translocation to the nucleus. In fact some of the non-nuclear effects of E_2 in the brain are sensitive to ICI 182 780, an inhibitor of both ERα and ERβ. Furthermore, membrane receptors can be immunostained with anti-ER antibodies suggesting that they may arise from splicing variants or post-translational modifications of the classical nuclear receptors.

THE REGULATION OF INTRACELLULAR CALCIUM, PHOSPHATASES AND KINASES

Membrane ERs (see Fig. 11.1) may be part of the macromolecular entities aggregated in specific plasma membrane domains, the caveolae, where they can hypothetically interact with G proteins, receptor tyrosine kinases, nonreceptor kinases and other signalling partners.[19] ERs can directly contact G proteins or transactivate other G protein-coupled receptors, leading to the stimulation of ion channels and phospholipase C.[13] Oestrogen-induced phospholipase C activation initiates a cascade of signals through increases in intracellular Ca^{2+} and the activation of protein kinase C (PKC) and protein kinase A (PKA), leading to the modulation of other ion channels and cyclic AMP-response element binding protein-dependent transcription.

Of particular relevance are glutamate-mediated increases in intracellular Ca^{2+} concentration that are potentiated by oestrogen,[3] because this has been proposed to modulate cognitive function. The risk of calcium overload in neurones exposed to E_2, which could occur in an excitotoxic condition, is attenuated through enhancing mitochondrial sequestration of Ca^{2+}. At the same time, Bcl-2 expression is increased, promoting mitochondrial calcium load tolerance.[11] It is important to consider, however, that the effects of E_2 on calcium balance are partly attenuated by progesterone. This may have important

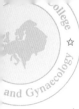

implications for the effective use of HRT to maintain cognitive function after menopause.[1]

Protein kinases and phosphatases are among the intracellular targets of Ca^{2+}. E_2 regulates, in a Ca^{2+}-dependent manner, the enzyme α-calcium-calmodulin-dependent protein kinase II (or α-CaMKII) and the Ser/Thr protein phosphatases calcineurin and protein phosphatase 1 (PP1). α-CaMKII is activated in the brain via a very rapid nongenomic mechanism that is blocked by the anti-oestrogen ICI 182 780. This is noteworthy because sustained activation of CaMKII localized at the postsynaptic density results in a series of short- and long-term events that culminate in synaptic potentiation. In parallel with CaMKII activation, E_2 elicits the inhibition of phosphatases; cytosolic levels of calcineurin are reduced while PP1 activity is lowered, thus reinforcing CaMKII activation.[1]

The E_2-elicited intracellular raise in calcium may result in a rapid stimulation of phosphatidylinositol-3-kinase (PI3K) signalling cascade.[3] Interestingly, PKA and the Ca^{2+}-dependent PKC isoform PKCδ enhance ERα activity. This reciprocal activation is also characteristic of the relationship between oestrogen and growth factors. IGF-I and other trophic factors can activate extracellular-regulated kinases (ERKs), members of the family of mitogen-activated protein kinases (MAPK), leading to the phosphorylation of ERs. In parallel, ERα, in an oestrogen-dependent process, can physically interact with the IGF-I receptor and with the downstream proteins IRS-1 and PI3K, enhancing IGF-I signalling in the brain.[5] The neuroprotective actions of E_2 may, in part, be mediated by the activation, through the IGF-I receptor-signalling cascade, of the anti-apoptotic kinase Akt. In addition, E_2 induces a transient activation of glycogen synthase kinase 3 (GSK3) in the adult female rat hippocampus, followed by a more sustained inhibition. This hormonal action may also promote neuronal survival since the inhibition of GSK3 is associated with the activation of surviving signalling pathways in neurones. E_2 also regulates the interaction of ERα with GSK3 and β-catenin, another molecule involved in the regulation of neuronal survival and the reorganization of the cytoskeleton. Furthermore, E_2 regulates the interaction of the microtubule associated protein Tau with GSK3, β-catenin and elements of the PI3 kinase complex and reduces the hyperphosphorylation of Tau, one of the molecular markers of Alzheimer's disease. All these actions may be involved in the plastic and neuroprotective effects of the hormone.

The ability of E_2 to activate members of the MAPK family, extracellular signal-regulated protein kinase 1 (ERK1) and 2 (ERK2), has been demonstrated in cultured neurones from different brain regions. In addition, a robust ERK1/2 activation is detected in the brain after oestrogen administration *in vivo*.[5] The response *in vitro* is rapid and mediated by both E_2 and E_2 conjugated to BSA and hence it can be considered a membrane-associated response. Moreover, most authors concur that the ER antagonist ICI 182 780 does not block MAPK activation by E_2.

MAPK activation by E_2 in the brain is a physiological process that can be demonstrated across the oestrous cycle in rats. The levels of activation in the hippocampus, a brain region involved in cognition, directly reflect the levels of circulating oestrogen, and phosphorylation of ERK2 reaches its maximum value during pro-oestrus. The principal consequences of oestrogen-dependent MAPK activation in the hippocampus are related to neuroprotection and synaptic plasticity which may modulate learning and memory. Both E_2-induced neuroprotection and E_2-induced synaptic plasticity are blocked by treatment with MAPK inhibitors.[1]

THE REGULATION OF NEUROTRANSMITTER RECEPTORS

E_2 regulates the expression of neurotransmitter receptors and the synthesis and release of neurotransmitters. As a result, E_2 modulates the communication between brain cells. This has important implications for brain physiology and pathology. For instance, effects on dopamine levels and receptors may contribute to the beneficial hormonal actions on Parkinson's disease. In addition, E_2 may bind to neurotransmitter receptors and neurotransmitter transporters affecting their activity. For instance, E_2 allosterically regulates the function of serotonin receptors and exhibits a noncompetitive inhibition of serotonin transport. Related to cholinergic neurotransmission, E_2 binds to the $\alpha 4$ subunit of nicotinic cholinergic receptors, causing an allosteric potentiation of the nicotinic receptor. These hormonal actions may be highly relevant for hormonal effects on depression and affective disorders and on neurodegenerative diseases. However, their precise physiological and pathological relevance remains to be clarified.[1]

INTERACTIONS WITH GROWTH FACTORS

Several growth factors appear to be involved in the actions of E_2 in the brain. One such factor is IGF-I.[5] Within the brain there is abundant coexpression of nuclear ERs and IGF-I receptor in the same cell and many cell responses to E_2 or IGF-I appear to depend on direct interactions of the two receptors. E_2 and IGF-I have a synergistic effect on the activation of Akt, a kinase involved in the promotion of neuronal survival.[5] Both E_2 and IGF-I cooperate in neuroprotection in an excitotoxic *in-vivo* animal model of hippocampal injury and in an experimental model of Parkinson's disease. When the IGF-I receptor is inhibited by a specific antagonist, E_2 is unable to protect hippocampal or dopaminergic mesencephalic neurones from neurodegenerative damage. Conversely, IGF-I-mediated neuroprotection is blocked by the anti-oestrogen ICI 182 780. The interaction of IGF-I and E_2 in neuroprotection has also been demonstrated in primary neuronal cultures, in the absence of glial cells, indicating that the interaction of both factors occurs directly on neurones. However, glial cells may be a local source of E_2 and IGF-I.

Brain-derived neurotrophic factor (BDNF) is another growth factor modulated by E_2 in the brain. The BDNF gene contains an oestrogen response element in its promoter region and so oestrogens may modulate the transcription of the neurotrophin. Furthermore, ERs and BDNF are coexpressed in several neuronal cell types. E_2-dependent upregulation of BDNF transcription is involved in the survival of cholinergic neurones projecting to the hippocampus. A rise in BDNF mRNA levels in the intact female rat has been correlated with better hippocampal function. In this scenario, E_2 is an indispensable factor in many of the phenomena that elevate BDNF, such as physical exercise. Unexpectedly, the E_2-dependent rise in hippocampal BDNF mRNA levels is not followed by the augmentation of protein levels. Indeed, BDNF protein is somewhat reduced after E_2 or phyto-oestrogen administration. This apparently paradoxical regulation of BDNF has been interpreted as an indication that the protein is released by hippocampal neurones and carried by fast retrograde transport to another brain area: the septum. This hypothesis is corroborated by the fact that, after E_2 replacement, BDNF protein levels are increased while the message does not vary in the medial septum, the major source of cholinergic innervation to the hippocampus.

E_2 ACTS IN THE BRAIN ON MULTIPLE CELL TYPES

It is important to remember that some cells can respond to E_2 even in the absence of ERs, provided that they receive appropriate signals from cells that do express ERs. The great degree of cell-to-cell communication characteristic of the nervous system builds the appropriate network for such signalling – neural cells expressing ERs are intercommunicated with cells devoid of ERs and with other cells expressing ERs. These cells may be neurones or glial cells and may express ERα only, ERβ only, either ER forms or neither. The final functional outcome of oestrogen action will depend on the integration of the intercellular signalling into these neuronal–glial networks. One example is the regulation of synaptic plasticity.

E_2 INDUCES NEURONAL AND GLIAL PLASTICITY

The role of glia as a mediator of oestrogen-induced synaptic plasticity was first described in the arcuate nucleus of the hypothalamus. Astrocytes in the arcuate nucleus are able to modify their cytoskeleton in response to E_2, resulting in expanding astrocytic processes interposed between neurones and thus modifying the functional synaptic area and the number of synaptic contacts. In rats, in late pro-oestrus, the surge of E_2 induces a transient growth of astrocyte processes on the surface of arcuate neurones. As a consequence, there is a transient disconnection of inhibitory GABAergic synapses from the arcuate neuronal cell body by the interposed glial processes. These changes are also elicited by the administration of E_2 to adult ovariectomized rats. E_2 also increases the number of excitatory synapses on dendritic spines in the arcuate nucleus. The result of the decrease in the number of inhibitory inputs and the increase in the number of excitatory inputs is an increased neuronal firing.[10]

A similar situation is observed in the hippocampus,[15] where the level of glial fibrillary acidic protein immunoreactivity and the number of synaptic contacts also depends on oestrogen levels. E_2 induces an increase in the number of dendritic spines and their associated presynaptic contacts in hippocampal pyramidal neurones. This effect is associated with the hormonal phosphorylation of the kinase Akt and is mediated by the spine scaffolding protein, postsynaptic density 95. In addition, the synaptic changes are accompanied by an increased expression of tyrosine kinase A (TrkA) receptors in astrocytes. Since nerve growth factor (the ligand for TrkA) stimulates astrocytes to function as a substrates for axon growth, it has been proposed that E_2 may regulate axonal growth and synaptic plasticity in the hippocampus by the induction of TrkA receptors in astrocytes. In addition, soluble factors released by astrocytes from target brain areas have been shown to influence the neuritogenic effect of E_2 on cultured hypothalamic neurones. Finally, astrocytes secrete laminin in response to oestrogen, facilitating neurite extension when co-cultured with neurones.

E_2 ACTS ON NEURONES AND GLIA TO REGULATE HORMONAL SECRETION

Coordinated actions of E_2 on neurones and glial cells are also important for neuroendocrine regulation.[10] Astrocytes and tanycytes (specialized glial cells of the mediobasal hypothalamus and the median eminence) modulate the function of the hypothalamic neurones synthesizing and secreting the luteinizing hormone-releasing hormone (LHRH). The most important molecules, released from glial cells and apparently responsible for these effects, are transforming growth factor α (TGF-α), transforming growth factors β1 and β2 (TGF-β1 and TGF-β2), bFGF and insulin-like growth factor I (IGF-I). The astrocytic involvement provides an additional and new mode of control of LHRH secretion, which is also regulated by neuronal inputs, as well as by steroid hormones acting via positive or negative feedback signals. The possibility of functional cooperation between growth factors and E_2 at the level of astrocytes and tanycytes in the control of the LHRH-secreting neurones has recently been considered.[10] E_2 influences the release of TGF-β1 and IGF-I from astrocytes and regulates local IGF-I levels in the hypothalamus. In addition, E_2 is able to induce an increase in TGF-α and bFGF mRNA levels in cultures of hypothalamic astrocytes. It is interesting to note that in hypothalamic astrocytes, E_2 is also able to facilitate the effect of prostaglandin PGE_2, one of the humoral factors intervening in the control of the secretion of LHRH.

E_2 ACTS ON NEURONES, AND GLIAL AND BRAIN ENDOTHELIAL CELLS TO PROMOTE NEUROPROTECTION

Many studies have demonstrated neuroprotective effects of E_2 in different experimental models of neurodegenerative diseases. E_2 promotes neuronal survival by inducing the transcription and repression, respectively, of anti- and pro-apoptotic genes in neurones, and activating intracellular signalling cascades that converge with those of growth factors.[11] In addition to direct hormonal effects on neurones, E_2 may also exert neuroprotective effects by the mediation of glial cells. E_2 may promote neuronal survival inducing the release of growth factors, such as

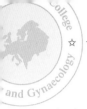
The menopause

TGF-β1 or IGF-I, by astrocytes. The hormone may also affect brain responses to pathological conditions by regulating reactive gliosis and the expression of molecules in reactive astroglia that are part of the response of astrocytes to injury. For instance, oestrogen downregulates the expression of bFGF in astrocytes and increases the expression of apolipoprotein E (ApoE), a molecule involved in neuroregulation after injury, in astrocytes and microglia. A very interesting finding with implications for reactive astroglia is that E_2 in cultured astrocytes reduces the activation of NF-κB induced by amyloid Aβ(1–40) and lipopolysaccharide. Since NF-κB is a potent immediate–early transcriptional regulator of numerous pro-inflammatory genes, the hormonal regulation of this molecule in astrocytes may play a crucial role in the neuroprotective effects of oestrogen.

Other effects of E_2 on astrocytes may also be relevant under neuropathological conditions. For instance, E_2 increases the expression of heat shock proteins in astrocytes, an effect that has also been observed after global ischaemia in gerbils and that may be related to the protective effects of the hormone in animal models of brain ischaemia. Furthermore, E_2 increases glutamate uptake in astrocytes derived from Alzheimer's patients, which may contribute to the potential protective hormonal effect against this neurodegenerative disease, where the extracellular glutamate concentration appears to be increased.

Other brain cells that are highly relevant in the neuroprotective effects of E_2 are microglia.[16] Microglia are specialized macrophages of the brain that are activated by neuronal injury and are involved, directly or indirectly, in most neurological disorders. Several studies have analysed the effect of E_2 on microglia, in the search for a basis for the neuroprotective effects of the hormone. E_2 enhances ApoE secretion by microglia *in vivo* and inhibits apoptosis in microglia cultures by a receptor-mediated enhancement of Nip2 protein production. In addition, E_2 inhibits the induction of inducible nitric oxide synthase, and the consequent production of nitric oxide, in response to lipopolysaccharide and to the pro-inflammatory cytokines interferon-γ and tumour necrosis factor α. Furthermore, E_2 also reduces lipopolysaccharide-induced production in microglia of other inflammatory mediators, such as PGE_2, and metalloproteinase 9. E_2 can also enhance the uptake of amyloid beta protein (Aβ) by microglia derived from the human cortex, an effect that may be relevant for the protective effect of this hormone against Alzheimer's disease. The mechanisms involved in the antiinflammatory actions of E_2 on microglia are under study. It is known that ER-dependent activation of MAPK is involved in hormonal action. This opens the possibility for a coordinated regulation of microglia by E_2 and growth factors via activation of the MAPK-signalling pathway.

Finally, it is important to consider that part of the neuroprotective effects of oestrogen may be due to hormonal actions on brain endothelium. For instance, oestrogen increases rat brain endothelial nitric oxide synthase via ERs, increases the endothelial cell glucose transporter GLUT1 and protects against brain capillary endothelial cell loss, which may in turn reduce focal ischaemic brain damage. E_2 may also exert protective effects in cerebral ischaemia by the blockade of leucocyte adhesion in cerebral endothelial cells, an effect that is a consequence of the hormonal downregulation of the expression of adhesion molecules in cerebral endothelium.

THE LOCAL PRODUCTION OF E_2 IS NEUROPROTECTIVE

In addition to being a target for hormonal oestrogens, the CNS is also affected by E_2 synthesized locally. The CNS is a steroidogenic tissue that expresses enzymes for steroid synthesis and metabolism. Steroidogenesis in the nervous system is altered under neurodegenerative conditions as indicated by the increase in the levels of steroids, such as pregnenolone and progesterone, which is observed following traumatic injury in the brain and spinal cord. Furthermore, proteins involved in the intramitochondrial trafficking of cholesterol, such as the steroidogenic acute regulatory protein (StAR) and the peripheral-type benzodiazepine receptor (PBR), are upregulated in the CNS after injury. Among other possibilities, the increased expression of StAR and PBR after injury may be associated with increased steroidogenesis, since these proteins allow the transfer of cholesterol from the outer to the inner mitochondrial membranes, allowing cholesterol to be transformed into pregnenolone by the enzyme P450scc. In this regard, it is interesting to note that PBR ligands promote neuronal survival and repair in axotomy and neuropathy models, suggesting that the modulation of PBR-mediated steroidogenesis may be neuroprotective. In addition, neurodegenerative conditions are associated with an increase in the expression of aromatase, the enzyme that converts testosterone and other C19 steroids into E_2.[12]

Under physiological conditions, aromatase is expressed in specific neuronal subpopulations of the mammalian brain, where it is involved in the regulatory effects of androgens, via conversion to oestrogens, on neural differentiation, neural plasticity, neuroendocrine function and sexual behaviour. In addition, different forms of brain lesion, in male and female animals, result in the induction of aromatase in reactive astrocytes located near neurodegenerative foci. Studies using specific aromatase inhibitors or aromatase knock-out mice indicate that aromatase activity reduces neuronal death in different experimental neurodegenerative models *in vivo*. Furthermore, the specific inhibition of the enzyme in the brain increases neurodegeneration after brain injury, indicating that brain aromatase is neuroprotective.[12] Therefore, aromatase is a potential target for therapeutic approaches. The aromatase gene is under the control of different tissue-specific promoters and it is therefore conceivable to develop selective aromatase modulators that will enhance the expression of the enzyme and the consequent increase in oestrogen formation, in the brain but not in other tissues.

CONCLUSION

The information reviewed here indicates that, in recent years, our knowledge on the mechanisms of action and effects of E_2 in the brain has noticeably increased. However, there are still many important issues that need to be adequately addressed in future experiments in order to predict and interpret the outcomes of

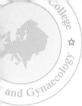
HRTs for the human brain. Although there is extensive literature showing that E_2 is neuroprotective, there is much less knowledge on the reparative properties of the hormone. It is necessary to define, with precision, the timing and duration of hormonal treatments that improve brain function under physiological and pathological conditions. It should be taken into consideration that neuroprotective effects of the hormone in a healthy brain might contribute to maintaining an appropriate brain function. However, regenerative actions in a neuronal circuit that is already damaged might have a negative rather than a positive impact on brain function. The mechanisms involved in the hormonal action in the brain should be explored in more detail. Rapid membrane effects of E_2 in the brain and their impact on physiology and pathology are not fully understood. The putative membrane ERs involved in these rapid actions of E_2 in neurones and glial cells remain to be characterized. The balance and interaction between the actions of E_2 on neurones, glial cells and endothelial cells need to be explored in more detail. In particular, the role of each cell within the neuroprotective effects of the hormone needs to be clarified. Although we know that E_2 is locally produced in the brain, we have very little information on the factors that regulate local E_2 formation and how these factors may interfere with the neuroprotective, cognitive and affective qualities of HRT. Similarly, our knowledge of the factors that regulate the expression and activity of ERs in the brain is also deficient. In particular, it is important to explore how ageing and long-term hormonal deprivation may affect the responsiveness of neural tissue to E_2. In this regard it is essential to determine whether there are windows during the perimenopausal or postmenopausal periods in which the brain has an altered sensitivity to the hormone.

References

1. Azcoitia I, Garcia-Segura L M, DonCarlos L L 2004 Oestradiol signalling in the hippocampus. Current Neuropharmacology 2:245–259
2. Behl C 2002 Oestrogen as a neuroprotective hormone. Nature Reviews. Neuroscience 3,6:433–442
3. Beyer C, Pawlak J, Karolczak M 2003 Membrane receptors for oestrogen in the brain. Journal of Neurochemistry 87(3):545–550
4. Brinton R D 2004 Impact of estrogen therapy on Alzheimer's disease: a fork in the road? CNS Drugs 18(7):405–422
5. Cardona-Gomez G P, Mendez P, DonCarlos L L et al 2002 Interactions of estrogen and insulin-like growth factor-I in the brain: molecular mechanisms and functional implications. The Journal of Steroid Biochemistry and Molecular Biology 83:211–217
6. Cyr M, Calon F, Morissette M et al 2002 Estrogenic modulation of brain activity: implications for schizophrenia and Parkinson's disease. Journal of Psychiatry & Neuroscience 27:12–27
7. Dhandapani K M, Brann D W 2002 Protective effects of estrogen and selective estrogen receptor modulators in the brain. Biology of Reproduction 67:1379–1385
8. Dluzen D, Horstink M 2003 Estrogen as neuroprotectant of nigrostriatal dopaminergic system: laboratory and clinical studies. Endocrine 21:67–75
9. Fillit H M 2002 The role of hormone replacement therapy in the prevention of Alzheimer's disease. Archives of Internal Medicine 162:1934–1942
10. Garcia-Segura L M, McCarthy M M 2004 Minireview: role of glia in neuroendocrine function. Endocrinology 145:1082–1086
11. Garcia-Segura L M, Azcoitia I, DonCarlos L L 2001 Neuroprotection by estradiol. Progress in Neurobiology 63:29–60

12. Garcia-Segura L M, Veiga S, Sierra A et al 2003 Aromatase: a neuroprotective enzyme. Progress in Neurobiology 71:31–41

13. Kelly M J, Ronnekleiv O K, Ibrahim N et al 2002 Estrogen modulation of K$^+$ channel activity in hypothalamic neurons involved in the control of the reproductive axis. Steroids 67:447–456

14. McCullough L D, Hurn P D 2003 Estrogen and ischemic neuroprotection: an integrated view. Trends in Endocrinology and Metabolism 14:228–235

15. McEwen B 2002 Estrogen actions throughout the brain. Recent Progress in Hormone Research 57:357–384

16. Maggi A, Ciana P, Belcredito S et al 2004 Estrogens in the nervous system: mechanisms and nonreproductive functions. Annual Review of Physiology 66:291–313

17. Resnick S M, Maki P M 2001 Effects of hormone replacement therapy on cognitive and brain aging. Annals of the New York Academy of Sciences 949:203–214

18. Saunders-Pullman R 2003 Estrogens and Parkinson's disease: neuroprotective, symptomatic, neither, or both? Endocrine 21:81–87

19. Toran-Allerand C D 2004 Minireview: a plethora of estrogen receptors in the brain. Where will it end? Endocrinology 145:1069–1074

20. Wise P M 2003 Estrogens: protective or risk factors in brain function? Progress in Neurobiology 69:181–191

12

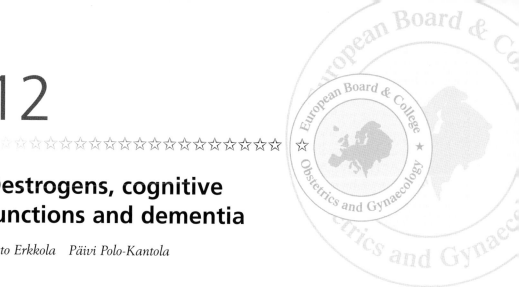

Oestrogens, cognitive functions and dementia

Risto Erkkola   Päivi Polo-Kantola

ABSTRACT

Oestrogen receptors are present in many brain areas. In animal and cell culture studies it has been shown that oestrogen has a strong positive effect on many brain functions. In the menopause, it has been shown that cognitive functions may be dependent on circulating oestrogen levels; with a low free oestrogen level cognitive functions may be impaired. In prospective randomized trials it has not been conclusively shown that hormone replacement therapy (HRT) for postmenopausal women would improve the cognitive ability.

The other important issue is whether HRT has any role in inhibiting the development of dementia. The information is conflicting: there is convincing evidence that HRT is not an effective treatment for dementia. However, there are many observational studies that suggest that Alzheimer's disease could be prevented by HRT. The new information from the Women's Health Initiative (WHI) suggests that this is not the case. It is of extreme importance to conduct more research on this issue, which has a great impact on health economics.

KEYWORDS

Alzheimer's disease, cognition, dementia, hormone replacement therapy (HRT), oestrogen

INTRODUCTION

The molecular and metabolic effects of oestrogen on brain function have been the subject of many review articles.[2,4,12] We will refer to these and briefly present the central view on the mechanisms by which oestrogen exerts its action in the brain and neurones.

Intracellular oestrogen receptors (ERs) exist in several brain areas – ERsα receptors are present in the hypothalamus, pituitary gland and amygdale; ERsβ receptors are probably present throughout the brain including the cortex, hippocampus, amygdala, thalamus, hypothalamus, basal forebrain and preoptic area. These areas are involved in several cognitive functions, particularly attention and memory. However, some oestrogen actions are very rapid indicating action via specific membrane receptors or via the same membrane receptors as neurotrophins or other growth factors. Some of the effects may also occur independently of a membrane receptor.[3]

Oestrogen modulates several neurotransmitter systems including the synthesis and activation of choline acetyltransferase, the rate-limiting enzyme in acetylcholine formation, as well as potassium-stimulated acetylcholine release in certain brain areas. By inducing the degradation of monoamine oxidase, oestrogen enhances the activity of noradrenaline and dopamine in neural pathways involved in cognitive functions. Furthermore, oestrogen regulates serotonin (5-hydroxytryptamine or 5-HT) transport and binding in the brain. It also upregulates 5-HT_1 receptors and downregulates 5-HT_2 receptors. Oestrogen also upregulates dopamine receptors and interferes with catechol O-methyltransferase, the enzyme catabolizing dopamine and noradrenaline. The exact nature of oestrogen effect on γ-aminobutyric acid (GABA) is not completely clear but changes in both the release and reuptake of GABA appear to be involved. Oestrogen also lowers the levels of glutamate, which is toxic in high concentrations.[2,3,4,12]

Oestrogen has direct effects on neurones by stimulating axonal sprouting and dendritic spine formation. In hippocampal neurones oestrogen increases dendritic spine density by reducing GABA neurotransmission. Evidence is also available to suggest that oestrogen could prevent neuronal atrophy. Oestrogen may protect against cerebral ischaemia by inducing cerebral vasodilatation, and probably slowing cerebral atherosclerosis.[2,3,4,12] Hence there is a wealth of evidence making it biologically plausible to suggest the benefit of oestrogen on brain function.

COGNITIVE FUNCTIONS

Cognitive functioning includes processes and actions related to knowing and finding. Cognitive efficiency refers to actions related to memory, perception, identification, voluntary action (among other things the performance of striped muscles), perception as an ability to holistic and spatial thinking, speed of reaction, ability to produce speech or writing, and actions related to vigilance and observation. Therefore cognitive functioning is a great determinator of the ability to function in day-to-day activities. Working and socializing make great demands on cognitive efficiency.

HOW ARE COGNITIVE FUNCTIONS INVESTIGATED?

Cognition is investigated by using subjective questionnaires, semi-objective psychological tests and, nowadays, with computer technology based on reaction times and the rates of mistakes committed.

Some widely used memory tests have been created for:

- verbal memory – Paired Associate Learning and Paragraph Recall, or Logical Recall from the Wechsler Memory Scale (WMS);
- visuospatial recall – visuospatial retention tests from the WMS, the Benton Visual Retention Test and Figure of Rey, Semantic Memory (verbal fluency both with animals and letters) and short-term memory retention/concentration (Digit Span).

There are also tests measuring information processing, such as Trail Making Tests A and B, the Digit Symbol Substitution Test, Reaction Time tests, the Stroop Interference test, abstract reasoning and mental rotation tests, clerical speed and accuracy tests, and letter cancellation tests.

THE EFFECT OF OESTROGEN LEVEL ON COGNITION IN POSTMENOPAUSAL WOMEN

Yaffe et al studied the relationship between non-protein bound or bioavailable oestradiol and cognitive performance assessed with the Modified Mini-Mental State Examination (3MSE) of women aged 65 or older.[23] The testing was carried out at baseline and after 6 years. The non-protein bound and bioavailable oestradiol levels were determined from the baseline-stored serum. Cognitive impairment occurs about three times more often in the lowest tertile in comparison with the highest tertile (15% vs. 5%). Total or non-protein-bound testosterone level was not associated with a risk of cognitive impairment. In an earlier study they did not find any benefit from the high total oestradiol level.

In our own study we compared two groups, one with an oestrogen level of 25–50 pmol/l (mean 43 pmol/l) and another with a higher oestrogen level of 105–424 pmol/l (mean 249 pmol/l). Cognitive performance was not dependent on oestrogen level.[15]

Oestrogen receptor polymorphism may affect the receptor function, hence women who have a p or at least one x allele show cognitive impairment slightly more often than women without receptor polymorphism.[23]

THE EFFECTS OF HORMONE REPLACEMENT THERAPY ON COGNITION

During the last decade, many investigations have addressed the effect of ageing with or without HRT on cognitive functions in postmenopausal women. Therefore we investigated the effect of the severity of climacteric symptoms on cognitive functioning. Despite subjective complaints of memory impairment in association with climacteric vasomotor symptoms, our results did not support a direct cause-and-effect relationship.[13] We also designed a prospective, randomized, placebo-controlled, crossover study of 70 healthy postmenopausal women. Three months' oestrogen replacement therapy (ET) had no effect on cognitive function. In that group, oestrogen was not superior to placebo in any task of our very comprehensive test battery. In those healthy and relatively young postmenopausal women, cognitive performance was well preserved. Observed cognitive changes were mild and primarily age-related, and not reversible by oestrogen therapy (ET).[14]

In recent meta-analyses of the current literature the following conclusions were reached:

1. There is evidence that oestrogen therapy improves cognitive performance in recently menopausal women, but no evidence of beneficial effect in asymptomatic women.[24]
2. Women with menopausal symptoms had improvements in verbal memory, vigilance, reasoning and motor speed, but no enhancement in other cognitive functions. Asymptomatic women did not benefit from HRT.[9]
3. There was little evidence regarding the effect of HRT or ET on overall cognitive function in healthy postmenopausal women. There was some effect on some verbal memory functions (immediate recall), on the test of abstract reasoning and a test of speed and accuracy in relatively young (47 years) surgically menopausal women receiving i.m. oestrogen injections.[7]

The lack of consistency between the studies included in meta-analyses has been attributed to factors such as: small numbers of subjects recruited, differences in the oestrogen preparations and their doses, the differences in the ages or symptomatologies of the subjects in the study populations, as well as the differences in the types of menopause (natural or surgical). Furthermore, there has frequently been a failure to distinguish between the effects of the hormone on the mood and depressive symptoms from an independent effect on cognition.

In a recent observational study from Cache County, Utah, USA, 2073 nondemented women of more than 65 years old were distributed to never users (n = 839, mean age 77.03 years), past users (n = 390, mean age 74.57 years) and current users (n = 763, mean age 72.32 years). As an assessment method, the MMSE was used. Lifetime HRT/ET exposure with conjugated equine oestrogen (CEE) with or without medroxyprogesterone acetate (MPA) was associated with improved global cognition and attenuated decline over a 3-year interval. Improvement was greatest among the oldest old, i.e. women of more than 85 years of age. No meaningful association of HRT with cognitive trajectory was found before the age of 75.[1]

The Women's Health Initiative Memory Study (WHIMS) is an ancillary study of the WHI. It includes 2145 women in the HRT arm and 2236 women in the placebo arm. All participants were over 65 years old and free of dementia. HRT consisted of 0.625 mg CEE and continuous combined 2.5 mg MPA. The 3MSE mean total scores were better over the mean follow-up of 4.2 years in both groups. On the other hand, 6.7% of women in the HRT group and only 4.8% in the placebo group had a clinically important (>2 standard deviations) decline in the 3MSE total score. The results of this study do not support the beneficial effect of HRT on cognitive function among women older 65 years of age.[16]

Similar results were achieved from the cognition part of the Heart and Estrogen/progestin Replacement Study, where it was found that CEE + MPA combination or placebo for 4 years did not result in better cognitive function as measured on six standardized tests. The participants had coronary heart disease and they were 71 ± 6 years old at the time of cognitive testing.[5]

THE PREVALENCE AND DEVELOPMENT OF DEMENTIA

Alzheimer's disease (AD) is the major obstacle against healthy ageing. Globally, it is estimated that some 18 million people suffer from dementia, but with the demographic changes caused by the increase in expected lifespan, the prevalence of AD can be expected to rise. By 2025, the number of AD patients is expected to approach 34 million. Among women, the prevalence of AD is expected to double every 5 years from 1% at 65 years of age to 15% at 85.[20] According to calculations (see http://www.iiasa.ac.at/collections/IIASA/_Research/) the number of female patients suffering from AD will rise in western, southern and Nordic European countries from 2 million in 1995 to more than 4 million in 2050.

A family history of dementia and increasing age are proven risk factors for AD. Also, poor education, the allele ε4 of the apolipoprotein E gene, mutations at specific loci in chromosomes 1, 14 and 21, Down's syndrome, head trauma, depression, vascular factors, hypothyroidism, aluminium and solvents have been proposed as risk factors. Further, the female gender seems to be a risk factor by itself: the age-specific prevalence of AD is 1.5–3 times greater for women than men. And, due to the long life expectancy, the total prevalence among ageing women is much higher than among ageing men.[2–4,12]

AD significantly limits the capabilities for everyday living. A decline of cognitive functions, especially memory, orientation, visuospatial abilities, language and thinking, is central and it leads to changes in personality and emotional abilities. Neuropathologically, AD is characterized by the destruction of cholinergic neurones, particularly in the basal forebrain, and by the accumulation of intracellular neurofibrillar tangles and extracellular senile plaques in the hippocampus and association neocortex. However, the motor cortex is spared. The central core of the senile plaque consists of β-amyloid peptide, which is a part of the intracellular amyloid precursor protein. β-Amyloid is also detected in the vessel walls.[2–4,12]

Regarding possible protective factors for AD the following have been suggested: allele ε2 of the apolipoprotein E gene, smoking, antioxidants, red wine and antiinflammatory drugs.[2–4,12]

Concerning the role of HRT/ET, there is a substantial body of biological evidence, whereby surrogate end-points suggest that ET might enhance brain functioning and prevent AD and vascular dementia.[2–4,12]

HORMONE REPLACEMENT THERAPY AND THE PREVENTION OF DEMENTIA

Some observational studies suggested that the prevalence of AD among ET users was lower than among non-users.[11,21] For example, Tang et al found that the relative risk of AD was 0.13 (95% CI; range 0.02–0.92) for women who had taken

ET/HRT for more than one year (mean 13.6 years) when compared to never users.[21] The use of oestrogen for more than one year reduced the development of AD by about 5% annually. In contrast, a recent UK study showed no relation of AD to HRT prescriptions within a 10-year period of observation.[21]

In a meta-analysis on the development of AD among ET/HRT users, Yaffe et al examined eight case-control and two prospective cohort studies.[24] The results were conflicting: some of the studies showed a lowered risk, some no change and some an elevated risk for AD. One of the first placebo-controlled studies found a greater improvement with ERT on one test for dementia but not in two other tests.[26]

In the Cache County study, 1889 women over 65 years of age (mean 74.5 years) had a 3-year follow-up.[25] The added risk for women appeared to be greatest among those with no reported use of HRT. The increase of risk disappeared entirely with more than 10 years of treatment (hazard ratio, HR 0.41; CI 0.17–0.86). Current use did not reduce the risk except in those women who had used HRT for more than 10 years. Interestingly, the former use of HRT was associated with a greatly lowered risk (HR 0.33; CI 0.15–0.65). This suggests that HRT is more efficient in preventing AD when used at menopause with a precipitous decline of endogenous oestrogen than when used near the onset of dementia.

In WHIMS, 2229 women aged more than 65 years received CEE + MPA and 2303 received placebo with a follow-up time of 4.05 years on average.[19] The risk of development of any type of dementia in the HRT group was 2.05–fold (CI 1.21–3.48) when compared with the placebo group. The increased risk would result in an additional 23 cases of dementia per 10 000 women per year. In the HRT and placebo groups, about half of the dementia patients had AD, it being the commonest form of dementia. The conclusion was that HRT cannot prevent the development of dementia in women having patient characteristics described in the WHI study and WHIMS. The conclusion does not necessarily apply to younger, healthy postmenopausal women.

HORMONE REPLACEMENT THERAPY IN WOMEN WITH LATENT OR ESTABLISHED DEMENTIA

The first randomized, double-blind, placebo-controlled study to address the effects of HRT on cognitive function in patients with mild or moderate AD, showed no therapeutic effect of CEE (either 0.625 or 1.25 mg) in comparison to placebo within a 1-year follow-up.[10] There is still a possibility that oestrogen may be useful as adjuvant therapy with anticholinesterases.[6]

Hence, the above-mentioned clinical studies showed similar yet weak positive results in favour of the use of ET, yet the level of evidence is not very high. However, as the biological evidence was plausible, most observational studies were unanimous, and the small prospective randomized trials showed positive results, the clinical community was rather anxious to accept the beneficial effect of ET in the primary and secondary prevention of AD.

Mulnard et al investigated 120 women who had had a hysterectomy and who had mild-to-moderate AD.[10] They were randomized into three arms receiving CEE 0.625 mg or 1.25 mg per day, or placebo. The follow-up time was 12 months. The conclusion of the study was that ET for one year did not slow disease progression, nor did it improve the global, cognitive or functional outcomes of the subjects. On the contrary, the only difference observed was in the Clinical Dementia Rating Scale favouring placebo. The conclusion that ET produced no global changes in the cognition of women with AD was further supported by the study by Henderson et al with, originally, 42 women with mild-to-moderate AD.[6] In that randomized, double-blind, placebo-controlled, parallel-group trial unopposed CEE 1.25 mg per day for 16 weeks showed no difference over placebo on the cognitive outcome measures, mood, clinician-rated global impression of change or caregiver-rated functional status.

The conclusion from these two studies is that ET cannot be used for the management of AD although the biological evidence for the utility of oestrogen is rather strong. Therefore, a new set of *in-vitro* or *in-vivo* studies might be needed. They should focus on the use of combinations and possible synergetic effects. There are, in fact, reports showing that cholinesterase inhibitors, such as tacrine, in combination with oestrogen gives a better therapeutic effect than tacrine alone.[17] Also, various neural growth factors (neurotrophins) should probably be tried in association with oestrogen.

References

1. Carlson M C, Zandi P P, Plassmann B L et al 2001 Hormone replacement therapy and reduced cognitive decline in older women. The Cache County Study. Neurology 57:2210–2216
2. Compton J, van Amelsvoort T, Murphy D 2001 HRT and its effect on normal ageing of the brain and dementia. British Journal of Clinical Pharmacology 52:647–653
3. Compton J, van Amelsvoort T, Murphy D 2002 Mood, cognition and Alzheimer's disease. Best Practice & Research. Clinical Obstetrics & Gynaecology 16:357–370
4. Fillitt H M 2002 The role of hormone replacement therapy in the prevention of Alzheimer's disease. Archives of Internal Medicine 162:1934–1942
5. Grady D, Yaffe K, Kristof M et al 2002 Effect of postmenopausal hormone therapy on cognitive function: the Heart and Estrogen/progestin Replacement Study. The American Journal of Medicine 113:543–548
6. Henderson V W, Paganini-Hill A, Miller B L et al 2000 Estrogen for Alzheimer's disease in women: randomized, double-blind, placebo-controlled trial. Neurology 54:295–301
7. Hogervorst E, Yaffe K, Richards M et al 2002 Hormone replacement therapy for cognitive function in postmenopausal women The Cochrane Database of Systematic Reviews, Issue 2. Article CD003122. DOI: 10.1002/14651858.CD003122
8. Hogervorst E, Yaffe K, Richards M et al 2002 Hormone replacement therapy to maintain cognitive function in women with dementia The Cochrane Database of Systematic Reviews, Issue 3. Article CD003799. DOI: 10.1002/14651858.CD003799
9. LeBlanc E S, Janowsky J, Chan B K et al 2001 Hormone replacement therapy and cognition: systematic review and meta-analysis. The Journal of the American Medical Association 285:1489–1499
10. Mulnard R A, Cotman C W, Kawas C et al for the Alzheimer's Disease Cooperative Study 2000 Estrogen replacement therapy for treatment of mild to moderate Alzheimer's disease. A randomized controlled trial. The Journal of the American Medical Association 283:1007–1015

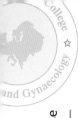

11. Paganini-Hill A, Henderson V W 1994 Estrogen deficiency and risk of Alzheimer's disease in women. American Journal of Epidemiology 140:256–261

12. Polo-Kantola P, Erkkola R 2001 Alzheimer's disease and estrogen replacement therapy. Where are we now? Acta Obstetricia et Gynaecologica Scandinavica 80:679–682

13. Polo-Kantola P, Portin R, Koskinen T et al 1997 Climacteric symptoms do not impair cognitive performances in postmenopause. Maturitas 27:13–23

14. Polo-Kantola P, Portin R, Polo O et al 1998 The effect of short-term estrogen replacement therapy on cognition. A randomized, double-blind, cross-over trial in postmenopausal women. Obstetrics and Gynecology 91:459–466

15. Portin R, Polo-Kantola P, Polo O et al 1999 Serum estrogen level, attention, memory and other cognitive functions in middle-aged women. Climacteric 2:115–123

16. Rapp S R, Espeland M A, Shumaker S A et al 2003 Effect of estrogen plus progestin on global cognitive function in postmenopausal women. The Women's Health Initiative Memory Study: a randomized controlled trial. The Journal of the American Medical Association 289:2663–2672

17 Schneider L S, Farlow M R, Henderson V W et al 1996 Effects of estrogen replacement therapy on response to tacrine in patients with Alzheimer's disease. Neurology 46:1580–1584

18. Seshadri S, Zomberg G L, Derby L E et al 2001 Postmenopausal estrogen replacement therapy and the risk of Alzheimer's disease. Archives of Neurology 58:435–440

19. Shumaker SA, Legault C, Rapp S R et al 2003 Estrogen plus progestin and the incidence of dementia and mild cognitive impairment in postmenopausal women. The Women's Health Initiative Memory Study: a randomized controlled trial. The Journal of the American Medical Association 289:2651–2662

20. Skoog I, Nilsson L, Palmertz B et al 1993 A population-based study of dementia in 85-year-olds. The New England Journal of Medicine 328:153–158

21. Tang M-X, Jacobs D, Stern Y et al 1996 Effect of oestrogen during menopause on risk and age at onset of Alzheimer's disease. The Lancet 348:429–432

22. Yaffe K, Lui L Y, Grady D et al 2000 Cognitive decline in women in relation to non-protein-bound oestradiol concentrations. The Lancet 356:708–712

23. Yaffe K, Lui L Y, Grady D et al 2002 Estrogen receptor 1 polymorphisms and risk of cognitive impairment in older women. Biological Psychiatry 51:677–682

24. Yaffe K, Sawaya G, Lieberburg I et al 1998 Estrogen therapy in postmenopausal women. Effects on cognitive function and dementia. The Journal of the American Medical Association 279:688–695

25. Zandi P P, Carlson M C, Plassmann B L et al 2002 Hormone replacement therapy and the incidence of Alzheimer's disease in older women. The Cache County Study. The Journal of the American Medical Association 288:2123–2129

13

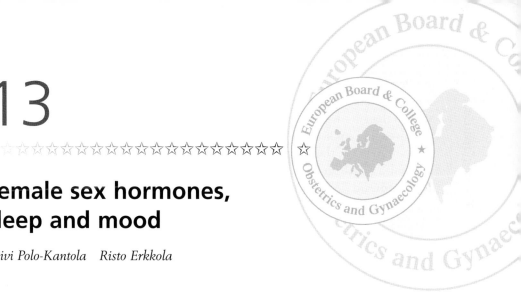

☆☆☆☆☆☆☆☆☆☆☆☆☆☆☆☆☆☆☆☆ ☆

Female sex hormones, sleep and mood

Päivi Polo-Kantola   Risto Erkkola

ABSTRACT

This review illustrates the effects of the menopause on sleep and mood, and evaluates whether hormone replacement therapy (HRT) may improve sleep quality and mood. Sleeping problems, as well as mood symptoms, are frequently reported during menopausal transition, but neither objectively measured sleep quality or prevalence of mood disorders show any specific changes brought about by the menopause. According to women's own judgement, HRT significantly improves sleep quality, although objective studies have reported inconsistent results. HRT effectively alleviates mood symptoms during the menopause, but if depressive disorder is in question the treatment of choice is not HRT but a standard psychiatric approach by either pharmacological or psychological means, or both.

Sleeping problems and mood symptoms are serious public health issues, imposing a substantial burden on the individual and society. HRT can be considered as a first-line therapy for these symptoms. However, if no relief has been achieved after a few months, other underlying causes should be ruled out by further medical examinations.

KEYWORDS

Breathing, female menopause, hormone replacement therapy (HRT), mood, oestrogen, sleep

INTRODUCTION

Little is known about the natural history of sleep complaints, as well as about worldwide epidemiology. The prevalence of sleep complaints reveals a range of results (10–49%), most probably reflecting differences in the definition of sleep complaints and in survey methodology. Sleep complaints are more common in women than in men across all age ranges. Insomnia is reported by 25% of women and severe insomnia by 15%. Between the ages of 50 and 64 years, and in the age group of over 65, the prevalences are 25% and 16%, respectively.[18]

Besides female gender, low income, poor education and living alone also predispose toward sleep complaints.[21] Patients suffering from chronic insomnia have poor work performance, memory problems and twice the frequency of fatigue-related car accidents than controls.[8]

Sleep complaints and disturbances related to different endocrinological states in women's lives (such as in menstruation, pregnancy and menopause) are common but they are poorly documented. Although women report sleeping problems more often than men,[21] the majority of sleep studies have been conducted on men.

Mood symptoms, such as depression and anxiety, occur more frequently in women than men.[14,22] While mood symptoms often coincide with sleeping problems, it may be assumed that they have a causal relationship.

THE PHYSIOLOGY OF SLEEP

THE STRUCTURE AND IMPORTANCE OF SLEEP

Sleep is a cyclical or episodic state, alternating with wakefulness. The characteristics of sleep are reduced awareness and responsiveness, as well as motor inhibition. Sleep is, however, promptly reversible, which differentiates it from other states of altered consciousness. Most adults have 7 or 8 hours of sleep per night and so sleep occupies approximately one-third of each person's lifetime. Nevertheless, the impact of good sleep on health remains largely overlooked and the importance of sleep is better understood through sleep deprivation or sleep disorders, which may cause excessive daytime sleepiness and related problems.

In electrophysiological terms, wakefulness and sleep are differentiated by changes in electroencephalogram (EEG), electro-oculogram (EOG) and electromyogram (EMG). Sleep state is characterized by increased synchrony of the EEG and low muscle tone. Depending on the presence or absence of rapid eye movements (REMs), the sleeping state is divided into REM sleep and non-rapid eye movement (NREM) sleep. NREM sleep and REM sleep continue to alternate through the night in cyclic fashion (Fig 13.1). In sleep studies, total sleep time, sleep efficiency (i.e. time spent asleep as a fraction of the total time in bed), the proportion of different sleep stages, sleep latencies and the number of awakenings are the variables that are usually evaluated.

NREM sleep is conventionally subdivided into four stages (stages 1, 2, 3 and 4), of which stages 3 and 4 are usually combined and called slow wave sleep (SWS) or deep sleep. Although the importance of different sleep stages is not fully understood, NREM sleep seems to be related to energy conserving, as the motor inhibition and lower body temperature occurring during that state lower the metabolic rate. In NREM sleep, anabolic activities dominate. NREM sleep

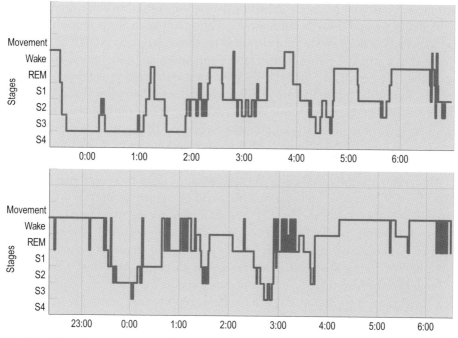

Fig 13.1 Sleep hypnograms: good regular sleep pattern (upper panel); disturbed sleep pattern (lower panel). REM, rapid eye movement sleep; S1–S4, stages 1–4 sleep.

provides time for both the central nervous and other systems to recover from previous activities during wakefulness and to be prepared for future challenges.[29] During REM sleep, information obtained during wakefulness is processed, modified and matured. REM sleep seems to be important, at least for memory functions and emotions.[29]

THE REGULATION OF SLEEP

Sleep is regulated by two major factors: the circadian factor (which facilitates falling asleep at a certain time of day – usually in the evening) and the homeostatic factor (which explains why falling asleep is easier after prolonged wakefulness). The most important brain areas involved in sleep regulation include the medulla oblongata, pons, formatio reticularis, midbrain, thalamus, hypothalamus, preoptic area, basal forebrain, hippocampus and cerebral cortex. Most of these areas are included in a reticular activation system.[9]

Several neurotransmitters are involved in the regulation of the sleep–wake state.[29] Acetylcholine and monoamines, especially dopamine, noradrenaline and adrenaline, are particularly important during wakefulness and cortical activation. Noradrenergic, serotoninergic and histaminergic neurones are important for sleep. The key role of serotonin for sleep has become evident as monoamine oxidase inhibitors, which primarily block serotonin catabolism, enhance and prolong SWS. Conversely, compounds that prevent the synthesis of serotonin lead to severe insomnia. Melatonin is closely linked to the circadian rhythm and suppressed by light. Prolactin and growth hormone are also involved in sleep regulation. Prolactin activity is sleep-related not circadian rhythm-related. As growth hormone is secreted as a series of pulses shortly after sleep onset and in temporal association with the first period of SWS, the sleep–wake homeostasis is determined by its release. Recent literature has provided much evidence that adenosine is also critically involved in sleep regulation. An increase of adenosine in the brain decreases the activation of neurones. γ-aminobutyric acid (GABA) is an inhibitory neurotransmitter. An increase in brain GABA levels by inhibiting its degradation results in an increase in SWS.[29]

Oestrogen may be involved in the regulation of sleep by several mechanisms. The effect of oestrogen on brain functions and on neurotransmitters is described elsewhere in this book (see Ch. 12). In a study comparing the diurnal characteristics of pulsatile prolactin secretion among postmenopausal women, young women and young men, the serum prolactin levels and secretory pulse frequency were higher during the night than the day in all groups and they were higher in younger women than in either postmenopausal women or young men.[10] Increased growth hormone levels have been reported in oestrogen users even after many years of treatment.[20]

SLEEP AND BREATHING

Breathing during sleep plays an essential role in sleep quality, thus, in sleep studies, nocturnal breathing cannot be dismissed. The control of breathing is critically and characteristically different during wakefulness, NREM sleep and REM sleep. During NREM sleep, the tidal volume and frequency of breathing are stable whereas REM sleep is characterized by irregular breathing.[15] The respiratory muscles receive impulses from the respiratory centre, which is situated in the medulla oblongata. The respiratory centre receives and responds to three general types of information: chemical information (from chemoreceptors responding to PaO_2, $PaCO_2$ and pH); mechanical information (from receptors in the lungs and chest wall); and behavioural information (from the higher cortical centres).[4]

HORMONES AND SLEEP

MENOPAUSE AND SLEEP

Several questionnaire studies have been carried out to assess the subjective sleep complaints associated with menopause. Perimenopausal women report more frequent and longer arousals resulting in significantly less sleep than in premenopausal women. They also experience more mood symptoms, which are associated with, or even mediated by, sleep disturbance.[2] A survey of 100 participants attending a menopause clinic indicated that 77% complained of insomnia and 91% suffered from fatigue; typical complaints were early morning awakenings or intermittent sleep.[1] After controlling for age, the odds ratio for sleep disturbance in a group of 1000 French women was 1.5 in postmenopausal women as compared to menstruating women.[17] According to another study with over 1200 responders in the UK, the risk for sleeping problems was 1.5 in perimenopausal women and 3.4 in postmenopausal women as compared with premenopausal women.[16]

There is often a difference between subjective and objective sleep quality, which makes it difficult to determine the prevalence of sleep disturbance not only in menopausal women but also in the general population. In our own study with 63 postmenopausal women, sleep complaints were strongly associated with climacteric vasomotor and mood symptoms but not with specific abnormalities in polygraphic sleep recordings.[24] In a recent large study by Young and colleagues, peri- and postmenopausal women were less satisfied with their sleep as compared to premenopausal women, although menopause was not associated with diminished sleep quality measured by polysomnography.[34] However, intensive hot flushes may cause arousals and have been found to be associated with increases in stage 4 sleep, a shortened first REM sleep period and disrupted sleep with reduced sleep efficiency.[33]

HORMONE REPLACEMENT THERAPY AND SLEEP

Previous studies have shown a beneficial effect of oestrogen therapy (ET) or HRT on subjective sleep quality. In an open, multicentre study with 249 women, oestradiol patches twice a week for 6 months removed sleep disturbances from 95% of those women who had reported sleep disturbance prior to treatment.[5] In another study, transdermal oestrogen for 2 weeks followed by transdermal oestrogen/norethisterone acetate for the next 2 weeks led to a reduction in sleep disturbance. The follow-up time was one year. Relief of the vasomotor symptoms strongly correlated with improvements in sleep quality.[32] In our study, ET alleviated several kinds of sleep problems: it facilitated falling asleep and decreased nocturnal restlessness and awakenings. Women reported less tiredness in the morning and during the day.[23] Again, in that study, the degree of improvement in vasomotor symptoms was the most important predictor of the degree of alleviation of sleep disturbance, providing further evidence that these two complaints are linked. However, the subgroup of menopausal women who reported insomnia in the absence of vasomotor symptoms, also markedly benefited from ET.[23]

There is some contradiction about the effects of HRT/ET on objectively measured sleep quality.[25] The main outcomes of the previous studies in healthy women are presented in Table 13.1. HRT has been reported to decrease awakenings and nocturnal wakefulness and increase REM sleep. A shortening of sleep latency, an improvement in sleep efficiency, a reduction of the rate of cyclic alternating patterns of sleep, as well as a reduced time spent awake during the first two sleep cycles have all been reported. Studies with no improvement in polygraphic sleep variables have also been reported.

The lack of consistency between these studies has been attributed to several reasons.[25] The age range in different studies has been wide. Including perimenopausal

Table 13.1 Previous studies on the effect of HRT on sleep polysomnography in healthy women[a]

Author(s)	Study design	Subjects	Treatment	Findings	Comment
Thomson and Oswald 1977	Prospective, placebo-controlled, double-blind	34 perimenopausal women	Piperazine oestrone sulphate. Study duration 14 weeks.	Decrease of wakefulness and awakenings. Increase in REM sleep	Oestrogen effect on hot flushes, mood or anxiety similar to placebo
Schiff et al 1979	Prospective, placebo-controlled, randomized, double-blind crossover	16 hypogonadal women	Conjugated equine oestrogen 0.625 mg per day. Study duration 100 days	Shorter sleep latency. Increase in REM sleep	Decrease in serum FSH and vasomotor symptoms
Erlik et al 1981 awakenings	Case-control No placebo group	4 postmenopausal women	Ethinyl oestradiol 50 µg × 4 per day. Study duration 30 days	Decrease in awakenings	Decrease of hot flushes
Purdie et al 1995	Prospective, randomized, placebo-controlled, single-blind	33 postmenopausal women	Conjugated equine oestrogen 0.625 mg per day + norgestrel 0.15 mg per day (days 17–28). Study duration 12 weeks	No improvement in polysomnographic parameters	Decrease of menopausal symptoms and improvement of psychological well-being
Scharf et al 1997	Prospective, placebo-controlled, single-blind	7 postmenopausal women	Conjugated equine oestrogen 0.625 mg per day. Study duration 4 weeks	Improvement of sleep efficiency. Reduction of cyclic alternating patterns of sleep and awakening	Decrease of hot flushes

Polo-Kantola et al 1999	Prospective, randomized placebo-controlled, double-blind crossover	62 postmenopausal women	Oestradiol 50 µg per 24 hours patches or gel 2.5 g per day. Study duration 7 months	Decrease of movement arousals	Decrease of serum FSH and vasomotor symptoms
Antonijevic et al 2000	Prospective	11 postmenopausal women	Oestradiol 50 µg per 24 hours patches. Study duration 4 weeks	Increase of REM sleep. Reduced time awake during first two sleep cycles	Decrease of serum FSH and LH levels. No placebo group
Montplaisir et al 2001	Prospective, randomized, two group-treatment study	21 postmenopausal women	Conjugated equine oestrogen 0.625 mg per day + either MPA 5 mg per day or micronized progesterone 200 mg per day. Study duration 6 months	Improvement in sleep efficiency and reduction of time spent awake after sleep onset during oestrogen + micronized progesterone but not during oestrogen + MPA	Decrease of menopausal symptoms and improvement in subjective sleep quality during both treatments. No placebo group

FSH, follicle-stimulating hormone; LH, luteinizing hormone; MPA, medroxyprogesterone acetate; REM, rapid eye movement.

[a] A detailed reference list is available from the contributor.

women instead of postmenopausal women may also have affected the results, and some studies have included both naturally and surgically menopausal women. While natural menopause normally causes gradual changes in biological and clinical symptoms, surgically menopausal women typically have more severe symptoms. The presence or absence of climacteric, especially vasomotor symptoms, has not been an exclusion criterion in the previous studies. Thus the women included may have been very different regarding their symptoms. Finally, the hormone treatment used has varied in its form, dose and duration from one study to another. The duration of the treatments has generally been short, lasting 6 months in the longest study.

HORMONES AND BREATHING DURING SLEEP

MENOPAUSE AND BREATHING DURING SLEEP

Of the breathing abnormalities during sleep, obstructive sleep apnoea syndrome (OSAS) is the most frequent and thus clinically most important. It occurs in 1–2% of the general population and is characterized by repeated episodes of upper airway obstruction often accompanied by severe snoring, leading either to an apnoea or a marked airflow limitation (hypopnoea). The major subjective daytime consequence is excessive sleepiness. OSAS is accompanied by a considerable increase in pulmonary and cardiovascular morbidity, and has previously been considered as a male disease. However, more recently, observations that women are also susceptible to this syndrome have been established. In a recent study, the prevalence of OSAS was 3.9% in men and 1.2% in women when the apnoea/hypopnoea index[10] or more and daytime sleepiness were considered as definition criteria.[3]

In women, partial upper airway obstruction, which contributes to hypoventilation and CO_2 retention during sleep, seems to be even more common than sleep apnoea. In our own study, a significant partial obstruction was found in 17% of an asymptomatic study population.[26] In partial upper airway obstruction, symptoms resemble those of sleep apnoea. Heavy snoring is frequent but not necessarily present. Other symptoms, such as excessive sleepiness, an irresistible tendency to fall asleep, sweating, morning headache, lack of energy, low initiation capacity, difficulties in concentration, poor memory and low mental tolerance, may be interpreted as climacteric symptoms.

HORMONE REPLACEMENT THERAPY AND BREATHING DURING SLEEP

The incidence of sleep-disordered breathing increases after menopause suggesting that hormonal factors may also be involved. Progestins, which have respiratory stimulant properties,[30] may protect women from the condition until menopause. The efficacy of either ET or plain progestin replacement therapies has been studied. Whereas there is only little if any improvement of nocturnal ventilation with oestrogen treatment alone,[12,26] the use of HRT[3,28] as well as high doses of medroxyprogesterone acetate (60 mg per day)[27] have significantly improved ventilation in postmenopausal women. However, nasal continuous positive airway pressure remains the treatment of choice in sleep-disordered breathing until convincing evidence of efficacy with alternative treatment options, including HRT, is available.

HORMONES AND MOOD

MENOPAUSE AND MOOD

Mood symptoms, such as depression and anxiety, are more frequent in women than men.[14,22] Factors, such as psychosocial vulnerability, unemployment, excessive stress and somatic diseases, have been proposed, as well as genetic transmission to explain gender differences. As mood symptoms seem to be related to the female reproductive cycle (premenstrual tension syndrome, postpartum depression or climacteric depression) the influence of hormonal fluctuations has also been attributed.

Depressive symptoms, anxiety, irritability and lack of initiative are frequent among climacteric women seeking treatment; a prevalence as high as 70–90% has been reported.[1] In a large epidemiological study by McKinlay, depressive symptoms in premenopause predicted hot flushes and sweating, as well as other climacteric symptoms.[19] However, contradictory results have also been presented. Kaufert et al observed that chronic somatic illnesses, shifts and stresses with family or with other relationships, rather than hormonal changes, triggered depression.[11] It is essential to differentiate between depressed mood and depressive disorder since the frequency of severe psychiatric diseases, depressive disorders or suicide attempts has not been found to be increased around menopause.[7] Psychiatric morbidity during menopause is greatest among women with a history of mood disorders.[7]

HORMONE REPLACEMENT THERAPY AND MOOD

A lowered oestrogen level may cause depression either directly by biochemical effects in brain or indirectly via climacteric symptoms, such as flushes, sweating and sleep disturbance. Several direct biochemical pathways are plausible. Lack of oestrogen reduces brain serotonin concentration, a critical neurotransmitter affecting mood. Also, adrenergic and dopaminergic activity can be altered by oestrogen, suggesting a potency of oestrogen to act as an antidepressive agent (see Ch. 12).

There is some controversy between psychiatrists and gynaecologists about whether any menopausal depression exits. Furthermore, studies about the effect of HRT in depression have produced conflicting results. However, in placebo-controlled trials an alleviation of climacteric mood symptoms has been reported by HRT/ET. In studies by Erkkola et al[5] and Wiklund et al[32] a significant improvement was observed. Klaiber et al[13] reported a beneficial effect of large-dose ET compared to placebo for premenopausal and postmenopausal women with severe depression resistant to conventional treatments. However, the risks of high doses of oestrogen, as used in that study, may exceed the benefits achieved. Soares and colleagues[31] conducted a randomized, placebo-controlled, double-blind study in 50 perimenopausal women, of whom 26 met the DSM-IV criteria for major depressive disorder, 11 for dysthymic disorder and 13 for minor depressive disorder. Transdermal ET (17β-oestradiol, 100 μg patches) effectively relieved the depression and patients receiving oestrogen sustained the antidepressant benefit of treatment after a 4-week wash-out period although somatic complaints returned. Despite these encouraging results, several other studies showing no improvement in depression have also been published.[6]

Whether depression in menopausal transition requires special treatment remains unsolved. If the diagnosis is depressive disorder, the treatment of choice is not oestrogen but standard psychiatric techniques – either pharmacological, psychological or both. In women with vasomotor symptoms, HRT/ET as an adjuvant therapy certainly improves compliance and possibly even recovery from depression. If the diagnosis is solely depressive mood, no specific drug should be initiated before treatment response to HRT/ET has been evaluated. If depression persists for 3 months under successful HRT, the indications for hormone should be re-evaluated and other forms of therapy considered.

References

1. Anderson E, Hamburger S, Liu J H et al 1987 Characteristics of menopausal women seeking assistance. American Journal of Obstetrics and Gynecology 156:428–433
2. Baker A, Simpson S, Dawson D 1997 Sleep disruption and mood changes associated with menopause. Journal of Psychosomatic Research 43(4):359–369
3. Bixler E O, Vgontzas A N, Lin H-M et al 2001 Prevalence of sleep-disordered breathing in women. Effect of gender. American Journal of Respiratory and Critical Care Medicine 163:608–613
4. Douglas N J 1994 Control of ventilation during sleep. In: Kryger M H, Roth T, Dement W C (eds) Principles and Practice of Sleep Medicine, 2nd edn. W B Saunders, Philadelphia, p 204–211
5. Erkkola R, Holma P, Järvi T et al 1991 Transdermal oestrogen replacement therapy in a Finnish population. Maturitas 13:275–281
6. Halbreich U 1997 Role of estrogen in postmenopausal depression. Neurology 48:S16–S20
7. Hällström T, Samuelsson S 1985 Mental health in the climacteric: the longitudinal study of women in Gothenburg. Acta Obstetricia et Gynecologica Scandinavica 130:13–18
8. Jacquinet-Salord M C, Lang T, Fouriaud C et al 1993 Sleeping tablet consumption, self-reported quality of sleep, and working conditions. Journal of Epidemiology and Community Health 47:64–68
9. Jones B E 1994 Basic mechanisms of sleep–wake states. In: Kryger M H, Roth T, Dement W C (eds) Principles and Practice of Sleep Medicine, 2nd edn. W B Saunders, Philadelphia, p 145–162
10. Katznelson L, Riskind P N, Saxe V C et al 1998 Prolactin pulsatile characteristics in postmenopausal women. The Journal of Clinical Endocrinology and Metabolism 83:761–764
11. Kaufert P A, Gilbert P, Tate R 1992 The Manitoba Project: a re-examination of the link between menopause and depression. Maturitas 14:143–155
12. Keefe D L, Watson R, Naftolin F 1999 Hormone replacement therapy may alleviate sleep apnea in menopausal women: a pilot study. Menopause 6:196–200

13. Klaiber E L, Broverman D M, Vogel W et al 1979 Estrogen replacement therapy for severe persistent depressions in women. Archives of General Psychiatry 36:550–554

14. Kornstein S G 1997 Gender differences in depression: Implications for treatment. The Journal of Clinical Psychiatry 58:12–18

15. Krieger J, Turlot J C, Mangin P et al 1983 Breathing during sleep in normal young and elderly subjects: hypopneas, apneas, and correlated factors. Sleep 6:108–120

16. Kuh D L, Wadsworth M, Hardy R 1997 Women's health in midlife: the influence of the menopause, social factors and health in earlier life. British Journal of Obstetrics and Gynaecology 104(8):23–33

17. Ledesert B, Ringa V, Breart G 1994 Menopause and perceived health status among the women of the French GAZEL cohort. Maturitas 20:113–120

18. Leger D, Guilleminault C, Dreyfus J P et al 2000 Prevalence of insomnia in a survey of 12,778 adults in France. Journal of Sleep Research 9:35–42

19. McKinlay J B 1987 Do menopausal symptoms cause depression, or does depression cause more reported symptoms? American Journal of Epidemiology 126:748

20. Moe K E, Prinz P N, Larsen L H et al 1998 Growth hormone in postmenopausal women after long-term oral estrogen replacement therapy. The Journals of Gerontology. Series A, Biological Sciences and Medical Sciences 53:B117–B124

21. Ohayon M 1996 Epidemiological study on insomnia in the general population. Sleep 19 Suppl 3):7–15

22. Pigott T A 1999 Gender differences in the epidemiology and treatment of anxiety disorders. The Journal of Clinical Psychiatry 60:4–15

23. Polo-Kantola P, Erkkola R, Helenius H et al 1998 When does estrogen replacement therapy improve sleep quality? American Journal of Obstetrics and Gynecology 178:1002–1009

24. Polo-Kantola P, Erkkola R, Irjala K et al 1999 Climacteric symptoms and sleep quality. Obstetrics and Gynecology 94:219–224

25. Polo-Kantola P, Saaresranta T, Polo O 2001 Aetiology and treatment of sleep disturbances during perimenopause and postmenopause. CNS Drugs 15(6):445–452

26. Polo-Kantola P, Rauhala E, Helenius H et al 2003 Breathing during sleep in menopause: a randomized, controlled, crossover trial with estrogen therapy. Obstetrics and Gynecology 102:68–75

27. Saaresranta T, Polo-Kantola P, Irjala K et al 1999 Respiratory insufficiency in postmenopausal women: sustained improvement of gas exchange with short-term medroxyprogesterone acetate. Chest 115:1581–1587

28. Shahar E, Redline S, Young T et al 2003 Hormone replacement therapy and sleep-disordered breathing. American Journal of Respiratory and Critical Care Medicine 167(9):1186–1192

29. Shneerson J M (ed) 2000 Handbook of Sleep Medicine. Blackwell Science, Oxford

30. Skatrud J B, Dempsey J A, Kaiser D G 1978 Ventilatory responses to medroxyprogesterone acetate in normal subjects: time course and mechanism. Journal of Applied Physiology 44:939–944

31. Soares C N, Almeida O P, Joffe H et al 2001 Efficacy of estradiol for the treatment of depressive disorders in perimenopausal women. Archives of General Psychiatry 58:529–534

32. Wiklund I, Berg G, Hammar M et al 1992 Long-term effect of transdermal hormonal therapy on aspects of quality of life in postmenopausal women. Maturitas 14:225–236

33. Woodward S, Freedman R R 1994 The thermoregulatory effects of menopausal hot flashes on sleep. Sleep 17(6):497–501

34. Young T, Rabago D, Zgierska A et al 2003 Objective and subjective sleep quality in pre-, peri- and postmenopausal women in the Wisconsin sleep cohort study. Sleep 26(6):667–672

14

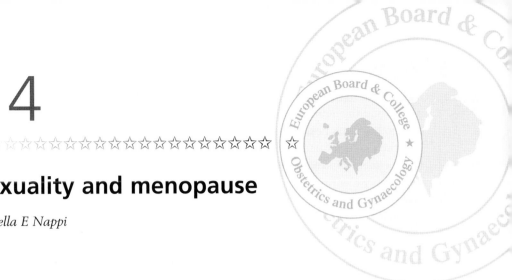

Sexuality and menopause

Rossella E Nappi

ABSTRACT

Sexuality is a critical issue at menopause for many women. A large number of biological, psychological and sociorelational factors are related to women's sexual health and they may negatively affect the entire sexual response cycle inducing significant changes in sexual desire, arousal, orgasm and satisfaction. Sex steroids, mainly low levels of oestradiol (E_2), physical and mental well-being and, very importantly, feelings for the partner are extremely relevant to women's sexuality in natural menopause. Even a significant lack of androgens, as frequently occurs in surgical menopause, has a negative impact on women's libido and sexual responsiveness. Therefore, the clinician should try to restore the hormonal balance, which modulates the sexual response, to improve the quality of life and to rule out any other factor affecting the sense of femininity and the sexual relationship. An accurate assessment and an individualized management of sexual symptoms is mandatory in routine menopause practice.

KEYWORDS

Arousal, assessment, disease, health, libido, management, menopause, orgasm, partner, sex steroids, sexual function

INTRODUCTION

Sexual complaints and problems in women are highly prevalent during the entire reproductive lifespan. However, our understanding of the pathophysiology of female sexual dysfunction (FSD) is still limited, mainly due to methodological difficulties deriving from the multidimensionality of the sexual response cycle. Women's sexual health comprises a well-balanced female sexual identity, a normal sexual function and a satisfactory sexual relationship. That not withstanding, animal models have been extremely helpful to investigate the neuroendocrine mechanisms and the neuroanatomical substrates that underlie sexual desire, arousal and orgasm but it has been very difficult to translate this growing body of basic research into the practical management of women with sexual dysfunction that may range from a mere dissatisfaction to a real pathology. The inadequacy of our clinical approach is confirmed by the several shortcomings and problems of the current classification systems for the diagnosis of FSD, very elegantly outlined by an international multidisciplinary expert group, and by the paucity of available treatments specifically designed for women with FSD.[12]

The menopause transition is a period of considerable biological, psychological and sociorelational changes for the majority of women who may be more vulnerable to developing sexual symptoms because of a complex interplay of peculiar individual factors variably affecting their sense of well-being.[10] That being so, in this chapter I will briefly summarize the current knowledge of sexuality and menopause and will try to provide diagnostic and therapeutic clues relevant to clinical practice.

WOMEN'S SEXUAL RESPONSE

Normal sexual functioning (basically an intact libido and the capacity to achieve satisfactory intercourse) is guaranteed by the integrity of neural (autonomic, somatosensory, somatomotor) and muscular substrates, of vascular supplies (arterial and venous), of hormonal environment and of modulating mechanisms depending on cortical and hypothalamic–limbic structures. An impairment of both peripheral and central pathways involved in the sexual response cycle may lead to FSD, which includes disorders of libido, arousal and orgasm, and sexual pain. Stages in reproductive life, age, partner and other contextual factors significantly affect the clinical expression of FSD.[3]

Sexual desire or libido is the physical and mental need to behave sexually in order to experience a sense of reward. It may be activated by endogenous and/or exogenous stimuli and its nature in humans is highly integrated being the result of several entangled biological, psychorelational and sociocultural issues. Multiple neuroendocrine messages are basically involved in promoting the instinctive component of libido (lust) which is modulated by emotional (attraction) and cognitive (attachment) aspects. A constant interaction among these factors gives rise to passion, affection and commitment, the key words of loving a specific mate, spirit and body.[11] Sexual arousal, a critical step in women's sexual response cycle, has been elegantly described as a mixture of subjective physical and mental feelings of sexual excitement and of objective awareness of non-genital and genital sensations due to vulvovaginal engorgement and lubrication. According to the most recent conceptualization, women are more likely to activate desire and arousal or to be responsive to sexual stimulation and to become physically aware of peripheral genital tension and excitement by mentally feeling motivations and incentives to be sexually intimate and to go ahead with sexual activity rather than perceiving a spontaneous drive not related to personal, relational and other contextual factors.[4] Sexual orgasm is a sensorimotor reflex, triggered by several physical and mental stimuli, which requires adequate neurovascular and neuro-muscular substrates and can create a sense of well-being and satisfaction modulated by neuroendocrine pathways. It constitutes an important reinforcing factor of sexual motivation, particularly when the quality of emotional intimacy and the degree of commitment with a sexual partner are very high.[3]

AGE AND MENOPAUSE

A recent comprehensive review of population-based studies reported an age-related decline of sexual functioning and an additional adverse effect of menopausal status. Ageing *per se* interferes with the level of sexual performance but the sexual behaviour of midlife and older women is highly dependent on several factors such as general physical and mental well-being, quality of relationship and life situation. The level of former sexual functioning, social class, education, employment, stressors, personality factors, sociocultural environment and negative attitude towards the menopause also play a significant role.[2] The longest population-based study – the Melbourne Women's Midlife Health Project – found a significant decrease of women's desire, arousal, orgasm and frequency of sexual activity and a significant increase in vaginal dryness/dyspareunia throughout the menopausal transition. Both age and declining E_2 (but not testosterone, which was already low in these middle-aged women) had significant detrimental effects on sexual functioning, libido and sexual responsiveness: arousal; sexual pleasure; and orgasm.[9,10] A number of other observational studies, both cross-sectional and longitudinal, have suggested that surgical menopause has a more negative impact on sexual function than hysterectomy alone, and there is a consensus (particularly for younger women) in which premature menopause may occur spontaneously or be induced medically.[2] It is important to note that the climacteric syndrome, especially physical, psychological and genital symptoms, significantly affects the clinical relevance of sexual symptoms after menopause.[16]

HEALTH-RELATED ISSUES

Apart from being menopausal and having had hysterectomy, many other medical and surgical conditions can exert a negative impact on women's sexuality. While there is no consensus on the effect of removing the uterus on sexual response depending on the pre-existing clinical, sexual and emotional situation, mastectomy is considered a major insult to the sense of femininity and to the perception of being a healthy operating female body with severe consequences on libido, arousal and sexual pleasure. Even abdominal/pelvic surgery for malignancies has a strong impact on women's sexual function, as well as any systemic disease and other surgery that challenges the perception of physical and mental well-being. In addition, mood disorders, especially depression, have been linked to poor sexual function as a result of the use of selective serotonin reuptake inhibitors, which are frequently prescribed for middle-aged women. Several common medical conditions, such as hypertension and diabetes, and many drugs frequently used in clinical practice may interfere with women's sexual response around menopause and beyond.[2,19]

PARTNER-RELATED ISSUES

The presence of a sexual partner, the partner's age and health, length of the relationship and most importantly feelings toward the partner, have a critical impact on women's sexual functioning in midlife. A significant increase in the partner's sexual problems is evident throughout the menopausal transition; changing the sexual partner may be considered a positive conditioner of sexual activity and response for menopausal women.[9,10] Focusing exclusively on the symptomatic woman without taking into account the quality of the partner's life and the presence of a satisfactory couple's relationship may be an omission responsible for treatment failure in routine menopausal practice.

HORMONAL CHANGES AND SEXUAL SYMPTOMS

Sex steroids exert both organizational and activational effects, which are relevant to sexual function, and their actions are mediated by nongenomic as well as direct and indirect genomic pathways. Oestrogens represent the core of womanliness and play a critical role in maintaining the physiological function of many tissues, including the central nervous system (CNS) and the genital apparatus, and of organs relevant to general health. Androgens are essential for the development of reproductive function and the growth and maintenance of secondary sex characteristics, directly or throughout their conversion to oestrogens; they influence many tissues and organs even in the female body. Sex steroids modulate cortical coordinating and controlling centres interpreting what sensations are to be perceived as sexual and issuing appropriate commands to the rest of the nervous system. In addition, sex steroids affect the threshold of sensitivity of both non-genital and genital organs and of hypothalamic–limbic structures where they elicit conscious perception and pleasurable reactions by influencing the release of specific neurotransmitters and neuromodulators.[13,18]

OESTROGENS

Within the nervous system, E_2 plays a permissive role on sexual receptivity by acting on its own receptor α (ERα) and by increasing progesterone receptor expression, which plays a part in the sexual response. Also, E_2 stimulates oxytocin release and the expression of its receptor, and facilitates the lordosis reflex by stimulating the noradrenaline α_1-receptor.

The importance of adequate oestrogen levels in preserving vaginal receptivity and preventing dyspareunia has long been established. Oestrogen deficiency causes urogenital ageing and vulvovaginal atrophy. Vaginal pH changes from acidic to alkaline, contributing not only to a change of vaginal flora but even to more infections. Over time, the vaginal vault becomes pale with loss of rogation and with tissue friability followed by progressive shortening and narrowing, while the clitoris becomes fibrosed. Urinary symptoms, such as frequency, urgency, nocturia, dysuria, incontinence and postcoital infection, may be present.

At a level of E_2 less than 50 pg/mL, women reported vaginal dryness, increased frequency and intensity of dyspareunia, pain with penetration and deep insertion, and burning. Women with higher E_2 levels had no complaints related to sexual desire, response or satisfaction. Indeed, E_2 levels below 35 pg/mL are associated with reduced coital frequency – a decline in E_2 is related to poor sexual functioning. To summarize, concerning vaginal vasocongestion and increased lubrication during objective genital arousal, it is likely that vaginal arteriolar dilatation – from vasoactive intestinal peptide, nitric oxide (NO) and other unknown neurotransmitters, and neuropeptide Y-associated venoconstriction – leads to increased interstitial fluid formation from vaginal submucosal capillaries. Neurogenic fluid filters through epithelial cells onto lumen with less potassium and more sodium than in the non-arousal state. This entire haemodynamic process is highly orchestrated by oestrogens. Similarly, the labia minora are able to release a transudate with the same modalities, while NO plays a dominant androgen- and oestrogen-dependent role in the clitoral cavernous body's vasocongestion by regulating, together with prostaglandins, clitoral smooth muscle tone.[2,15]

During the climacteric, when hormonal imbalance is highly dominant, the inadequate hormonal-dependent vaginal receptivity by precipitating dyspareunia may cause other sexual symptoms that contribute toward amplified pain during coitus. Indeed, it is extremely common to observe a lack of arousal and a decline of libido following a history of sexual pain; the consequent reduction of orgasmic capacity may then reduce sexual satisfaction, which negatively influences sexual motivation, activity and a couple's relationship. This model clearly explains the high degree of comorbidity of sexual symptoms in menopausal women and the importance of the timely recognition of the leader symptom to avoid such a cascade of negative events and of established appropriate treatments.[2]

PROGESTINS

Some neurosteroids such as allopregnanolone (a ring A-reduced pregnane derivative of progesterone) are involved in the lordosis reflex at hypothalamic levels by interfering with GABAergic function. In addition, progesterone and its metabolites may indirectly influence sexual receptivity by modulating mood and cognition together with oestrogens and androgens. The role of progesterone on

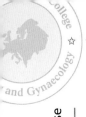

peripheral vaginal arousal is poorly understood, even though the use of progestins seems to blunt the positive effect on vaginal dryness and dyspareunia
exerted by oestrogen, an action that seems highly dependent on the biochemical
properties of progestins.[20]

ANDROGENS

The most potent androgen, testosterone, is secreted by the adrenal zona fascic-
ulata (25%) and the ovarian stroma (25%), while the remainder (50%) derives
from peripheral conversion of circulating androstenedione. Testosterone is converted to dihydrotestosterone (DHT) but it can also be aromatized to E_2 in
target tissues; DHT is the principal ligand to androgen receptors. Other androgens in women include dehydroepiandrosterone sulphate (DHEAS), dehydroepiandrosterone (DHEA) and androstenedione, which are considered as
pro-androgens because they have to be converted to testosterone to express their
effects.

While oestrogens decrease sharply at menopause, plasma testosterone levels
fall slowly with age. At physiological menopause, the cessation of follicular
activity is characterized by a significant decline of ovarian production of
androstenedione, more than testosterone; the progressive decrease in plasma
testosterone concentrations is the consequence of the reduced peripheral conversion from its major precursor and from DHEA and DHEAS, which decline
with age. Indeed, plasma testosterone and androstenedione levels in a woman's
60s are about half those in women aged 40 years. As far as surgical menopause
is concerned, bilateral oophorectomy (both premenopausally and postmenopausally) leads to a sudden 50% fall in circulating testosterone levels,
which are associated with the so-called androgen insufficiency syndrome, which
is an increasingly accepted clinical entity comprising specific symptoms such as
low libido, persistent and inexplicable fatigue, blunted motivation and a general
reduced sense of well-being. However, prospective data fail to demonstrate a
correlation between plasma testosterone levels and sexual symptoms during the
menopausal transition, even though low plasma androgen levels are significantly associated with poor libido. No cut-off level for a normal range of testosterone has been agreed on. The lack of consensus on the definition of low
testosterone levels depends on the difficulties with sensitive assays of total and
free testosterone in women, on the fluctuations during the menstrual cycle and
in different periods of life. In addition, sex hormone-binding globulin (SHBG)
levels fall with declining E_2, influencing free testosterone concentration during
the late menopausal transition.[8,18]

Testosterone directly or throughout aromatization to E_2 within the CNS contributes to the initiation of sexual activity and permission for sexual behaviour.
A further non-genomic action by testosterone metabolites on sexual receptivity
has been described at the hypothalamic level. Experimental data suggest that
androgens directly modulate vaginal and clitoral physiology by influencing the
muscular tone of erectile tissue and the vaginal walls. Androgens facilitate vaginal

smooth muscle relaxation, especially in the proximal vagina, producing distinct physiological responses in comparison with E_2. Testosterone may enhance lubrication, being converted to E_2. Therefore, androgen insufficiency may certainly contribute to poor genital engorgement and sensation, which contribute to arousal and orgasmic disorders.[17]

ASSESSMENT

Menopause is always – but particularly when it occurs prematurely or surgically and if vulvovaginal atrophy is evident – the 'golden moment' to bring up the topic of the quality of sexual life. Women may not be willing to start a conversation on such an issue themselves but they usually appreciate being questioned. Some very simple questions may help the clinician to establish a connection between the occurrence of sexual symptoms and the menopausal transition, while it may require skilled training to determine whether factors other than the hormonal changes enter the picture of sexual health. An accurate medical, urogynaecological and obstetric history, including use of medications and life-style risk factors, is part of the sexual history with the aim of identifying any possible organic factor affecting desire, arousal, orgasm and sexual pain. It is extremely important to bear in mind that even sexual symptoms that are strongly correlated to biological determinants always have a psychorelational counterpart which is much stronger depending on the duration of the symptoms and on the type of distress perceived by the woman and/or the couple.[2]

CLINICAL EVALUATION

A thorough pelvic examination is the critical step to identifying the signs and symptoms of genital involution, of introital and deep pain-triggering points, of hypertonic and hypotonic pelvic floor alterations and of any other urogynaecological conditions (recurrent urinary infections, urinary incontinence, fear of urine leakage during orgasm, etc.) possibly leading to sexual symptoms. Vaginal pH should always be measured because acidity highly correlates with oestrogenization. Determining the karyopycnotic index may also be useful. Other objective indicators of FSD, i.e. genital blood flow, genital sensation, etc., are not routinely performed and are presently used only for research purpose. An endocrine evaluation may be needed but it is not mandatory at present, apart from excluding hyperprolactinaemia states and thyroid dysfunction. On the basis of clinical history, other tests to investigate the potential impact of disease states such as hypertension, diabetes, hypercholesterolaemia, etc., may be indicated.[2,7]

PSYCHOSEXUAL AND SOCIORELATIONAL EVALUATIONS

It is not always easy to evaluate menopausal women from a psychological and sociorelational perspective in the clinical setting, mainly because of the limited length of consultations and of the need for particular expertise. However, many validation tools may be used in women reporting sexual complaints at menopause, even though the majority of them are still for research purposes. The most common self-rated questionnaires are McCoy's, the Brief Sexual Function Index for Women, the Female Sexual Function Interview and the Derogatis Interview for Sexual Functioning. Daily diaries and event logs quantify the frequency of sexual activity, attempts at intercourse and other forms of sexual activity. Semi-structured interviews, as well as qualitative assessments, can also be performed to diagnose FSD and gain information on sexual constructs of menopausal women and on a couple's relationship.[2,6]

MANAGEMENT

The management of sexual symptoms at menopause should be individualized and tailored to a woman's history and current needs. 'Pills' are not everythin in the field of FSD and offering unrealistic expectations may be extremely fru trating for women and their partners and can be a real 'boomerang' for the clnician. However, a well-balanced view of the biological components conditioningthe most common complaints such as vaginal dryness and lack of lubri cation, low libido and poor sexual pleasure, as well as the psychorelational aspects amplifying or initiating some of these symptoms, is always very helpful and those women who are effectively distressed by FSD may gain great benefits.

PHARMACOLOGICAL AGENTS

Systematic reviews including all randomized and placebo-controlled trials of treatment for FSD in postmenopausal women concluded that many hormonal therapies that are used in practice are not supported by adequate evidence.[1,14] Even though ET/HRT may be an effective treatment for vaginal atrophy, increasing vaginal lubrication and reducing dyspareunia, it has not been shown to increase sexual desire or activity consistently and many women with FSD remain unresponsive. There is a significant subgroup of women with sexual difficulties who respond initially to ET/HRT but subsequently revert to their initial problems, especially when symptoms include loss of libido, particularly in surgical menopause. In these cases, the addition of androgen therapy (AT) has proved helpful, even if on a short-term basis. However, the results available for ET/HRT need to be expanded taking into account the differences, mainly on plasma sex steroid and SHBG levels, existing between various schemes of conventional hormonal treatments in terms of type of molecules, routes of administration, mechanisms of action and metabolism.

As far as ET/AT is concerned, many data obtained with various combinations of systemically exogenous oestrogens and androgens, and even administered genitally, support a significant improvement in libido, enjoyment, ability to reach orgasm and initiation of sex. Similarly to ET/HRT, the type and route of

AT seem crucial, given the evidence of peculiar effects on bioavailable plasma sex steroid levels when combined with different types of ET. However, at present, the use of androgens in the clinical management of menopause awaits further confirmation and needs a certain degree of caution, mainly because the long-term effects of such preparations on women's general health are still partially unexplored.

Tibolone, a synthetic steroid with tissue-specific oestrogenic, progestagenic and androgenic properties, has been successfully used for the treatment of climacteric symptoms including low mood and libido. Apart from direct effects of its metabolites on vaginal tissue and brain areas relevant to well-being, tibolone increases bioavailable sex steroids (FreeT and DHEAS). In randomized studies against placebo and HRT, tibolone alleviates vaginal dryness and dyspareunia, improving libido, arousal and sexual satisfaction in postmenopausal women to a greater extent, while having a positive effect on sexual function which is better than that with HRT/AT.

Raloxifene, a selective oestrogen receptor modulator, used in the prevention of postmenopausal osteoporosis, does not seem to offer any benefit for urogenital ageing but its concomitant administration did not alter the effects of E_2 on alleviating signs and symptoms of genitourinary atrophy and did not counteract the improvement of vaginal atrophy observed by using either low-dose conjugated oestrogen cream or nonhormonal moisturizer in postmenopausal women.

DHEA supplement has been proposed for the treatment of low libido and mental well-being both pre- and postmenopausally with encouraging results, although well-controlled studies are needed.

Nonhormonal pharmacological vasoactive agents – sildenafil (a selective phosphodiesterase type 5 inhibitor used in the treatment of male erectile dysfunction), yohimbine (an α_2-adrenoceptor antagonist), phentolamine (a non-specific adrenoceptor antagonist), alprostadil (a naturally occurring form of the hormone prostaglandin E_1), etc. – have been tested in postmenopausal FSD with mixed results and are a promising field of research alone or in association with hormonal therapies.[2,5]

OTHER THERAPEUTIC STRATEGIES

The most important task of the caring clinician is to promote women's general sense of well-being and the pleasure of being into their 50s. Lifestyle changes (e.g. stopping smoking, aerobic exercise) have positive impacts on sexuality by improving energy, decreasing depression, enhancing body image and self-esteem, etc. Helping women to understand the physiological changes of the sexual response associated with the ageing process in both sexes and how to counteract them (e.g. genital caring, pelvic floor exercises, more foreplay), to communicate sexual preferences between partners and to improve intimacy by spending more time sharing pleasurable activities with their partner is extremely valuable in sexual counselling. Potential psychotherapeutic treatment options may include education and cognitive restructuring favouring a better understanding of the impact of emotions on sexual functioning, body image desensitization and refocus on pleasure sensations and sexual fantasies, psycho-dynamic exploration and a couple's therapy, etc. Specific training in sexual medicine and a multidisciplinary approach are critical for long-lasting successful results in the most difficult cases.[6]

CONCLUSION

Sexual health is relevant for physical and emotional well-being throughout menopause and beyond. Apart from preserving the biological substrate of sexual response, it is mandatory to explore the psychorelational universe of midlife and older women in order to design effective interventions. Well-defined end-points and outcomes and a general consensus on a diagnostic framework for the assessment and management of FSD are important goals for the future of sexual health in order to develop hormonal and nonhormonal treatments, and psychosexual strategies specifically designed for menopausal women with sexual symptoms.

References

1. Alexander J L, Kotz K, Dennerstein L et al 2004 The effects of postmenopausal hormone therapies on female sexual functioning: a review of double-blind, randomized controlled trials. Menopause 11:749–765
2. Bachmann G A, Leiblum S R 2004 The impact of hormones on menopausal sexuality: a literature review. Menopause 11:120–130
3. Basson R, Berman J, Burnett A et al 2000 Report of the International Consensus development conference on female sexual dysfunction: definitions and classifications. The Journal of Urology 163:888–893
4. Basson R, Leiblum SL, Brotto L et al 2003 Definitions of women's sexual dysfunctions reconsidered: advocating expansion and revision. Journal of Psychosomatic Obstetrics and Gynecology 24:221–229
5. Basson R 2004 Pharmacotherapy for sexual dysfunction in women. Expert Opinion on Pharmacotherapy 5:1045–1059
6. Basson R 2004 Introduction to special issue on women's sexuality and outline of assessment of sexual problems. Menopause 11:709–713
7. Berman J R, Adhikari S P, Goldstein I 2000 Anatomy and physiology of female sexual function and dysfunction: classification, evaluation and treatment options. European Urology 38:20–29
8. Davis S, Tran J 2001 Testosterone influences libido and well-being in women. Trends in Endocrinology and Metabolism 12:33–37
9. Dennerstein L, Dudley E C, Hopper J L et al 2000 A prospective population-based study of menopausal symptoms. Obstetrics and Gynecology 96:351–358
10. Dennerstein L, Randolph J, Taffe J et al 2002 Hormones, mood, sexuality, and the menopausal transition. Fertility and Sterility 77:S42–S48
11. Levine S B 2003 The nature of sexual desire: a clinician's perspective. Archives of Sexual Behavior 32:279–285
12. Lue T F, Basson R, Rosen R et al (eds) 2004 Sexual Medicine: Sexual dysfunctions in men and women. Editions 21, Paris
13. Meston C M, Frohlich P F 2000 The neurobiology of sexual function. Archives of General Psychiatry 57:1012–1030
14. Modelska K, Cummings S 2003 Female sexual dysfunction in postmenopausal women: systematic review of placebo-controlled trials. American Journal of Obstetrics and Gynecology 188:286–293
15. Munarriz R, Kim N N, Goldstein I et al 2002 Biology of female sexual function. The Urologic Clinics of North America 29:685–693
16. Nappi R E, Verde J B, Polatti F et al 2002 Self-reported sexual symptoms in women

attending menopause clinics. Gynecologic and Obstetric Investigations 53:181–187

17. Nappi R E, Detaddei S, Ferdeghini F et al 2003 Role of testosterone in feminine sexuality. Journal of Endocrinological Investigation 26:97–101

18. Rosen R, Bachmann G, Leiblum S et al 2002 Androgen insufficiency in women: the Princeton Conference. Fertility and Sterility 77 (Suppl 4):S1–S107

19. Salonia A, Munarriz R M, Naspro R et al 2004 Women's sexual dysfunction: a pathophysiological review. British Journal of Urology International 93:1156–1164

20. Sarrel P M 1990 Sexuality and menopause. Obstetrics and Gynecology 75:26S–35S

15

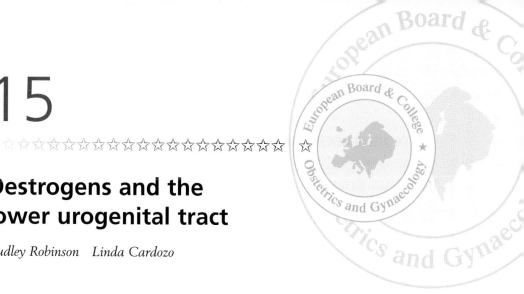

Oestrogens and the lower urogenital tract

Dudley Robinson   Linda Cardozo

ABSTRACT

The urogenital tract is sensitive to the effect of oestrogen and progesterone throughout adult life. Epidemiological studies have implicated oestrogen deficiency in the aetiology of lower urinary tract symptoms occurring following the menopause. Although to date the role of oestrogen (replacement) therapy (ET) in the management of postmenopausal urinary incontinence remains controversial, its use in the management of women complaining of urogenital atrophy is now well-established.

   This chapter reviews the recent evidence regarding the urogenital effects of hormone replacement therapy (HRT) with a particular emphasis on the management of postmenopausal urinary incontinence, recurrent lower urinary tract infections (UTIs) and urogenital atrophy.

KEYWORDS

Oestrogen, urinary incontinence, urogenital atrophy, urogenital tract

INTRODUCTION

The female genital and lower urinary tract share a common embryological origin from the urogenital sinus and both are sensitive to the effects of female sex steroid hormones. Oestrogen is known to have an important role in the function of the lower urinary tract throughout adult life, and oestrogen and progesterone receptors have been demonstrated in the vagina, urethra, bladder and pelvic floor musculature.[4,5,19,37] Oestrogen deficiency occurring following the menopause is known to cause atrophic changes within the urogenital tract[36] and is associated with urinary symptoms such as frequency, urgency, nocturia, incontinence and

155

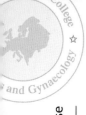
The menopause

recurrent infection. These may coexist with symptoms of vaginal atrophy such as dyspareunia, itching, burning and dryness.

OESTROGEN RECEPTORS

The effects of the steroid hormone 17β-oestradiol are mediated by ligand-activated transcription factors known as oestrogen receptors (ERs), which are glycoproteins sharing common features with androgen and progesterone receptors. The classic oestrogen receptor ERα was first discovered by Elwood Jensen in 1958 and cloned from uterine tissue in 1986[30] although it was not until 1996 that the second oestrogen receptor ERβ was identified.[45]

ERs have been demonstrated throughout the lower urinary tract and are expressed in the squamous epithelium of the proximal and distal urethra, vagina and trigone of the bladder[10] although not in the dome of the bladder, reflecting its different embryological origin. The pubococcygeus and the musculature of the pelvic floor have also been shown to be oestrogen sensitive[35,68] although ERs have not yet been identified in the levator ani muscles.[9]

More recently, the distribution of ERs throughout the urogenital tract has been studied with α and β receptors being found in the vaginal walls and uterosacral ligaments of premenopausal women, although the latter was absent in the vaginal walls of postmenopausal women.[20] In addition, α receptors are localized in the urethral sphincter and when sensitized by oestrogens are thought to help maintain muscular tone.[64] Interestingly, ERs have also been identified in mast cells in women with interstitial cystitis[52] and in the male lower urinary tract.

LOWER URINARY TRACT FUNCTION

In order to maintain continence the urethral pressure must remain higher than the intravesical pressure at all times except during micturition.[1] Oestrogens play an important role in the continence mechanism with bladder and urethral function becoming less efficient with age.[57] Elderly women have been found to have a reduced flow rate, increased urinary residuals, higher filling pressures, reduced bladder capacity and lower maximum voiding pressures.[48] Oestrogens may affect continence by increasing urethral resistance, raising the sensory threshold of the bladder or by increasing α-adrenoreceptor sensitivity in the urethral smooth muscle.[41,75] In addition, exogenous oestrogens have been shown to increase the number of intermediate and superficial cells in the vagina of postmenopausal women[69] and these changes have also been demonstrated in the bladder and urethra.[62]

BLADDER FUNCTION

ERs, although absent in the transitional epithelium of the bladder, are present in the areas of the trigone which have undergone squamous metaplsia.[21] Oestrgen is known to have a direct effect on detrusor function through modificatios in muscarinic receptors[3,65] and by the inhibition of movement of extracellular calcium ions into muscle cells.[21] Consequently, oestradiol (E_2) has been shown to reduce the amplitude and frequency of spontaneous rhythmic detrusor contractions[66] and there is also evidence that it may increase the sensory threshold of the bladder in some women.[25]

NEUROLOGICAL CONTROL

Sex hormones are known to influence the central neurological control of micturition although their exact role in the micturition pathway has yet to be elucidated. ERs have been demonstrated in the cerebral cortex, limbic system, hippocampus and cerebellum.[47,71]

URETHRA

ERs have been demonstrated in the squamous epithelium of the proximal and distal urethra,[21] and oestrogen has been shown to improve the maturation index of urethral squamous epithelium.[8] It has been suggested that oestrogen increases urethral closure pressure and improves pressure transmission to the proximal urethra, both of which promote continence.[28,54,58,76] Oestrogens have been shown to cause vasodilatation in the systemic and cerebral circulation and these changes are also seen in the urethra.[28,54] The vascular pulsations seen on urethral pressure profilometry secondary to blood flow in the urethral submucosa and urethral sphincter have been shown to increase in size following oestrogen administration,[76] while the effect is lost following oestrogen withdrawal at the menopause.

COLLAGEN

Oestrogens are known to have an effect on collagen synthesis and they have been shown to have a direct effect on collagen metabolism in the lower genital tract.[24] Changes found in women with urogenital atrophy may represent an alteration in systemic collagenase activity.[46] Urodynamic stress incontinence and urogenital prolapse have been associated with a reduction in both vaginal and periurethral collagen.[18,39,60]

UROGENITAL ATROPHY

Withdrawal of endogenous oestrogen at the menopause results in climacteric symptoms such as hot flushes and night sweats in addition to the less commonly reported symptoms of urogenital atrophy. Symptoms do not usually develop until several years following the menopause when levels of endogenous oestrogens fall below the level required to promote endometrial growth.[60] This temporal relationship would suggest oestrogen withdrawal as the cause.

Vaginal dryness is commonly the first reported symptom and is caused by a reduction in mucus production within the vaginal glands. Atrophy within the

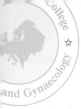

vaginal epithelium leads to thinning and an increased susceptibility to infection and mechanical trauma. Glycogen depletion within the vaginal mucosa following the menopause leads to a decrease in lactic acid formation by Döderlein's lactobacillus and a consequent rise in vaginal pH from around 4 to between 6 and 7. This allows bacterial overgrowth and colonization with Gram-negative bacilli compounding the effects of vaginal atrophy and leading to symptoms of vaginitis such as pruritis, dyspareunia and discharge.

LOWER URINARY TRACT SYMPTOMS

Epidemiological studies have implicated oestrogen deficiency in the aetiology of lower urinary tract symptoms with 70% of women relating the onset of urinary incontinence to their final menstrual period.[36] Lower urinary tract symptoms have been shown to be common in postmenopausal women attending a menopause clinic with 20% complaining of severe urgency and almost 50% complaining of stress incontinence.[18] Urge incontinence in particular is more prevalent following the menopause; this prevalence would appear to rise with increasing years of oestrogen deficiency.[44] There is, however, conflicting evidence regarding the role of oestrogen withdrawal at the time of the menopause. Some studies have shown a peak incidence in perimenopausal women[40,73] while other evidence suggests that many women develop incontinence at least 10 years prior to the cessation of menstruation with significantly more premenopausal women than postmenopausal being affected.[13,61]

Cyclical variations in the levels of oestrogen and progesterone during the menstrual cycle have been shown to lead to changes in urodynamic variables and lower urinary tract symptoms with 37% of women noticing a deterioration in symptoms prior to menstruation.[33] Measurement of the urethral pressure profile in nulliparous premenopausal women shows that there is an increase in functional urethral length midcycle and early in the luteal phase corresponding to an increase in plasma E_2.[74]

Urinary tract infection is also a common cause of urinary symptoms in women of all ages. This is a particular problem in the elderly with a reported incidence of 20% in the community and over 50% in institutionalized patients.[11,63] Pathophysiological changes, such as impairment of bladder emptying, poor perineal hygiene and faecal and urinary incontinence, may partly account for the high prevalence observed. Also, changes in the vaginal flora due to oestrogen depletion lead to colonization with Gram-negative bacilli, which, in addition to causing local irritating symptoms, also act as uropathogens.

OESTROGENS IN THE MANAGEMENT OF INCONTINENCE

Oestrogen preparations have been used for many years in the treatment of urinary incontinence[59,79] although their precise role remains controversial. Many of the studies performed have been uncontrolled observational series examining the use of a wide range of different preparations, doses and routes of administration.

The inconsistent use of progestogens to provide endometrial protection is a further confounding factor making interpretation of the results difficult.

In order to clarify the situation, a meta-analysis from the Hormones and Urogenital Therapy (HUT) Committee has been reported.[27] Of 166 articles identified that were published in English between 1969 and 1992 only six were controlled trials and 17 were uncontrolled series. Meta-analysis found an overall significant effect of ET on subjective improvement in all subjects and for subjects with genuine stress incontinence alone. Subjective improvement rates with ET in randomized controlled trials ranged from 64% to 75% although placebo groups also reported an improvement of 10% to 56%. In uncontrolled series, subjective improvement rates were 8% to 89% with subjects with genuine stress incontinence showing improvement of 34% to 73%. However, when assessing objective fluid loss there was no significant effect. Maximum urethral closure pressure was found to increase significantly with ET although this outcome was influenced by a single study showing a large effect.[32]

A further meta-analysis performed in Italy has analysed the results of randomized controlled clinical trials on the efficacy of ET in postmenopausal women with urinary incontinence.[80] A search of the literature (1965–96) revealed 72 articles of which only four were considered to meet the meta-analysis criteria. There was a statistically significant difference in subjective outcome between oestrogen and placebo although there was no such difference in objective or urodynamic outcome. The authors conclude that this difference could be relevant although the studies may have lacked objective sensitivity to detect this.

The role of ET in the prevention of ischaemic heart disease has recently been assessed in a four-year randomized trial, the Heart and Estrogen/progestin Replacement Study (HERS) involving 2763 postmenopausal women younger than 80 years with intact uteri and ischaemic heart disease.[29] In this study, 55% of women reported at least one episode of urinary incontinence each week, and were randomly assigned to oral conjugated oestrogen plus medroxyprogesterone acetate or placebo daily. Incontinence improved in 26% of women assigned to placebo as compared to 21% receiving HRT, while 27% of the placebo group complained of worsening symptoms compared with 39% in the HRT group ($P = 0.001$). The incidence of incontinent episodes per week increased an average of 0.7 in the HRT group and decreased by 0.1 in the placebo group ($P < 0.001$). Overall, combined HRT was associated with worsening stress and urge urinary incontinence although there was no significant difference in daytime frequency, nocturia or number of UTIs.

These findings have also been confirmed in the Nurses' Health Study, which followed 39 436 postmenopausal women aged 50–75 years over a 4-year period. The risk of incontinence was found to be elevated in those women taking HRT when compared to those who had never taken it. There was an increase in risk in women taking oral oestrogen (relative risk, RR 1.54; 95% confidence interval, CI; range 1.44–1.65), transdermal oestrogen (RR 1.68; 95% CI; range 1.41–2.00), oral oestrogen and progesterone (RR 1.34; 95% CI; range 1.24–1.34) and transdermal oestrogen and progesterone (RR 1.46; 95% CI; range 1.16–1.84). In addition, while there remained a small risk after the cessation of HRT (RR 1.14; 95% CI; range 1.06–1.23) by 10 years the risk was identical (RR 1.02; 95% CI; range 0.91–1.41) and was identical to those women who had never taken HRT.[31]

More recently the effects of oral oestrogens and progestogens on the lower urinary tract have been assessed in 32 female nursing home residents with an average age of 88 years.[51] Subjects were randomized to oral oestrogen and progesterone or placebo for 6 months. At follow-up there was no difference between severity of incontinence, prevalence of bacteriuria or the results of vaginal cultures although there was an improvement in atrophic vaginitis in the placebo group.

The most recent meta-analysis of the effect of ET on the lower urinary tract was performed by the Cochrane Group.[50] Overall, 28 trials were identified, including 2926 women. In the 15 trials comparing oestrogen to placebo there was a higher subjective impression of improvement rate in those women taking oestrogen, and this was the case for all types of incontinence (RR for cure 1.61; 95% CI; range 1.04–2.49). Equally, when subjective cure and improvement were taken together there was a statistically higher cure and improvement rate for both urge (57% vs. 28%) and stress (43% vs. 27%) incontinence. In those women with urge incontinence the chance of improvement was 25% higher than in women with stress incontinence and, overall, about 50% of women treated with oestrogen were cured or improved compared to 25% on placebo. The authors concluded that oestrogens can improve or cure incontinence and that the effect may be most useful in women complaining of urge incontinence.

OESTROGENS IN THE MANAGEMENT OF STRESS INCONTINENCE

In addition to the studies included in the HUT meta-analysis, several authors have also investigated the role of ET in the management of urodynamic stress incontinence only. Oral oestrogens have been reported to increase the maximum urethral pressures and lead to symptomatic improvement in 65–70% of women,[14,58] although other work has not confirmed this.[77,78] More recently, two placebo-controlled studies have been performed examining the use of oral oestrogens in the treatment of urodynamic stress incontinence in postmenopausal women. Neither conjugated equine oestrogens and medroxyprogesterone acetate,[26] or unopposed E_2 valerate[39] showed a significant difference in either subjective or objective outcomes. Furthermore, a review of eight controlled and 14 uncontrolled prospective trials concluded that ET was not an efficacious treatment for stress incontinence but may be useful for symptoms of urgency and frequency.[72]

A recently reported meta-analysis has helped determine the role of oestrogen replacement in women with stress incontinence.[2] Of the papers reviewed, 14 were nonrandomized studies, six were randomized trials (of which four were placebo-controlled) and two were meta-analyses. Interestingly, there was only a symptomatic or clinical improvement noted in the nonrandomized studies while there was no such effect noted in the randomized trials. The authors concluded that currently the evidence would not support the use of oestrogen replacement alone in the management of stress incontinence.

From the available evidence, oestrogen does not appear to be an effective treatment for stress incontinence although it may have a synergistic role in combination therapy. Two placebo-controlled studies have examined the use of oral and vaginal oestrogens with the α-adrenergic agonist phenylpropanolamine used separately and in combination. Both studies found that combination therapy was superior to either drug given alone although while there was subjective improvement in all groups,[6] there was only objective improvement in the combination therapy group.[34]

OESTROGENS IN THE MANAGEMENT OF URGE INCONTINENCE

Oestrogens have been used in the treatment of urinary urgency and urge incontinence for many years although there have been few controlled trials to confirm their efficacy. A double-blind placebo-controlled crossover study using oral oestriol (E_3) in 34 postmenopausal women produced subjective improvement in eight women with mixed incontinence and 12 with urge incontinence.[61] However, a double blind multicentre study of the use of E_3 (3 mg per day) in postmenopausal women complaining of urgency has failed to confirm these findings,[17] showing both subjective and objective improvement but not significantly better than placebo. E_3 is a naturally occurring weak oestrogen which has little effect on the endometrium and does not prevent osteoporosis although has been used in the treatment of urogenital atrophy. Consequently it is possible that the dosage or route of administration in this study was not appropriate in the treatment of urinary symptoms, and higher systemic levels may be required.

The use of sustained-release 17β-oestradiol vaginal tablets (Vagifem®, Novo Nordisk, Denmark) has also been examined in postmenopausal women with urgency and urge incontinence or a urodynamic diagnosis of sensory urgency or detrusor instability. Following a six-month course of treatment, the only significant difference between active and placebo groups was an improvement in the symptom of urgency in those women with a urodynamic diagnosis of sensory urgency.[7] A further double-blind, randomized, placebo-controlled trial of vaginal 17β-oestradiol vaginal tablets has shown lower urinary tract symptoms of frequency, urgency, urge and stress incontinence to be significantly improved although there was no objective urodynamic assessment performed.[23] In both of these studies the subjective improvement in symptoms may simply represent local oestrogenic effects reversing urogenital atrophy rather than a direct effect on bladder function.

To try to clarify the role of ET in the management of women with urge incontinence a meta-analysis of the use of oestrogen in women with symptoms of 'overactive bladder' has been reported by the HUT Committee (unpublished data, 2001). In a review of ten randomized placebo-controlled trials, oestrogen was found to be superior to placebo when considering symptoms of urge incontinence, frequency and nocturia, although vaginal oestrogen administration was found to be superior for symptoms of urgency. In those taking oestrogens there was also a significant increase in first sensation and bladder capacity as compared to placebo.

OESTROGENS IN THE MANAGEMENT OF RECURRENT URINARY TRACT INFECTION

Oestrogen therapy has been shown to increase vaginal pH and reverse the micro-biological changes that occur in the vagina following the menopause.[12] Initial small uncontrolled studies using oral or vaginal oestrogens in the treatment of recurrent UTI appeared to give promising results[53,55] although unfortunately this has not been supported by larger randomized trials.

Kjaergaard and colleagues[43] compared vaginal E_3 tablets with placebo in 21 postmenopausal women over a five-month period and found no significant dif-ference between the two groups. However, a subsequent randomized, double-blind, placebo-controlled study assessing the use of E_3 vaginal cream in 93 postmenopausal women during an eight-month period did reveal a significant effect.[56]

Kirkengen et al randomized 40 postmenopausal women to receive either placebo or oral E_3 and found that although initially both groups had a signifi-cantly decreased incidence of recurrent infections, after 12 weeks E_3 was shown to be significantly more effective.[42] These findings, however, were not con-firmed subsequently in a trial of 72 postmenopausal women with recurrent UTIs randomized to oral E_3 or placebo. Following a six-month treatment period and a further six-month follow-up, E_3 was found to be no more effective than placebo.[16]

More recently a randomized, open, parallel-group study assessing the use of an E_2-releasing silicone vaginal ring (Estring®, Pharmacia and Upjohn, Sweden) in postmenopausal women with recurrent infections has been performed which showed the cumulative likelihood of remaining infection free was 45% in the active group and 20% in the placebo group.[22] Estring was also shown to decrease the number of recurrences per year and to prolong the interval between infec-tion episodes.

OESTROGENS IN THE MANAGEMENT OF UROGENITAL ATROPHY

Symptoms of urogenital atrophy do not occur until the levels of endogenous oestrogen are lower than that required to promote endometrial proliferation.[62] Consequently, it is possible to use a low dose of ET to alleviate urogenital symp-toms while avoiding the risk of endometrial proliferation and removing the necessity of providing endometrial protection with progestogens.[49] The dose of E_2 commonly used in systemic oestrogen replacement is usually 25–100 µg although studies investigating the use of oestrogens in the management of uro-genital symptoms have shown that 8–10 µg of vaginal E_2 is effective.[67] Thus only 10–30% of the dose used to treat vasomotor symptoms may be effective in the management of urogenital symptoms. Since 10–25% of women receiving systemic HRT still experience symptoms of urogenital atrophy,[70] low-dose local preparations may have an additional beneficial effect.

A recent review of ET in the management of urogenital atrophy has been performed by the HUT Committee.[15] Ten randomized trials and 54 uncontrolled series were examined from 1969 to 1995 assessing 24 different treatment regimens. Meta-analysis of ten placebo-controlled trials confirmed the significant effect of oestrogens in the management of urogenital atrophy.

The route of administration was assessed and oral, vaginal and parenteral (transcutaneous patches and subcutaneous implants) were compared. Overall the vaginal route of administration was found to correlate with better symptom relief, greater improvement in cytological findings and higher serum E_2 levels.

With regard to the type of oestrogen preparation, E_2 was found to be most effective in reducing patient symptoms although conjugated oestrogens produced the most cytological change and the greatest increase in serum levels of E_2 and oestrone (E_1).

Finally, the effect of different dosages was examined. Low-dose vaginal E_2 was found to be the most efficacious according to symptom relief although oral E_3 was also effective; E_3 had no effect on the serum levels of E_2 or E_1 while vaginal E_3 had minimal effect. Vaginal E_2 was found to have a small effect on serum oestrogen although not as great as systemic preparations. In conclusion it would appear that oestrogen is efficacious in the treatment of urogenital atrophy and low-dose vaginal preparations are as effective as systemic therapy.

More recently, the use of a continuous low-dose E_2-releasing silicone vaginal ring (Estring) releasing E_2 (5–10 µg per day) has been investigated in postmenopausal women with symptomatic urogenital atrophy.[22] There was a significant effect on symptoms of vaginal dryness, pruritis vulvae, dyspareunia and urinary urgency with improvement being reported in over 90% of women in an uncontrolled study. The patient acceptability was high, and while the maturation of vaginal epithelium was significantly improved there was no effect on endometrial proliferation.

CONCLUSION

Oestrogens are known to have an important physiological effect on the female lower genital tract throughout adult life leading to symptomatic, histological and functional changes. Urogenital atrophy is the manifestation of oestrogen withdrawal following the menopause, presenting with vaginal and/or urinary symptoms. The use of ET has been examined in the management of lower urinary tract symptoms as well as in the treatment of urogenital atrophy although only recently has it been subjected to randomized placebo-controlled trials and meta-analysis.

ET alone has been shown to have little effect in the management of genuine stress incontinence although when used in combination with an α-adrenergic agonist may lead to an improvement in urinary leakage. When considering the irritating symptoms of urinary urgency, frequency and urgeincontinence, ET may be of benefit although this may simply represent a reversal of urogenital atrophy rather than a direct effect on the lower urinary tract. The role of ET in the management of women with recurrent lower UTI remains to be deteined although there is now some evidence that vaginaladministration may be efficacious. Finally, low-dose vaginal oestrogens have been shown to have a role in the treatment of urogenital atrophy in postmenopausal women and would appear to be as effective as systemic preparations.

References

1. Abrams P, Blaivas J G, Stanton S L et al 1990 The standardisation of terminology of lower urinary tract dysfunction. British Journal of Obstetrics and Gynaecology 97:1–16

2. Al-Badr A, Ross S, Soroka D et al 2003 What is the available evidence for hormone replacement therapy in women with stress urinary incontinence? Journal of Obstetrics and Gynaecology Canada 25:567–574

3. Batra S, Anderson K E 1989 Estrogen-induced changes in muscarinic receptor density and contractile responses in the female rat urinary bladder. Acta Physiologica Scandinavica 137:135–141

4. Batra S C, Fossil C S 1983 Female urethra: a target for estrogen action. The Journal of Urology 129:418–420

5. Batra S C, Iosif L S 1987 Progesterone receptors in the female urinary tract. The Journal of Urology 138:130–134

6. Beisland H O, Fossberg E, Moer A et al 1984 Urethral insufficiency in post-menopausal females: treatment with phenylpropanolamine and estriol separately and in combination. Urologia Internationalis 39:211–216

7. Benness C, Wise B G, Cutner A et al 1992 Does low-dose vaginal oestradiol improve frequency and urgency in postmenopausal women. International Urogynecology Journal 3:281

8. Bergman A, Karram M M, Bhatia N N 1990 Changes in urethral cytology following estrogen administration. Gynecologic and Obstetric Investigation 29:211–213

9. Bernstein I T 1997 The pelvic floor muscles: muscle thickness in healthy and urinary-incontinent women measured by perineal ultrasonography with reference to the effect of pelvic floor training. Oestrogen receptor studies. Neurourology and Urodynamics 16:237–275

10. Blakeman P J, Hilton P, Bulmer J N 1996 Mapping estrogen and progesterone receptors throughout the female lower urinary tract. Neurourology and Urodynamics 15:324–325

11. Boscia J A, Kaye D 1987 Asymptomatic bacteria in the elderly. Infectious Disease Clinics of North America 1:893–903

12. Brandberg A, Mellström D, Samsioe G 1987 Low-dose oral estriol treatment in elderly women with urogenital infections. Acta Obstetricia et Gynecologica Scandinavica 140:33–38

13. Burgio K L, Matthews K A, Engel B 1991 Prevalence, incidence and correlates of urinary incontinence in healthy, middle-aged women. The Journal of Urology 146:1255–1259

14. Caine M, Raz S 1973 The role of female hormones in stress incontinence. In: Proceedings of the 16th Congress of the International Society of Urology, Amsterdam, The Netherlands

15. Cardozo L D, Bachmann G, McClish D et al 1998 Meta-analysis of estrogen therapy in the management of urogenital atrophy in postmenopausal women. Second report of the Hormones and Urogenital Therapy Committee. Obstetrics and Gynecology 92:722–727

16. Cardozo L D, Benness C, Abbott D 1998 Low-dose oestrogen prophylaxis for recurrent urinary tract infections in elderly women. British Journal of Obstetrics and Gynaecology 105:403–407

17. Cardozo L D, Rekers H, Tapp A et al 1993 Oestriol in the treatment of postmeno-pausal urgency: a multicentre study. Maturitas 18:47–53

18. Cardozo L D, Tapp A, Versi E et al (eds) 1987 The lower urinary tract in peri- and postmenopausal women. In: The Urogenital Deficiency Syndrome. Novo Industri AS, Bagsverd, Denmark, p 10–17

19. Cardozo L D 1990 Role of oestrogens in the treatment of female urinary incontinence. Journal of the American Geriatrics Society 38:326–328

20. Chen G D, Oliver R H, Leung B S et al 1999 Estrogen receptor α and β expression in the vaginal walls and uterosacral ligaments of premenopausal and postmenopausal women. Fertility and Sterility 71:1099–1102

21. Elliott R A, Castleden C M, Miodrag A et al 1992 The direct effects of diethylstilboestrol and nifedipine on the contractile responses of isolated human and rat detrusor muscles. European Journal of Clinical Pharmacology 43:149–155

22. Eriksen B 1999 A randomised, open, parallel-group study on the preventive effect of an estradiol-releasing vaginal ring (Estring) on recurrent urinary tract infections in postmenopausal women. American Journal of Obstetrics and Gynecology 180:1072–1079

23. Eriksen P S, Rasmussen H 1992 Low dose 17β-estradiol vaginal tablets in the treatment of atrophic vaginitis: a double-blind placebo-controlled study. European Journal of Obstetrics, Gynecology, and Reproductive Biology 44:137–144

24. Falconer C, Ekman-Ordeberg G, Ulmsten U et al 1996 Changes in paraurethral connective tissue at menopause are counteracted by oestrogen. Maturitas 24:197–204

25. Fantl J A, Wyman J F, Anderson R L et al 1988 Postmenopausal urinary incontinence: comparison between non-estrogen and estrogen supplemented women. Obstetrics and Gynecology 71:823–828

26. Fantl J A, Bump R C, Robinson D et al 1996 Efficacy of estrogen supplementation in the treatment of urinary incontinence. Obstetrics and Gynecology 88:745–749

27. Fantl J A, Cardozo L D, McClish D K and the Hormones and Urogenital Therapy Committee 1994 Estrogen therapy in the management of incontinence in postmenopausal women: a meta-analysis. First report of the Hormones and Urogenital Therapy Committee. Obstetrics and Gynecology 83:12–18

28. Gangar K F, Vyas S, Whitehead R W et al 1991 Pulsatility index in the internal carotid artery in relation to transdermal oestradiol and time since the menopause. The Lancet 338:839–842

29. Grady D, Brown J S, Vittinghoff E et al 2001 Postmenopausal hormones and incontinence: the Heart and Estrogen/progestin Replacement Study. Obstetrics and Gynecology 97:116–120

30. Green S, Walter P, Kumar V et al 1986 Human estrogen receptor cDNA: sequence, expression and homology to v-erbA. Nature 320:134–139

31. Grodstein F, Lifford K, Resnick N M et al 2004 Postmenopausal hormone therapy and risk of developing urinary incontinence. Obstetrics and Gynecology 103:254–260

32. Henalla S M, Hutchins C J, Robinson P et al 1989 Non-operative methods in the treatment of female genuine stress incontinence of urine. British Journal of Obstetrics and Gynaecology 9:222–225

33. Hextall A, Bidmead J, Cardozo L et al 1999 Hormonal influences on the human female lower urinary tract: a prospective evaluation of the effects of the menstrual cycle on symptomatology and the results of urodynamic investigation. Neurourology and Urodynamics 18:282–283

34. Hilton P, Tweddel A L, Mayne C 1990 Oral and intravaginal estrogens alone and in combination with alpha adrenergic stimulation in genuine stress incontinence. International Urogynecology Journal 12:80–86

35. Ingelman-Sundberg A, Rosen J, Gustafsson S A 1981 Cytosol oestrogen receptors in urogenital tissues in stress incontinent women. Acta Obstetricia et Gynecologica Scandinavica 60:585–586

36. Iosif C, Bekassy Z 1984 Prevalence of genitourinary symptoms in the late menopause. Acta Obstetricia et Gynecologica Scandinavica 63:257–260

37. Iosif S, Batra S, Ek A et al 1981 Oestrogens receptors in the human female lower urinary tract. American Journal of Obstetrics and Gynecology 141:817–820

38. Jackson S, Avery N, Shepherd A et al 1996 The effect of estradiol on vaginal collagen in postmenopausal women with stress urinary incontinence. Neurourology and Urodynamics 15:327–328

39. Jackson S, Shepherd A, Brookes S et al 1999 The effect of estrogen supplementation on post-menopausal urinary stress incontinence: a double-blind, placebo-controlled trial. British Journal of Obstetrics and Gynaecology 106:711–718

40. Jolleys J 1988. Reported prevalence of urinary incontinence in a general practice. British Medical Journal 296:1300–1302

41. Kinn A C, Lindskog M 1988 Estrogens and phenylpropanolamine in combination

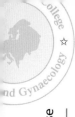

for stress incontinence. Urology 32:273–280

42. Kirkengen A L, Anderson P, Gjersoe E et al 1992 Estriol in the prophylactic treatment of recurrent urinary tract infections in postmenopausal women. Scandinavian Journal of Primary Health Care 10:142

43. Kjaergaard B, Walter S, Knudsen A et al 1990 Treatment with low-dose vaginal oestradiol in postmenopausal women. A double-blind controlled trial. Ugeskrift for Laeger 152:658–659

44. Kondo A, Kato K, Saito M et al 1990 Prevalence of hand washing incontinence in females in comparison with stress and urge incontinence. Neurourology and Urodynamics 9:330–331

45. Kuiper G, Enmark E, Pelto-Huikko M et al 1996 Cloning of a novel estrogen receptor expressed in rat prostate and ovary. Proceedings of the National Academy of Sciences of the USA 93:5925–5930

46. Kushner L, Chen Y, Desautel M et al 1999 Collagenase activity is elevated in conditioned media from fibroblasts of women with pelvic floor weakening. International Urogynecology Journal 10(S1):34

47. Maggi A, Perez J 1985 Role of female gonadal hormones in the CNS. Life Sciences 37:893–906

48. Malone-Lee J 1988 Urodynamic measurement and urinary incontinence in the elderly. In: Brocklehurst J C (ed) Managing and Measuring Incontinence. Proceedings of the Geriatric Workshop on Incontinence, July (Geriatric Medicine)

49. Mettler L, Olsen P G 1991 Long-term treatment of atrophic vaginitis with low-dose oestradiol vaginal tablets. Maturitas 14:23–31

50. Moehrer B, Hextall A, Jackson S 2003 Oestrogens for urinary incontinence in women. Cochrane Database of Systematic Reviews. Issue 2. CD001405. Article number DOI:10.1002/14651858

51. Ouslander J G, Greendale G A, Uman G et al 2001 Effects of oral estrogen and progestin on the lower urinary tract among female nursing home residents. Journal of the American Geriatrics Society 49:803–807

52. Pang X, Cotreau-Bibbo M M, Sant G R et al 1995 Bladder mast cell expression of high-affinity oestrogen receptors in patients with interstitial cystitis. British Journal of Urology 75:154–161

53. Parsons C L, Schmidt J D 1982 Control of recurrent urinary tract infections in postmenopausal women. The Journal of Urology 128:1224–1226

54. Penotti M, Farina M, Sironi L et al 1997 Long-term effects of postmenopausal hormone replacement therapy on pulsatility index of the internal carotid and middle cerebral arteries. Menopause 4:101–104

55. Privette M, Cade R, Peterson J et al 1988 Prevention of recurrent urinary tract infections in postmenopausal women. Nephron 50:24–27

56. Raz R, Stamm W E 1993 A controlled trial of intravaginal estriol in postmenopausal women with recurrent urinary tract infections. The New England Journal of Medicine 329:753–756

57. Rud T, Anderson K E, Asmussen M et al 1980 Factors maintaining the urethral pressure in women. Investigative Urology 17:343–347

58. Rud T 1980 The effects of estrogens and gestagens on the urethral pressure profile in urinary continent and stress incontinent women. Acta Obstetricia et Gynecologica Scandinavica 59:265–270

59. Salmon U L, Walter R I, Gast S H 1941 The use of estrogen in the treatment of dysuria and incontinence in postmenopausal women. American Journal of Obstetrics and Gynecology 14:23–31

60. Samsioe G 1998 Urogenital ageing – a hidden problem. American Journal of Obstetrics and Gynecology 178:S245–S249

61. Samsioe G, Jansson I, Mellström D et al 1985 Urinary incontinence in 75-year-old women. Effects of estriol. Acta Obstetricia et Gynecologica Scandinavica 93 (Suppl):57

62. Samsioe G, Jansson I, Mellström D et al 1985 Occurrence, nature and treatment of urinary incontinence in a 70-year-old female population. Maturitas 7:335–342

63. Sanford J P 1975 Urinary tract symptoms and infection. Annual Reviews of Medicine 26:485–505

64. Screiter F, Fuchs P, Stockamp K 1976 Estrogenic sensitivity of α–receptors in the urethral musculature. Urologia Internationalis 31:13–19

65. Shapiro E 1986 Effect of estrogens on the weight and muscarinic receptor density of the rabbit bladder and urethra. The Journal of Urology 135:1084–1087

66. Shenfield O Z, Blackmore P F, Morgan C W et al 1998 Rapid effects of estriol and progesterone on tone and spontaneous

rhythmic contractions of the rabbit bladder. Neurourology and Urodynamics 17:408–409

67. Smith P, Heimer G, Lindskog M et al 1993 Oestradiol-releasing vaginal ring for treatment of postmenopausal urogenital atrophy. Maturitas 16:145–154

68. Smith P 1993 Estrogens and the urogenital tract. Acta Obstetricia et Gynecologica Scandinavica 72:1–26

69. Smith P J B 1976 The effect of oestrogens on bladder function in the female. In: Campbell S (ed) The Management of the Menopause and Postmenopausal Years. MTP, Carnforth, p 291–298

70. Smith R J N, Studd J W W 1993 Recent advances in hormone replacement therapy. British Journal of Hospital Medicine 49:799–809

71. Smith S S, Berg G, Hammar M (eds) 1993 The modern management of the menopause. Hormones, mood and neurobiology – a summary. Parthenon Publishing, Carnforth, Lancs., UK, p 204

72. Sultana C J, Walters M D 1995 Oestrogen and urinary incontinence in women. Maturitas 20:129–138

73. Thomas T M, Plymat K R, Blannin J et al 1980 Prevalence of urinary incontinence. British Medical Journal 281:1243–1245

74. Van Geelen J M, Doesburg W H, Thomas C M G 1981 Urodynamic studies in the normal menstrual cycle: the relationship between hormonal changes during the menstrual cycle and the urethral pressure profile. American Journal of Obstetrics and Gynecology 141:384–392

75. Versi E, Cardozo L D 1988 Estrogens and lower urinary tract function. In: Studd J W W, Whitehead M I (eds) The Menopause. Blackwell Scientific, Oxford, p 76–84

76. Versi E, Cardozo L D 1986 Urethral instability: diagnosis based on variations in the maximum urethral pressure in normal climacteric women. Neurourology and Urodynamics 5:535–541

77. Walter S, Wolf H, Barlebo H et al 1978 Urinary incontinence in postmenopausal women treated with oestrogens: a double-blind clinical trial. Urologia Internationalis 33:135–143

78. Wilson P D, Faragher B, Butler B et al 1987 Treatment with oral piperazine oestrone sulphate for genuine stress incontinence in postmenopausal women. British Journal of Obstetrics and Gynaecology 94:568–574

79. Youngblood V H, Tomlin E M, Davis J B 1957 Senile urethritis in women. The Journal of Urology 78:150–152

80. Zullo M A, Oliva C, Falconi G et al 1998 Efficacy of estrogen therapy in urinary incontinence. A meta-analytic study. Minerva Ginecologica 50:199–205

16

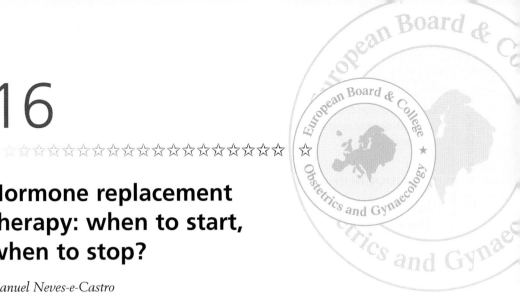

Hormone replacement therapy: when to start, when to stop?

Manuel Neves-e-Castro

ABSTRACT

Hormone replacement therapy (HRT) is the administration of hormones to individuals who, under normal conditions, should have them in circulation within a normal range. Concerning sex steroid hormones, the administration of oestrogens (with or without associated progestin) is an HRT in cases of ovarian agenesis, surgically induced or naturally occurring premature menopause.

Many postmenopausal women complain of vasomotor symptoms and atrophic changes of the genital tract which are due to oestrogen deficiency; treatment with systemic or local oestrogen is highly effective for treating those symptoms and signs. Under such circumstances oestrogens are being used as a specific treatment, as with any other drug. They are not aimed at restoring the plasma levels of the reproductive years – they are designed for the specific treatment of conditions that are due to their deprivation from the body.

Treatment should go on as long as it is needed, provided it is well-monitored for side-effects and there are no previous or new contraindications, e.g. a newly diagnosed breast cancer, deep vein thrombosis, etc. The doses should be adapted, from time to time, to determine if they are still needed.

True HRT is to be started as soon as the condition is present: an ovarian agenesis or surgically or prematurely occurring amenorrhoea before the age of the normal spontaneous menopause. For how long? Definitely until the age of 50–55 years, just as under normal conditions, after which decisions will be made whether to continue or to change to alternative treatments.

Therefore, it seems that the earlier a postmenopausal hormonal treatment, or an HRT, is started, the better protected will be the vascular endothelium, bone and the central nervous system (CNS).

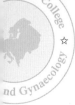

KEYWORDS

Cardiovascular disease prevention, central nervous system (CNS) disease prevention, hormone replacement therapy (HRT), hormone treatment, menopause

INTRODUCTION

Hormone replacement therapy (HRT) is the administration of hormones to individuals who, under normal conditions, should have them in circulation within a normal range. A typical example is type 1 diabetes, a disease characterized by a lack of insulin. Thus the administration of insulin is a hormone therapy in order to equilibrate the metabolic disturbances of such patients. The same applies to Addison's disease and hypothyroidism when cortisone or thyroxine are, respectively, administered.

EARLY MENOPAUSE

Concerning sex steroid hormones, the administration of oestrogens (with or without associated progestogen) is an HRT in cases of ovarian agenesis, surgically induced or naturally occurring premature menopause. Women should not be deprived of oestrogens when, under normal conditions, they should have higher plasma levels. These are the only cases when the administration of sex steroid hormone is replacing what should be in circulation. Thus, this is a true HRT.

NATURAL MENOPAUSE

However, after naturally occurring menopause, at around 50 years of age, what is normal is that both the exocrine and endocrine functions of the ovaries have come to an end. Despite the fact that some postmenopausal ovaries may still have a small secretion of oestrogens and androgens, the resulting plasma levels are definitely below what is found during reproductive years.

Many postmenopausal women complain of vasomotor symptoms and atrophic changes of the genital tract, which are due to oestrogen deficiency; treatment with systemic or local oestrogen is highly effective to treat those symptoms and signs. Under such circumstances oestrogens are being used as a specific treatment, as with any other drug. They are not aimed at restoring the plasma levels of the reproductive years. They are designed for the specific treatment of conditions which are due to their deprivation from the body.

This explanation may seem semantic but it is not. If one continues to accept HRT as the correct designation after the natural menopause then it may be equivalent to an obligation to 'replace' all women. Those who were not given the HRT would feel underprivileged. This is also important in order to differentiate symptomatic treatments from preventive treatments (primary and secondary).

There is no doubt that oestrogens are the best medication for relieving vaso-motor symptoms and atrophic changes of the genital tract at dose levels that are below those of the reproductive years.

Treatment should go on as long as it is needed, provided it is well-monitored for side-effects and there are no previous or new contraindications, e.g. a newly diagnosed breast cancer, deep vein thrombosis, etc. The doses should be adapted, from time to time, to determine if they are still needed.

HORMONE REPLACEMENT THERAPY FOR THE PREVENTION OF DISEASE

The other possible indication for a treatment with oestrogens after natural menopause would be for the primary prevention of cardiovascular diseases, osteoporosis, CNS disturbances, etc. After the recent epidemiological studies – the Heart and Estrogen/progestin Replacement Study (HERS)[2] and the Women's Health Initiative (WHI)[7] – the secondary prevention of such diseases is con-traindicated. However, those studies have shown that long-term oestrogen treat-ment could prevent bone fractures and colon cancer.

Then the question is: could or should HRT, be given to prevent cardiovascu-lar diseases, osteoporosis, colon cancer and CNS dysfunctions?

Extensive experimental studies in female monkeys have clearly demon-strated that if oestrogens are replaced early after castration, when the vascular endothelium is still intact, the subsequent administration of an atherogenic diet has a much weaker effect in the development of atheromatous plaques than would be observed if it is given during an oestrogen-depleted state.[4] Fur-thermore, it was also observed that the administration of oestrogens in mon-keys who had already developed a diet-induced atherosclerosis would neither be effective in terms of secondary prevention nor devoid of vascular negative side-effects.

This is precisely what was observed in the HERS and WHI trials, since most selected women were of an age when spontaneous atherosclerotic lesions were already very likely to be present. Thus, the occurrence of cardiovascular events was likely to be expected, as shown in the monkey model.

ALTERNATIVES TO OESTROGENS

Today, luckily, for the prevention of cardiovascular diseases, osteoporosis and colon cancer, one has access to very potent and specific drugs and strategies, such as the statin family, platelet anti-aggregants, bisphosphonates, SERMs, tibolone, a Mediterranean diet, exercise, etc. They are obligatory for disease prevention after the menopause, with or without the addition of oestrogens if indicated, and not contraindicated. It was concluded that postmenopausal women on HRT had fewer cardiovascular events if a statin was administered concomitantly.[1,3]

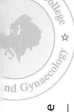
CONCLUSION

HORMONE REPLACEMENT THERAPY: WHEN TO START, WHEN TO STOP?

True HRT should be started as soon as the condition is presented: an ovarian agenesis, or surgically or prematurely occurring amenorrhoea before the age of normal spontaneous menopause. But for how long? Definitely until the age of 50–55 years, just as with normal conditions, after which decisions will be made as to whether to continue or to change to alternative treatments.

HRTs, after naturally occurring menopause around the age of 50, are to be started, if there is no contraindication, as soon as symptoms justify it, for as long as necessary and with proper monitoring. In the early postmenopause an oestrogen plus progestogen (E + P) sequential regimen (CSHRT) (or oestrogens alone on hysterectomized women) is to be preferred. Later, one may follow-up with low-dose continuous combined E + P (CCHRT) or with tibolone. SERMs are preferably used in the late postmenopause if indicated.

HORMONE REPLACEMENT THERAPY: FOR HOW LONG?

Again, proper monitoring of the response of the initial objective/targets is mandatory. The need for symptom relief should be assessed at regular intervals in an attempt to reduce the doses up to the point of concluding that HRT may no longer be needed for such an indication. If this is the case, then the question is to decide if HRT should go on for primary preventive purposes. This should be carefully discussed in comparison with other nonhormonal medications and non-drug-related interventions.

For the cardiovascular system and bone it is likely that HRTs are not indispensable or superior to other medicines. As for the CNS, the question is still unanswered. Oestrogens, at present, are the only molecules with a nerve growth effect; no other substances have been found to have such properties. They act at several levels of the brain as neurotransmitters. They can also prevent experimentally induced cerebral lesions. The recent conclusions of the WHI (on dementia showing a higher incidence of Alzheimer's in the hormone-treated group as compared with placebo) may also reflect, as in the cardiovascular studies, that healthy neurones can be protected by oestrogens and that already damaged brain nerve cells can be further altered by oestrogens.

Therefore it seems that the earlier a postmenopausal HRT is started the better it is at protecting the vascular endothelium, bone and the CNS.[5] HRTs are very good but treatments without hormones can be equally good for women's health. 'Preventing a woman from the benefits of a postmenopausal HRT because of the fear of rare side-effects does not seem to be satisfactory medicine'.[6] What is important is to know how to practice good medicine.

References

1. Herrington D M, Klein K P 2003 Randomized clinical trials of hormone replacement therapy for treatment or prevention of cardiovascular disease: a review of the findings. Atherosclerosis 166:203–212

2. Herrington D M, Vittinghoff E, Lin F et al 2002 Statin therapy, cardiovascular events, and total mortality in the Heart and Estrogen/progestin Replacement Study (HERS). Circulation 105:2962–2967

3. Hulley S, Grady D, Bush T et al 1998 Randomized trial of estrogen plus progestin for secondary prevention of coronary heart disease in postmenopausal women. Heart and Estrogen/progestin Replacement Study (HERS) Research Group. The Journal of the American Medical Association 180:605–613

4. Mikkola T, Clarkson T 2002 Estrogen replacement therapy, atherosclerosis, and vascular function. Cardiovascular Research 53:605–619

5. Neves-e-Castro M 2003 Menopause in crisis post-Women's Health Initiative? A view based on personal clinical experience. Human Reproduction 180:1–7

6. Neves-e-Castro M 2002 Is there a menopausal medicine? The past, the present and the future. Maturitas 43:S79–S84

7. Rossouw J E, Anderson G L, Prentice R L et al 2002 Risks and benefits of estrogens plus progestin in healthy postmenopausal women: principal results from the Women's Health Initiative randomized controlled trial. The Journal of the American Medical Association 288:321–333

Hormone replacement therapy: when to start, when to stop?

17

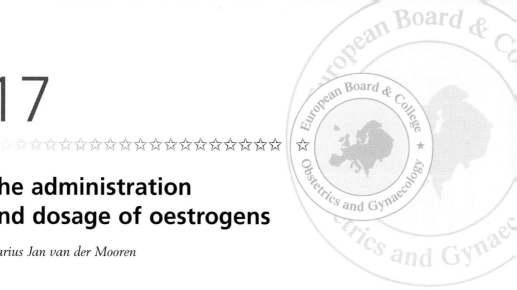

The administration and dosage of oestrogens

Marius Jan van der Mooren

ABSTRACT

A major misconception introduced by many scientific papers is that postmenopausal oestrogen therapy (ET) is just one therapeutic entity, regardless of its
dosage, its route of administration, and whether or not it is combined with a
progestogen. The controversies that have arisen in recent years regarding
postmenopausal hormone use appear largely related to the fact that high
hormone dosages as used in elderly women were not representative of the
patients we usually treat in our practice.

    This chapter illustrates that lowering the oestrogen dosage, and in specific
patients using non-oral routes of administration, will improve the benefit/risk
ratio.

    Therefore, in general, doctors should prescribe the lowest effective oestrogen
dosage and give it in the route of administration and for the duration that best
fits the woman's personal risk profile as well as her preferences.

KEYWORDS

Dosage, intranasal, oestrogen, oral, transdermal

INTRODUCTION

Postmenopausal ET is most effective in the treatment of vasomotor symptoms
as well as other oestrogen deficiency complaints.[15] It has also been shown to
help prevent chronic diseases such as osteoporosis.[1] The role of ET as a preventive strategy for coronary heart disease (CHD), Alzheimer's disease and cognitive function is currently under debate.[12,22] Contrary to these benefits of ET,
several disadvantages are known, and these may substantially limit patients' as

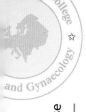

well as doctors' willingness to start or continue its use. Well-known disadvantages are unwanted side-effects such as [ir]regular vaginal bleeding, breast tenderness, fluid retention, nausea, headaches and bloating. Risks associated with ET are endometrial carcinoma (if unopposed oestrogen is given to nonhysterectomized women), venous thromboembolism (VTE), stroke, breast cancer and possibly ovarian cancer.[6,9,19] Excess risk of CHD, shortly after the initiation of treatment, should also be considered as a potential hazard. This chapter will discuss the influence of lower dosages and non-oral routes of oestrogen administration on balance between the benefits and potential disadvantages of postmenopausal ET.

DOSAGES

ET for climacteric complaints became popular in the 1960s but then it was very common to treat women with relatively high doses of 2.5 mg or more of oral conjugated equine oestrogens (CEE). However, since then there has been a trend toward lower oestrogen doses (Table 17.1). In general, one may expect that lowering the oestrogen dosage will reduce unwanted effects, but that it may also impair the effectiveness of symptom relief and preventing bone resorption. These two consequences of lowering the oestrogen dosage do not appear to run parallel.

ROUTES OF ADMINISTRATION

For decades, oral ET with (relatively) high oestrogen dosages has been the most widely used route of administration. As alternatives, subcutaneous and i.m. administrations were also available. Since the 1980s new forms of application, such as patches, gels, nasal spray, vaginal rings and tablets, have become available (Table 17.2). One of the main differences between oral and all non-oral forms of oestrogen administration is the avoidance of the hepatic first-pass effect. Orally

Table 17.1 Oral oestrogen formulations

Type	Daily dosage (mg)
Conjugated oestrogens	0.3, 0.625, 0.9, 1.25, 2.5
Esterified oestrogens	0.3, 0.625, 1.25, 2.5
Estropipate	0.75, 1.5
Micronized oestradiol	0.5, 1, 2, 4
Oestradiol valerate	1, 2
Oestriol	1, 2
Other	
Tibolone	2.5

Table 17.2 Non-oral oestrogen formulations

Route	Dosage (mg)[a]
Transdermal	
oestradiol gel	1
oestradiol patch	0.025, 0.0375, 0.05, 0.075, 0,1
Intranasal	
oestradiol spray	0.150 mg per puff
Subcutaneous	
oestradiol implant	20 mg per tablet every 4–8 months
Intramuscular	
oestradiol valerate depot	10 mg per depot every 2 weeks
Vaginal	
conjugated oestrogens creme	0.625 mg
dienoestriol creme	0.5 mg
oestradiol ring	2 mg per ring every 3 months
oestradiol tablet	0.025 mg
oestriol creme	0.5 mg
oestriol ovule	0.5 mg

[a] Daily dosage unless indicated otherwise.

administered oestrogens are largely metabolized by the liver to oestrone conjugates and excreted in the bile. Therefore, relatively high dosages are needed to obtain clinically relevant serum oestradiol concentrations. The hepatic exposure to oestrogens induces many metabolic effects, such as changes in concentrations of (sex hormone-) binding globulins, precursor proteins (e.g. angiotensinogen), lipids and lipoproteins, haemostatic and fibrinolytic factors, glucose and insulin, and probably of homocysteine. Non-orally administered oestrogens have a much lesser impact on hepatic metabolism but effects have also been reported after longer exposures. Another aspect of alternative routes of administration is the frequency of administration. Oral therapy is taken once daily, whereas for non-oral routes the frequency varies from once daily (transdermal gel, nasal spray) to once or twice weekly (transdermal patch) or even once every 4–8 months (subcutaneous implants). An important role of the route of administration is the impact on the woman's satisfaction – women may have their own personal preferences for a specific route of administration. So, with the ability to satisfy personal preferences, women's adherence to the treatment may be improved.

VASOMOTOR AND UROGENITAL SYMPTOMS

For the treatment of vasomotor symptoms, oral dosages of 2 mg 17β-oestradiol and 1.25 mg CEE have been shown to be equally effective, and the same was found for 1 mg 17β-oestradiol and 0.625 mg CEE.[3] The maximum effect is reached within 4–6 weeks with the higher dosages, whereas lowering the dosage from, for example, 2 to 1 mg 17β-oestradiol will result in 10–15% less effect but also more time needed to reach the maximum effect. Furthermore, one has to consider the very large interindividual as well as intra-individual bioavailability of one dose of oestrogen, meaning that a low dosage for one woman may be more effective than a high dosage for another. In general, starting with a low dosage may very well be sufficiently effective in vasomotor symptom relief with less chance of side-effects, and one can always increase the dosage in individual cases if indicated (Fig. 17.1).[24] Also, almost any route of administration can be used for the treatment of vasomotor symptoms as long as adequate serum oestrogen levels (comparable with the early follicular phase of the menstrual cycle) are achieved. Most of the presently marketed oestrogen preparations are available in different dosages and some are also available in combination with a progestogen.

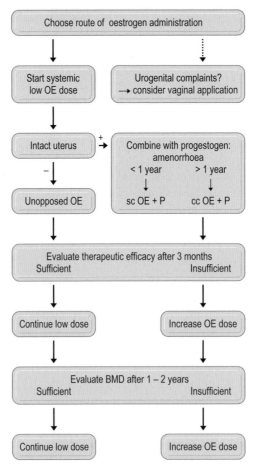

Fig 17.1 Flowchart postmenopausal hormone therapy. BMD, Bone mineral density; cc, continuous combined; E, oestrogen; P, progestogen; sc, sequential combined.

Urogenital symptoms may well respond to low-dose systemic oestrogen treatment but in the case of unsatisfactory improvement of symptoms it is recommended either to increase the systemic dosage, e.g. in the presence of unsatisfactory relief of vasomotor symptoms, or to combine systemic treatment with a vaginal application of oestrogens. In cases of urogenital complaints only, vaginal oestrogen treatment is a rational alternative to systemic treatment.

OSTEOPOROSIS

Since the first publication of the results of the Women's Health Initiative (WHI) trial, there is no longer any reason to doubt the effectiveness of ET to prevent osteoporotic fractures.[1] The reduction in such fractures is confirmed by the preventive effects of systemic ET on postmenopausal bone mineral density (BMD) loss. Therefore, even in the absence of large randomized controlled trials investigating fractures during other hormone formulations and other routes of administration, one may consider BMD studies quite reliable in predicting population-based preventive effects of such therapies.

Lower systemic oestrogen dosages may be less potent in preventing osteoporotic fractures. However, from dose-response BMD studies it appears that there is no proportional relation. Oral 17β-oestradiol 1 mg and 2 mg were comparable in their increasing BMD effects on the lumbar spine and femoral neck.[9] The oldest women showed the greatest treatment response with low oestrogen dosages. So, also from the point of osteoporosis prevention there is no absolute need to start with a high dosage. However, with lower dosages the percentage of nonresponders may be slightly higher. Therefore, it is recommended that the clinician follows up bone densitometry measurements to monitor the effectiveness of especially low-dose treatment in high-risk women (see Fig. 17.1).

No large, randomized, controlled trials have been carried out to study osteoporotic fractures and non-oral oestrogen treatments, but BMD studies have shown that the effects of, for example, transdermal patches on the prevention of bone resorption in postmenopausal women are comparable with oral oestrogen administration.[8] So, obviously the route of oestrogen administration is of much less concern than the dosage when considering the need for follow-up BMD investigations in women at risk of osteoporotic fractures.

COLON CANCER

With respect to colon cancer, results from observational studies have recently been confirmed by the WHI trial showing a risk reduction of 37% in women using postmenopausal HRT.[20] These studies were all using CEE (in combination with medroxyprogesterone acetate, MPA) and results may therefore not be equal for other oestrogenic compounds. At present no data are available on the impact of lower oestrogen dosages or non-oral routes of oestrogen administration on colon cancer risk.

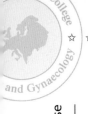
CORONARY ARTERY DISEASE

For many years, a vast amount of evidence, based on observational studies, as well as on cardiovascular disease (CVD) surrogate end-point and animal studies, was reason to believe that postmenopausal ET could prevent CHD, especially in high-risk women. The Heart and Estrogen/progestin Replacement Study (HERS) and the WHI trial have shown that elderly women, either with established CHD or apparently healthy, are not protected from a (recurrent) cardiovascular event and may even be put at risk early after the initiation of HRT, when treated with oral CEE 0.625 mg plus MPA 2.5 mg daily.[12,20] Since the publications of these negative results, postmenopausal HRT is considered not indicated for the prevention of CHD only. Presently, there still is much debate whether or not these results can be extrapolated to younger and healthier women, and if lower oestrogen dosages or non-oral oestrogen administration may be safer or even protective. Also, the introduction of MPA to the observed cardiovascular event rate is unclear. Interestingly, in the oestrogen-only WHI trial, evidence was found that unopposed ET does not increase coronary risk and may be protective in women between 50 and 60 years of age.[1]

In contrast to the randomized controlled trials, the observational Nurses' Health Study reported a comparable reduction of CHD events in relatively young women treated with 0.3 mg CEE (–42%) when compared with 0.625 mg CEE (–46%).[10] No large randomized controlled trials investigating clinical cardiovascular end-points during low-dose ET are yet available. However, small studies indicate that lower oestrogen dosages may be safe or even protective. The Women's Hormone Intervention Secondary Prevention (WHISP) pilot study indicated that less CVD-related events may occur during one year's treatment with 1 mg 17β-oestradiol plus 0.5 mg norethisterone (norethindrone) acetate in women who have suffered an acute myocardial infarction.[7] Furthermore, CVD surrogate end-point studies have shown that lowering the oestrogen dosage may maintain effects related to risk reduction, whereas it may attenuate unfavourable effects related to an increased risk.[11,14,17,18,23]

With lower oestrogen dosages the direction of changes in lipids and lipoproteins are comparable with the standard dosage.[11] Also, the lipoprotein(a) concentration, a factor with both atherogenic as well as thrombogenic properties, is reduced by low-dose therapy.[11] In comparison with 2 mg oestradiol combinations, which are known to impair the procoagulant–anticoagulant balance, a 1 mg oestradiol combination resulted in a null effect toward a potential anticoagulant effect.[14,18,25] Reductions in homocysteine observed during 1 mg oestradiol were almost comparable with 2 mg oestradiol.[23] C-reactive protein (CRP), an inflammation factor and independent risk factor for CVD, is increased more than three times during orally administered 2 mg oestradiol whereas the increase during 1 mg oestradiol was less.[17] However, the role of progestogens when combined with oestrogen, and the route of oestrogen administration, appear to be more important in modulating the oestrogenic effect on CRP concentrations. Future studies should clarify the clinical relevance of changes in CRP concentrations during HRT. Endothelial function, as assessed by ultrasound parameters as well as plasma markers, appears to be influenced beneficially by standard oestrogen dosages as well as by lower dosages. Oral ET appears not to influence glucose metabolism although it may induce a slight improvement in insulin sensitivity, both by standard and low-dose therapies.

As indicated above, one of the main differences between the various routes of oestrogen administration is the impact on liver metabolism, and therefore especially on metabolic and haemostatic risk factors for CVD. In general, one can make a distinction between oral and non-oral administration although this may be too simplistic. Due to avoiding hepatic first-pass effects, non-oral treatments will expose the liver less, resulting in fewer or no changes in the synthesis or clearance of proteins involved in, for example, lipid metabolism and coagulation.

Non-oral oestrogen administration also results in decreased levels of total and low-density lipoprotein cholesterol.[11] Lipoprotein(a) levels decrease, as well during non-oral therapy,[11] whereas high-density lipoprotein cholesterol and triglyceride levels are usually unchanged.[11] Homocysteine levels are not affected by transdermal oestrogen administration;[23] also, coagulation factors are not or only slightly affected.[18] C-reactive protein is another important risk factor that is not influenced by transdermal ET, in contrast to the observed increases during oral administration.[17] The effects of the different routes of oestrogen administration on CVD surrogate end-points sometimes contradict each other, and therefore any interpretation remains complicated. These effects may prove to be of particular importance to explain clinical observations. Knowledge of these effects may be helpful in therapeutic decisions in individual patients, especially in those with metabolic abnormalities.

Despite the potential cardiovascular benefit of non-oral oestrogen administration, as suggested by surrogate end-point studies, the Papworth HRT Atherosclerosis Study in elderly women with established CHD who were treated with transdermal oestradiol 80 μg daily, reported negative results similar to HERS.[5] The relatively high oestradiol dosage could be an explanation for the observed overall null-effect and the early excess risk in this study.

ALZHEIMER'S DISEASE

The role of menopause and ET in Alzheimer's disease is still unclear. Although it was suggested that oestrogen deficiency may cause memory loss after menopause, this was not supported by data from the Rancho Bernardo Study. On the other hand, studies on specific cognitive functions, such as verbal memory, have demonstrated improvements during ET, and therefore are suggestive for a protective role of oestrogen. The recent Women's Health Initiative Memory Study (WHIMS) data, however, do not support a preventive effect of ET on Alzheimer's disease or cognitive function.[22] Nevertheless, one has to consider that the effects observed in the elderly women studied in WHIMS should not be extrapolated to younger early menopausal women or to women treated with

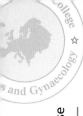

oestrogens in lower dosages or by non-oral routes of administration. Therefore, it is not possible to speculate on the effects of low oestrogen dosages or non-oral routes of oestrogen administration on Alzheimer's disease or cognitive function.

UNWANTED EFFECTS

SIDE-EFFECTS

Oestrogen-related side-effects such as [ir]regular vaginal bleeding, breast tenderness, fluid retention, nausea, headaches and bloating are less frequent and less severe when lowering the oestrogen dosage. Side-effects specifically related to the route of administration, e.g. skin irritation by a patch, can be solved by changing to another patch with other adhesive characteristics or to another route of administration.

BLEEDING

Irregular as well as scheduled bleeding episodes are an annoyance for many women on HRT. Bleeding is influenced by progestogen administration and oestrogen dosage; lowering the dosage reduces the incidence of bleeding in sequential and continuous combined regimens.[2] No specific differences in respect to the various routes of administration are reported for bleeding.

ENDOMETRIAL CANCER

Large meta-analyses have shown that the risk of endometrial cancer associated with unopposed ET is dose-dependent, and that even systemic treatment with low-dose and weak oestrogens, such as oestriol, may induce endometrial cancer.[9] For systemic treatment, the route of oestrogen administration does not influence endometrial cancer risk, whereas no increased risk has been reported in relation to the vaginal application of low-dose oestrogens.

VENOUS THROMBOEMBOLISM

Only a few studies have addressed the effect of lower oestrogen dosages on the risk of VTE. Observational studies have indicated a dose dependency, and plasma markers indicate that lowering the oestrogen dosage may attenuate the unfavourable effects of oral HRT on the procoagulant–anticoagulant balance.[14,18] Recently, resistance to activated protein C, one of the major risk factors for VTE, was found to increase only modestly during transdermal oestrogen administration, in contrast with a 100% increase during oral ET.[16] Such observations do fit well with the clinical observations performed by Scarabin et al who also observed less risk for VTE in women treated with transdermal oestrogen in comparison with oral administration.[21] These observations could be particularly important for women at risk of VTE.

STROKE

The Nurses' Health Study showed an increased risk of stroke during 0.625 mg CEE, which was confirmed by the WHI trial.[1,10] However, the Nurses' Health Study also showed that 0.3 mg CEE reduced stroke risk non-significantly.[10] No specific differences in respect to the various routes of administration are reported for stroke risk.

CORONARY HEART DISEASE

Coronary heart disease might have to be listed as a potential risk in specific populations as the HERS and WHI trials showed an early excess risk in elderly women with established CHD as well as in women with and without one or more CHD risk factors.[1,12,20] As described above, lower oestrogen dosages have been suggested to be less harmful but this needs to be studied more extensively.[10] The same uncertainty exists concerning the non-oral route of oestrogen administration, especially since the Papworth HRT Atherosclerosis Study showed the same negative results as HERS.[5]

BREAST CANCER

Little is known about the effect of lowering the oestrogen dosage on breast cancer risk. It was suggested that due to local oestrogen metabolism in the breast, tissue oestradiol levels are much higher than serum concentrations, and that therefore no relevant effects can be expected from lowering oestrogen dosages.[4] It has been suggested that weak oestrogens, such as oestriol, and that vaginal application of oestrogens, may not be associated with an increased breast cancer risk. However, there are no data to confirm this.

OVARIAN CANCER

In observational studies, the very long-term administration of postmenopausal HRT has been associated with ovarian cancer.[19] The implications of lower oestrogen dosages and non-oral oestrogen administration are not known.

PERSONAL PREFERENCE

The woman's personal opinion and preference obviously play an important role in menopausal care as she is the only one who will ultimately decide whether to start and continue treatment. Based on the information the woman gets from her friends, the media and her doctor, it is up to her to make these decisions. She should have the opportunity to decide on a specific route of administration, and to have a choice about changing the oestrogen dosage if she feels this may improve her balance between benefits and disadvantages. The woman's benefit/risk profile combined with her personal opinions and preferences will be a challenge for the doctor of today involved in patient-tailored menopausal care.

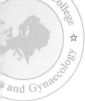

CONCLUSION

In comparison with two decades ago, many postmenopausal hormone preparations have become available, varying in oestrogen dosage and route of administration. Furthermore, an increasing number of preparations is being marketed combining oestrogen with a variety of progestogens. In general, we should choose the lowest possible dosage that is able to treat climacteric complaints and prevent bone resorption adequately, and which has as few unwanted effects as possible, and we should give it in the route of administration and for the duration that best fits the woman's personal risk profile as well as her preferences.

References

1. Anderson G L, Limacher M, Assaf A R et al for the Women's Health Initiative Steering Committee 2004 Effects of conjugated equine estrogen in postmenopausal women with hysterectomy: the Women's Health Initiative randomized controlled trial. The Journal of the American Medical Association 291:1701–1712
2. Archer D F, Dorin M, Lewis V et al 2001 Effects of lower doses of conjugated equine estrogens and medroxyprogesterone acetate on endometrial bleeding. Fertility and Sterility 75:1080–1087
3. Archer D F, Fischer L A, Rich D et al 1992 Estrace vs Premarin for treatment of menopausal symptoms. Dosage comparison study. Advances in Therapy 9:21–31
4. Blankenstein M A, van de Ven J, Maitimu-Smeele I et al 1999 Intratumoral levels of estrogens in breast cancer. The Journal of Steroid Biochemistry and Molecular Biology 69:293–297
5. Clarke S C, Kelleher J, Lloyd-Jones H et al 2002 A study of hormone replacement therapy in postmenopausal women with ischaemic heart disease: the Papworth HRT Atherosclerosis Study. British Journal of Obstetrics and Gynaecology 109:1056–1062
6. Collaborative Group on Hormonal Factors in Breast Cancer 1997 Breast cancer and hormone replacement therapy: collaborative reanalysis of data from 51 epidemiological studies of 52705 women with breast cancer and 108411 women without breast cancer. The Lancet 350:1047–1059
7. Collins P 2002 Clinical cardiovascular studies of hormone replacement therapy. The American Journal of Cardiology 90(1A):30F–34F
8. Delmas P D, Pornel B, Felsenberg D et al for the International Study Group 2001 Three-year follow-up of the use of transdermal 17beta-estradiol matrix patches for the prevention of bone loss in early postmenopausal women. American Journal of Obstetrics and Gynecology 184:32–40
9. Grady D, Gebretsadik T, Kerlikowske K et al 1995 Hormone replacement therapy and endometrial cancer risk: a meta-analysis. Obstetrics and Gynecology 85:304–313
10. Grodstein F, Manson J E, Colditz G A et al 2000 A prospective, observational study of postmenopausal hormone therapy and primary prevention of cardiovascular disease. Annals of Internal Medicine 133:933–941
11. Hemelaar M, van der Mooren M J, Mijatovic V et al 2003 Oral, more than transdermal, estrogen replacement therapy improves lipids and lipoprotein(a) in postmenopausal women: a randomized, placebo-controlled study. Menopause 10:550–558
12. Hulley S, Grady D, Bush T et al 1998 Randomized trial of estrogen plus progestin for secondary prevention of coronary heart disease in postmenopausal women. Heart and Estrogen/progestin Replacement Study (HERS) Research Group. The Journal of the American Medical Association 280:605–613
13. Lees B, Stevenson J C 2001 The prevention of osteoporosis using sequential low-dose hormone replacement therapy with estradiol-17β and dydrogesterone. Osteoporosis International 12:251–258
14. Lobo R A, Bush T, Carr B R et al 2001 Effects of lower doses of conjugated equine estrogens and medroxyprogesterone acetate

on plasma lipids and lipoproteins, coagulation factors, and carbohydrate metabolism. Fertility and Sterility 76:13–24

15. MacLennan A, Lester S, Moore V 2001 Oral estrogen replacement therapy versus placebo for hot flushes: a systematic review. Climacteric 4:58–74

16. Post M S, Christella M, Thomassen L G et al 2003 Effect of oral and transdermal estrogen replacement therapy on hemostatic variables associated with venous thrombosis. A randomized, placebo-controlled study in postmenopausal women. Arteriosclerosis, Thrombosis, and Vascular Biology 23:1116–1121

17. Post M S, van der Mooren M J, Stehouwer C D et al 2002 Effects of transdermal and oral oestrogen replacement therapy on C-reactive protein levels in postmenopausal women: a randomised, placebo-controlled trial. Thrombosis and Haemostasis 88:605–610

18. Post M S, van der Mooren M J, van Baal W M et al 2003 Effects of low-dose oral and transdermal estrogen replacement therapy on hemostatic factors in healthy postmenopausal women. A randomized placebo-controlled study. American Journal of Obstetrics and Gynecology 189:1221–1227

19. Rodriguez C, Patel A V, Calle E E et al 2001 Estrogen replacement therapy and ovarian cancer mortality in a large prospective study of US women. The Journal of the American Medical Association 285:1460–1465

20. Rossouw J E, Anderson G L, Prentice R L et al of the Writing Group for the Women's Health Initiative Investigators 2002 Risks and benefits of estrogen plus progestin in healthy postmenopausal women. Principal results from the Women's Health Initiative randomized controlled trial. The Journal of the American Medical Association 288:321–333

21. Scarabin P Y, Oger E, Plu-Bureau G for the EStrogen and THromboEmbolism Risk Study Group 2003 Differential association of oral and transdermal oestrogen-replacement therapy with venous thromboembolism risk. The Lancet 362:428–432

22. Shumaker S A, Legault C, Kuller L et al for the Women's Health Initiative Memory Study 2004 Conjugated equine estrogens and incidence of probable dementia and mild cognitive impairment in postmenopausal women: Women's Health Initiative Memory Study. The Journal of the American Medical Association 291:2947–2958

23. Smolders R G, van der Mooren M J, Teerlink T et al 2003 A randomized placebo-controlled study of the effect of transdermal vs. oral estradiol with or without gestodene on homocysteine levels. Fertility and Sterility 79:261–267

24. Utian W H, Shoupe D, Bachmann G et al 2001 Relief of vasomotor symptoms and vaginal atrophy with lower doses of conjugated equine estrogens and medroxyprogesterone acetate. Fertility and Sterility 75:1065–1079

25. Van Baal W M, Emeis J J, van der Mooren M J et al 2000 Impaired procoagulant–anticoagulant balance during hormone replacement therapy? A randomised, placebo-controlled 12-week study. Thrombosis and Haemostasis 83:29–34

18

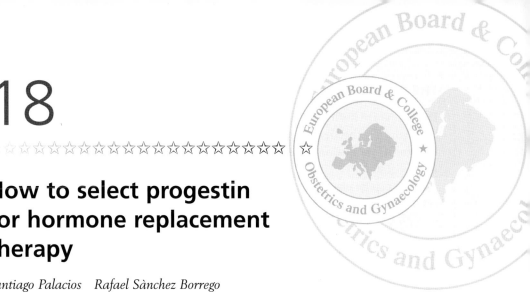

How to select progestin for hormone replacement therapy

Santiago Palacios   Rafael Sànchez Borrego

ABSTRACT

The role of progestins in hormone replacement therapy (HRT) is to give endometrial protection in oestrogen therapy (ET). Progestins that achieve endometrial protection (while maintaining oestrogen's beneficial effects with no side-effects) are needed. Every progestin has different androgenic, anti-androgenic, oestrogen, glucocorticoid and antimineral corticoid effects. Different progestins may produce different results. Most of the larger trials have selected the same HRT regimen, conjugated equine oestrogens (CEEs), and medroxyprogesterone acetate (MPA). Further data are needed to compare the effects of different progestins used in clinical practice.

KEYWORDS

Metabolic effects, progestins, receptor effects, selectivity

INTRODUCTION

Since 1975 when the use of oestrogens in the postmenopause was related to endometrial cancer,[24,33] progestins or progesterone have been used to diminish the risk of endometrial hyperplasia. With the use of unopposed oestrogens there is an incidence of 18–32% of endometrial hyperplasia, often with cytological atypias that indicate a premalignant lesion. By adding 7 days of treatment with progestins every month, the rate of hyperplasia was reduced to 3%. By increasing the length of administration of progestins from 12 to 13 days, the incidence of hyperplasia was reduced to less than 1%.[31]

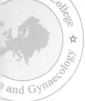
THE DEFINITION AND CLASSIFICATION OF PROGESTINS

Progestins are hormonal action molecules characterized, as their name indicates, by favouring the development of pregnancy in mammals. Any substance that transforms the endometrium stimulated by oestrogens toward a secretory phase is a progestin.[9]

They can be classified as natural and synthetic. There is a unique natural progestin with an important biological significance: progesterone. Despite the extensive protein binding of serum progesterone, its half-life is only about 5 minutes. Because of the poor oral absorption of progesterone and its susceptibility to rapid first-pass metabolism in the liver, a variety of oral, injectable and implantable synthetic analogs, called 'progestins', have been developed.[22] We can count on a large number of synthetic progestins, each one with its own characteristics. The synthetic progestins have been classified into three groups: C21 progestins; 19-nortestosterone; and one derived from 17α-spirolactone (Box 18.1).

PHARMACODYNAMICS AND SELECTIVITY

Once ingested, the steroids are absorbed in the small intestine from where they are transported by the hepatic portal system, where they can be modified and circulated in a systematic manner or they can be eliminated by biliary excretion. This is called pre-systemic effect or hepatic first-pass. From the gallbladder the molecules return to the small intestine, they are reabsorbed in the portal circulation or are excreted in the faeces. Norgestrel does not suffer the first-pass effect, unlike nearly all the other progestins, which produces variations in bioavailability among users.[25]

Box 18.1   The classification of progestogens

- Progestogen (identical to endogenous progestogen);

- Progestogens (not identical to endogenous progestogen):

  - C21 progestogen derivatives:

    - Pregnanes: medroxyprogesterone acetate; megestrol acetate; cyproterone acetate; dydrogesterone;

    - 19-Norpregnane derivatives: nomegestrol acetate; trimegestone; promegestone;

  - 19-Nortestosterone derivatives:

    - Estranes: norethisterone (e.g. norethynodrel); norethisterone acetate; ethynodiol acetate; lynestrenol; norethynodrel;

    - Gonanes: norgestrel; levonorgestrel; norgestimate; desogestrel; gestodene;

  - Spirolactone derivates:

    - Drospirenone.

The progestins can be absorbed via oral or vaginal routes, or through the skin. To be effectively absorbed by the oral route, a micronized form of progesterone should be ingested.

MODE OF ACTION

The effect of progesterone is mediated by progesterone intracellular receptor (PR) located in the nucleus of target cells, which is induced by oestradiol in most target tissues. In humans, two PR proteins, PR-A and PR-B, have been described although the biological importance of these different ratios of PR expression is not clear.

The progestins presently available for prescription interact with other steroidal receptors, including oestrogen receptor (ER), androgen receptor (AR), the glucocorticoid receptor and the mineralocorticoid receptor. Very small structural changes may induce considerable differences on the effects of the progestins (Table 18.1)

Progesterone has a moderate glucocorticoid and antimineralocorticoid effect. The 19-nortestosterone derivatives are shown to exert some androgenic activity but only norethisterone and lynestrenol exert an oestrogenic effect. The pregnane derivatives have varying activities: cyproterone acetate (CPA) is a potent anti-androgenic compound; trimegestone has a moderate anti-androgenic effect; while MPA has a slight androgenic activity and also exerts glucocorticoid activity. Drospirenone is essentially an antimineralocorticoid progestin with some anti-androgenic activity.[20,23]

METABOLIC EFFECTS

Referring to the metabolism of lipoproteins, the effects are derived to a great extent from their affinity to the ARs. The hepatic lipase is sensitive to this type of activity, in such a way that the reinforcement of the same supposes that a large number of high-density lipoproteins are eliminated from the circulation. This coexists with increases of total cholesterol and LDL-cholesterol, outlining an atherogenic profile.[12]

This situation is clearer with the nonderived progestins. For this reason, for some time now the use of derived progesterones is recommended and, more recently, that of micronized progesterone, with clearly improved results.

SIDE-EFFECTS

The majority of women do not have systematic symptoms related to the administration of progestins, with the exception of haemorrhage due to deprivation. Unwanted uterine bleeding is one of the most frequent factors in a post-menopausal woman's decision to discontinue HRT.[15] Many of these reported effects are based on limited data.[17] One of the most comprehensive placebo-controlled studies comparing HRT regimens in postmenopausal women

Table 18.1 Progestins: receptors effects

	Progestin	Oestrogen	Anti oestrogen	Androgen	Antiandrogen	Glucocorticoid	Antimineralocorticoid
Progesterone	−	+	−	±	+	+	+
Norethisterone	+	+	+	−	−	−	−
Lynestrenol	+	+	+	−	−	−	
Norethindrone	+	+	±	−	−	−	
Levonorgestrel		−	+	+	−	−	−
Norgestimate	−	+	+	−	−	+	
Medroxyprogesterone acetate		−	−	+	±	−	+
Cyproterone	−	+	−	+	+	−	
Megestrol	−	+	−	+	+	−	±
Dydrogesterone	−	−	+	−	−	−	
Etonogestrel	−	+	+	−	−	−	
Gestodene	−	+	+	−	±	+	+
Drospirenone	−	+	+	+	+	+	+
Desogestrel	−	+	+	−	−	−	
Dienogest	−	+	−	+	+	−	
Chlormadinone	−	−	+	−	+	+	−
Trimegestone	−	+	−	+	−	+	
Tibolone	+	+	+	−	−	−	

demonstrated that progestin-containing regimes did not result in weight gain, increased anxiety or cognitive and affective symptoms.[10] However, some women have disagreeable side-effects which include breast tenderness, oedema or bloating, symptoms similar to premenstrual syndrome, headache, irritability, depression or sleepiness. Sometimes it is useful to change from one formula to another, for example drospirenone can block the adverse effects of aldosterone on the cardiovascular system,[32] or to change from a cyclic to a continuous regimen.

ENDOMETRIAL EFFECTS

The primary role of progestin in postmenopausal HRT is endometrial protection. Progestins control the oestrogen-primed endometrial protection. They also regulate mitosis in fully differentiated endometrial cells.[5] It now appears that severely atypical endometrial lesions and early well-differentiated endometrial cancer can be reversed with high-dose progestin therapy in women of reproductive age.[18] Progestins can be prescribed each menstrual cycle, in a continuous form or in trimestral regimens (four times a year).

PROGESTIN GUIDELINES

At present, we have a wide range of progestin formulations whose pharmacological and metabolic characteristics are distinct. Moreover, not all guidelines for oestrogen–progestin have the same metabolic transcendence, essentially because the progestin-dependent effects maintain a direct relation with the dose of formulation.

Progestins can be used in two regimens to treat menopause, either continuous or cyclic forms. The addition of oral progestin to ET, administered either cyclically or continuously combined, is associated with reduced rates of hyperplasia.[13]

They can be added in continuous or cyclic form to convert the proliferative endometrium established by unopposed oestrogens into a secretory endometrium. This conversion usually requires at least 10 days of progestin administration (although the current recommendation is 12–14 days). With the cyclic administration of a progestin, the secretory transformation and endometrial disruption is achieved. Therefore protection against endometrial hyperplasia is double: on the one hand glandular secretion with a reduction of epitheliosis mitosis and, on the other, endometrial disruption.[7] Endometrial disruption is not a mechanism of absolute protection as zones with an endometrial pathology can be left in the depths of the endometrium. Nevertheless, when focal hyperplasia is noticed, there is no doubt that tissue disintegration could comprise a defence mechanism against endometrial proliferation. However, epidemiological studies of continuous therapy indicate no risk and may suggest some added protection against endometrial cancer.[11,29]

It has been shown that complete secretory gland maturation and subsequent withdrawal bleeding are not required for the prevention of endometrial hyperplasia.

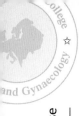
The appropriate doses and durations of progestin therapy are those that reduce secretory gland mitosis to a very low rate with marginal secretory gland transformation and those that induce a high incidence of amenorrhoea without irregular bleeding.

Studies have better defined the necessary doses and durations of the progestin course to oppose the oestrogen-induced risk of endometrial hyperplasia and adenocarcinoma. All progestin formulations will provide endometrial protection if the doses and durations are adequate. In this respect, the so-called minimum effective doses of progestin that assure the absence of hyperplasia have been established. Nevertheless this dose is merely orientative as there is already a wide variety of endometrial response (Table 18.2).

A basic consideration is that this dose of progestin is considered against a standard dose of 0.625 mg CEE. Larger or smaller oestrogen doses may require larger or smaller progestin doses, respectively. However, the risk of endometrial cancer is never eliminated in women with a uterus as women not using hormones can develop this disease. Long-term surveillance is necessary, even in women receiving

Table 18.2 Principal progestins and their suggested doses in HRT to assure endometrial protection

Route	Active ingredient	Doses	Days per cycle (28 days)
Oral	Cyproterone	1 mg	10
	Dienogest	1–2 mg	?[a]
	Dihydrogesterone	10 mg	14
	Drospirenone	1–3 mg	?[a]
	Gestodene	0.025–0.05 mg	12
	Levonorgestrel	0.075–0.25 mg	12
	Megestrol	5 mg	10
	Medroxyprogesterone	2.5–10 mg	12[b]
	Nomegestrol	5 mg	10
	Norethisterone	1 mg	10
	Progesterone	200–300 mg	14
	Trimegestone	0.25 mg	12
Transdermal	Levonorgestrel	0.02 mg	14
	Norethisterone	0.125–0.25 mg	14
Vaginal	Progesterone	100–200 mg	14[c]
Intrauterine	Levonorgestrel	0.02 mg	28

[a] Nothing has been published in any scientific journal about the number of days per cycle necessary for endometrial protection with this new progestin.
[b] The suggested dose of medroxyprogesterone is 10 mg administered for 12 days per cycle. For continuous combined treatment, it seems that a dose of 2.5 mg per day administered during every day of the cycle is sufficient for endometrial protection.
[c] The vaginal route in HRT is beginning to be used. Everything seems to indicate that the optimum dose for a continuous combined treatment regimen is 100 mg per day for 28 days of a cycle. For sequential treatments, the dose could be established in 200 mg per day for 14 days of the cycle.

appropriate doses of progestin. Because of concerns that adding progestin may increase breast cancer risk and may attenuate some benefits of ET, the lowest appropriate dose of progestin should be used. The use of oestrogen–progestin therapy (EPT) should be limited to the shortest duration consistent with treatment goals, benefits and risks for the individual woman.

From a biochemical point of view, the maximum effect of progestins on the synthesis of DNA and the ER is not achieved until after 6 days of administration. In the normal menstrual cycle this suppression continues until menstrual bleeding is produced. Therefore the length of treatment recommended with progestins is between 12 and 14 days each month. To date, the largest clinical trial in endometrial protection was published by the Menopause Study Group and established that a dose 10 mg MPA for 14 days has no incidence of hyperplasia.[16]

Retrospective trials have suggested that withdrawal uterine bleeding occurring after day 11 of a cyclic 12-day progestin course reflects the normal secretory pattern of endometrial tissue.[16,26] However, prospective trials have not confirmed these findings,[13] and no correlation has been established between day of bleeding onset and histological findings. Nevertheless, most studies with the cyclic administration of progestins have shown a high percentage of regular withdrawal uterine bleeding in women with a normal secretory endometrium.[2,13]

With the continuous administration of progestin, endometrial atrophy is achieved after a few months of administration. Continuously administered combined EPT (CCHRT) can provide the same endometrial protection as cyclic HRT,[13] yet avoid withdrawal bleeding.[8] Bleeding pattern is a less reliable indicator of endometrial safety when continuous combined regimens are used.[16,28,30]

Breakthrough uterine bleeding has been observed in 40% of women on a CCHRT during the first 3–6 months.[16] The probability of achieving amenorrhoea is greater if CCHRT is started 12 months or more after menopause – women who are recently postmenopausal exhibit more breakthrough bleeding.[2,21] Most women (75–89% of all users) who continue therapy become amenorrhoeic within 12 months. However, bleeding may persist intermittently for months or years. Persistent breakthrough bleeding with CCHRT may necessitate changing to another regimen.

The 19-nortestosterone derivatives – e.g. norethisterone (NET), norethisterone acetate (NETA), levonorgestrel (LNG) and norgestimate – tend to produce less breakthrough uterine bleeding during the first few months of use because of atrophy resulting from increased progestational activity. Conversely, micronized oral progesterone, when given cyclically, may lead to quantitatively more uterine bleeding than progestins. In this setting, the endometrium is weakly proliferative and does not exhibit a strong progestational effect.

The administration of progestin for 3 days of therapy and 3 days off (i.e. an intermittent regimen) has not been described. In agreement with the knowledge about the changes in the PRs, and with the lowest dose of progestin based on the said receptor, a greater hormonal action is sought to be achieved.[4] There is no doubt that more experience is required to ensure that there is an antihyperplasia action in the long term for this type of therapy.

Intrauterine-administerd progestin (IUD, Mirena®, Schering AG, Berlin, Germany) is an option to avoid systemic side-effects. This method, which releases LNG at a rate of 20 μg per day, seems to be effective in postmenopausal women in opposing the proliferative effects of ET on the endometrium.[127]

THERAPEUTIC MANAGEMENT

The clinical goal of progestin therapy when added to ET is to provide endometrial protection while minimizing unwanted side-effects. As with any pharmaceutical agent, therapy should be tailored to the woman's individual needs. The only menopause-related indication for chronic progestin use seems to be endometrial protection from unopposed ET.

Some progestins, with a higher androgenic potency than others, may attenuate the beneficial effects of oestrogens on the lipid profile as well as the effects on the vessels. On the other hand, other progestins devoid of androgenic properties do not exert these deleterious effects.

In the last WHI trial,[19] the relative risk of breast cancer with the use CEE + MPA was 1.26. In the Million Women Study,[3] the authors found an increase of relative risk of breast cancer with the use of combined HRT in continuous and combined regimens, but no differences were found between different kinds of progestin. In a recent French cohort study,[6] the relative risk was 1.1 (range 0.8–1.6) for oestrogen use alone and 1.3 (1.1–1.5) when used in combination with oral progestogens. The risk was significantly greater ($P < 0.001$) with HRT containing micronized progesterone, the relative risks being 1.4 (1.2–1.7) and 0.9 (0.7–1.2), respectively.

In combined therapy analysis, there have been studies of progestins with a slight androgenic profile. The results cannot be applied to recently developed progestins with better pharmacological profiles as compared to the ones included in the study.

It is recommended that clinicians prescribe adequate progestins for all postmenopausal women with an intact uterus who are using ET; postmenopausal women without a uterus should not be prescribed progestins.

CONCLUSION

The clinical goal of progestins in HRT is to provide endometrial protection while maintaining oestrogen benefits and minimizing progestin-induced side-effects, particularly uterine bleeding.

There is no consensus on the preferred regimen.[14] However, by changing the progestin type, route or regimen, clinicians can help minimize any attenuation of oestrogen's benefits, decrease side-effects and reduce uterine bleeding while providing adequate endometrial protection.

Progestins exhibit effects on organ systems other than the endometrium. These effects vary depending on the progestin type, dose and route of administration, and the EPT regimen. Further data are needed to compare the effects of various progestins used in clinical practice.

References

1. Andersson B, Mattsson L A, Rybo G et al 1992 Intrauterine release of levonorgestrel: a new way of adding progestogen in hormone replacement therapy. Obstetrics and Gynecology 79:963–967

2. Archer D F, Pickar J H, Bottiglioni F for the Menopause Study Group 1994 Bleeding patterns in postmenopausal women taking continuous combined or sequential regimens of conjugated estrogens with medroxyprogesterone acetate. Obstetrics and Gynecology 83:686–692

3. Beral V for the Million Women Study Collaborators 2003 Breast cancer and hormone replacement therapy in the Million Women Study. The Lancet 362:419–427

4. Casper R F, Chapdelaine A 1993 Estrogen and interrupted progestin: a new concept for menopausal hormone replacement therapy. American Journal of Obstetrics and Gynecology 168:1188–1196

5. Ferenczy A, Gelfand M 1989 The biologic significance of cytologic atypia in progesterone-treated endometrial hyperplasia. American Journal of Obstetrics and Gynecology 160:126–131

6. Fournier A, Berrino F, Riboli E et al 2005 Breast cancer risk in relation to different types of hormone replacement therapy in the E3N-EPIC cohort. International Journal of Cancer 2005 114(3):448–454

7. Gambrell R D Jr 1997 Strategies to reduce the incidence of endometrial cancer in postmenopausal women. American Journal of Obstetrics and Gynecology 177:1196–1207

8. Gillet J Y, Andre G, Faguer B et al 1994 Induction of amenorrhea during hormone replacement therapy: optimal micronized progesterone dose. Maturitas 19:103–115

9. González Merlo J 1997 Hormonoterapia en ginecología. In: González Merlo J (ed) Ginecología, 7th edn. Editorial Masson SA, Barcelona

10. Greendale G A, Reboussin B A, Hogan P et al 1998 Symptom relief and side-effects of postmenopausal hormones. Results from the Postmenopausal Estrogen/Progestin Interventions Trial. Obstetrics and Gynecology 92:982–988

11. Hill D A, Weiss N S, Beresford S A et al 2000 Continuous combined hormone replacement therapy and risk of endometrial cancer. American Journal of Obstetrics and Gynecology 183:1456–1461

12. Kuhl H 1996 Comparative pharmacology of the newer progestogens. Drugs 51(2):188–215

13. Lethaby A, Farquhar C, Sarkis A et al 2000 Hormone replacement therapy in postmenopausal women: endometrial hyperplasia and irregular bleeding. Cochrane Database Systematic Reviews 2:CD000402

14. North American Menopause Society 2003 Role of progestogen in hormone therapy for postmenopausal women: position statement of the North American Menopause Society. Menopause 10(2)113–132

15. Ödmark I S, Jonsson B, Bäckström T 2001 Bleeding patterns in postmenopausal women using continuous combination hormone replacement therapy with conjugated estrogen and medroxyprogesterone acetate or with 17β-estradiol and norethindrone acetate. American Journal of Obstetrics and Gynecology 184:1131–1138

16. Pickar J H, Archer DF 1997 Is bleeding a predictor of endometrial hyperplasia in postmenopausal women receiving hormone replacement therapy? Menopause Study Group. American Journal of Obstetrics and Gynecology 177:1178–1183

17. Prior J C, Alojado N, McKay D W et al 1994 No adverse effects of medroxyprogesterone treatment without estrogen in postmenopausal women: double-blind, placebo-controlled, crossover trial. Obstetrics and Gynecology 83:24–28

18. Randall T C, Kurman R J 1997 Progestin treatment of atypical hyperplasia and well-differentiated carcinoma of the endometrium in women under age 40. Obstetrics and Gynecology 90:434–440

19. Rossouw J E, Anderson G L, Prentice R L et al of the Writing Group for the Women's Health Initiative Investigators 2002 Risks and benefits of estrogen plus progestin in healthy postmenopausal women. The Journal of the American Medical Association 288:321–333

20. Schindler A E, Campagnoli C, Druckmann R et al 2003 Classification and pharmacology of progestins. Maturitas 46 (Suppl 1):S7–S16

21. Shau W-Y, Hsieh C-C, Hsieh T-T et al 2002 Factors associated with endometrial bleeding in continuous hormone replacement therapy. Menopause 9:188–194

22. Simon J A 1995 Micronized progesterone: vaginal and oral uses. Clinical Obstetrics and Gynecology 38:902–914

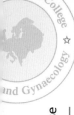
The menopause

23. Sitruk-Ware R 2002 Progestogens in hormonal replacement therapy: new molecules, risks, and benefits. Menopause 9(1):6–15

24. Smith D C, Prentice R, Thompson D J et al 1975 Association of exogenous estrogen and endometrial carcinoma. The New England Journal of Medicine 293:1164–1167

25. Stancyk F Z, Roy S 1990 Metabolism of levonorgestrel, norethindrone and structurally related compounds. Contraception 42:67–96

26. Sturdee D W, Barlow D H, Ulrich L G et al 1994 Is the timing of withdrawal bleeding a guide to endometrial safety during sequential oestrogen–progestogen replacement therapy? UK Continuous Combined HRT Study Investigators. The Lancet 344:979–982

27. Suvanto-Luukkonen E, Malinen H, Sundstrom H et al 1998 Endometrial morphology during hormone replacement therapy with estradiol gel combined to levonorgestrel-releasing intrauterine device or natural progesterone. Acta Obstetricia et Gynecologica Scandinavica 77:758–763

28. Udoff L, Langenberg P, Adashi E Y 1995 Combined continuous hormone replacement therapy: a critical review. Obstetrics and Gynecology 86:306–316

29. Weiderpass E, Adami H-O, Baron J A et al 1999 Risk of endometrial cancer following estrogen replacement with and without progestins. Journal of the National Cancer Institute 91:1131–1137

30. Wells M, Sturdee D W, Barlow D H et al 2002 Effect on endometrium of long-term treatment with continuous combined oestrogen–progestogen replacement therapy: follow-up study. British Medical Journal 325:239–244

31. Whitehead M I, Hillard T C, Crook D et al 1990 The role and use of progestogens. Obstetrics and Gynecology 75 (Suppl 4):59S–76S

32. Williams G H 2003 Cardiovascular benefits of aldosterone receptor antagonists. Climacteric 6 (Suppl 3):29–35

33. Zeil H K, Finkle W D 1975 Increased risk of endometrial carcinoma among users of conjugated estrogens. The New England Journal of Medicine 293:1167–1170

19

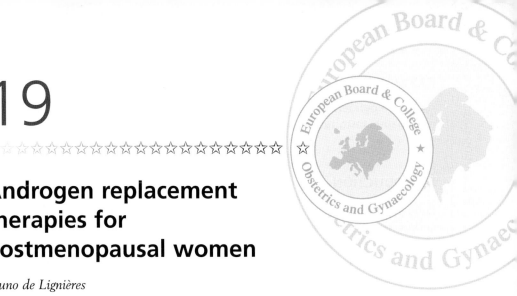

★☆★☆★☆★☆★☆★☆★☆★☆★☆★★ ☆   ★

Androgen replacement therapies for postmenopausal women

Bruno de Lignières

ABSTRACT

If the occurrence in some postmenopausal women of an androgen deficiency inducing target tissue dysfunction is plausible, then there is still no consensus on the way to select candidates for various androgen replacement therapies (ATs), neither on their main clinical and biological characteristics nor on guidelines to monitor the treatments. Most of the controversy comes from the present difficulty of evaluating androgen activities in target tissues by using only serum measurements. Compared to total testosterone, the measurement of bioavailable testosterone (BT) is an important improvement in laboratory tests for the identification of androgen deficiency in men over 50 but not in women. Assuming that, in women, the most important part of active testosterone and dihydrotestosterone (DHT) is synthesized directly within the target tissue and does not circulate, the most informative serum measurements already feasible are the levels of the major physiological DHT precursor, androstenedione, and DHT metabolite, androstane-3α,17β-diol-glucuronide (3α-Adiol-G). They have been documented in hyperandrogenic states and should be included in future androgen deficiency studies. Only substantial progress in the biochemical investigations of aromatase and 5α-reductase activities may improve the screening and treatment of postmenopausal women suspected to be androgen deficient. The typical candidates for AT complain of loss of libido and have a relatively low body mass index (BMI) and bone mineral density (BMD) despite a careful individual adjustment of a non-oral oestradiol replacement therapy. Treatments with several formulations of testosterone or dehydroepiandrosterone (DHEA) have often been associated with oral oestrogen therapy (ET) increasing the difficulties of detecting androgen deficiency, and no impressive benefits have been documented within the physiological range of a true replacement therapy. AT remains largely empirical and should not be recommended in current practice.
Dr Bruno de Lignières died on 4 July 2004. His friends and colleagues throughout the world feel great sorrow about this loss of an internationally well-known colleague.

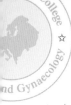

KEYWORDS

Androgen deficiency, androgens, dehydroepiandrosterone (DHEA), female menopause, testosterone

INTRODUCTION

Following ageing and menopause, the adrenal and ovarian production of androgens decreases and, for most investigators, the occurrence in some women of an androgen deficiency, inducing clinical symptoms and target tissue dysfunctions, is plausible. However, there is still no consensus on the way to select such candidates for various ATs, neither on their main clinical and biological characteristics nor on guidelines to monitor the treatments. For some experts, because the expected benefits seem far larger than potential side-effects, AT should be prescribed to any postmenopausal woman complaining of low sexual desire and poor energy despite ET, mostly if she is ovariectomized or hysterectomized and/or treated with oral oestrogens.[15,34,56] For others, on the contrary, the potential long-term side-effects of overtreatment are worrying, even more so after the disappointing results of classical oral ET; not one of the proposed ATs has yet convincingly demonstrated a favourable efficacy/safety ratio.[19,38,43] Therefore, investigators do not recommend prescribing AT to post-menopausal women in current practice until identifying androgen deficiency and preventing side-effects can be clarified. Most of the controversy comes from the present difficulty of evaluating androgen activities in target tissues by serum measurements only.

ANDROGEN DEFICIENCY IN POSTMENOPAUSAL WOMEN: BIOLOGY

SERUM TESTOSTERONE

A popular concept is that postmenopausal androgen deficiency can be simply put down to low serum testosterone, which is expected to reflect the full set of changes occurring in androgen synthesis by the adrenals, ovaries and peripheral tissues. Total testosterone is most often assessed with sufficient precision by radioimmunoassays but it does not, by itself, allow for the detection of androgen deficiencies in women (or in men) over 50 years of age.[34,43] Total testosterone levels tend to decline slightly between the ages of 40 and 70 in most studies. A decrease of the sex hormone-binding globulin (SHBG) is also observed after menopause, which leads to a lower retention of testosterone in the plasma and an increase in its bioavailability for the target tissues.[8] Therefore the measurement of SHBG seems mandatory to allow an estimate of the circulating portion of BT. The assessment of the BT concentration depends on two independent measurements of testosterone and SHBG, each with its own potential inaccuracies, and it assumes that the molecular behaviour of SHBG and of serum albumin is homogenous in all women, an assumption that is probably partially incorrect. Since this measurement only gives information on the quantity of circulating SHBG (and not on its quality as a steroid carrier) optimal information should come from the direct measurement of BT, i.e. the addition of albumin-bound testosterone and of free testosterone, both of which are not bound to SHBG. Several laboratories use various analytical approaches requiring control of the precipitation procedure by the ammonium sulphate of SHBG and the steroids that are bound to it, and of the standardization of the assessment of free and albumin-bound testosterone in the supernatant. To be reliable, each laboratory must establish its own reference values along with its own coded procedure based on a sufficient number of normal premenopausal asymptomatic women. There is, as yet, no validated commercial method for directly measuring serum BT, and the indirect estimation on the basis of a combined measurement of total testosterone and SHBG is still the most common practice, even if there is still no consensus on threshold values establishing both androgen deficiency and androgen excess in ageing women.[34]

Based on BT estimations, normal menopause does not induce androgen deficiency nor justify AT.[8] In the most convincing longitudinal study, not only is there no average decrease in BT during the untreated menopause transition but also no correlation between changes in BT and the rapidly increasing occurrence of symptoms supposedly related to androgen deficiency, such as sexual dysfunction.[16] Similarly, almost all hysterectomized women (with or without oophorectomy) and those treated with oral oestrogens have a reduced BT.[30,34,49] In the latter group it is due to an increased liver synthesis of SHBG because of the first-pass effect. However, the individuals complaining of sexual dysfunction cannot be identified by their BT levels.

Neither total testosterone, SHBG nor BT measurements appear to be the appropriate tools to find potential androgen deficiency in most post-menopausal women and then to monitor a testosterone replacement. This situation occurs because changes in serum concentration of testosterone (and oestradiol) may not reflect similar changes in the target tissues of post-menopausal women.[28,50] To the changes in production and transport of these sex steroids related to ageing and menopause can be added changes of metabolism in the target tissues, changes which become the most significant modulators of actual androgen effects, although they mostly escape current serum measurements.

5α-REDUCTASE AROMATASE

The main effect of androgens on their targets depend on their binding either to the ER after aromatization or to the androgen receptor (AR), with or without 5α-reduction (Fig. 19.1).

The local 5α-reductase activity dramatically amplifies the binding of testosterone to the ARs via DHT synthesis, and then the actual activity of the same amount of bioavailable androgen. 5α-reductases of either type 1 or 2 have been

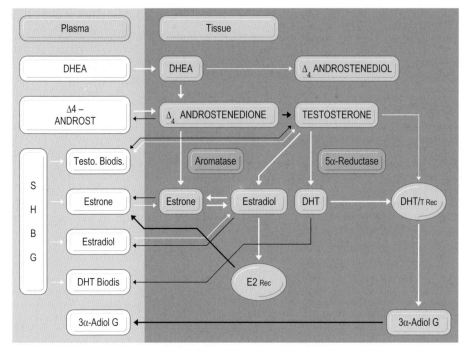

Fig 19.1 Androgens in the plasma and tissues of postmenopausal women.

identified in most female targets of androgens; their activities are probably pivotal for the androgen effects not only on the skin[34,37] but also on mood, sex organs, body composition and bone.[5,22,24,25,37,57] They control the intensity of the specific androgenic effects and inhibit aromatization of androgens to oestrogens and subsequent binding to ERs. Since a small amount of DHT is enough to fully activate an androgen receptor, the local 5α-reductase activity may more easily become a limiting factor than the relatively large serum reservoir of androgens. The main reason to suspect a relative decrease in 5α-reductase activities related to ageing, at least in some women, is that aromatization of the reduced amount of androgenic substrates increases.[30,35,46,49,50,56]

As for testosterone, the serum levels of total DHT (and even of bioavailable DHT) do not closely reflect the quantity of DHT formed from either testosterone or androstenedione in female target tissues.[28,37,56] About 85% of the locally synthesized DHT is also locally metabolized after binding to ARs, and less than 15% of intact DHT reaches the general circulation. Almost all of this circulating intact DHT (and 40–50% of circulating testosterone) comes from target cells via several precursors but has not been used by ARs and then its measurement is not very informative. The strong binding affinity of DHT for SHBG renders this serum measurement even more inaccurate in postmenopausal women.

Because DHT is metabolized mostly to androstane-3α,17β-oestradiol by target tissues and then circulates in serum as water-soluble 3α-Adiol-G, this metabolite is theoretically the best candidate for evaluating the portion of androgens actually used by the DHT/testosterone receptors in women.[7,13,17,28,37,51]

Therefore tissue levels of testosterone and DHT, as for oestradiol, are determined more by local synthesis, via serum precursors and metabolism, than by their own plasma levels in untreated postmenopausal women.[28,37,50,56]

ANDROSTENEDIONE AND DHEA

Serum androstenedione, 90% reflecting the adrenal and ovarian secretions, is the major substrate for both aromatase and 5α-reductase activities. More than 90% of serum androstenedione is bioavailable and independent of SHBG levels. The *in-vivo* conversion rate to 3α-Adiol-G is four or five times higher from radiolabelled androstenedione than from DHEA and equivalent from testosterone and androstenedione in women.[37] Because the blood production of androstenedione is almost ten times that of testosterone, the circulating amount of androstenedione is clearly the most important precursor of DHT synthesis in the tissues of postmenopausal women.[20,37,56] By contrast with BT, serum androstenedione levels tend to decrease in most postmenopausal women,[34,56] with a limited influence of oral ET[49] and hysterectomy.[30] In one cross-sectional study of androgen status and sex life in perimenopausal women the most frequent and strong reverse correlation was found between serum androstenedione and sexual desire in untreated postmenopausal women.[20] No such correlation was found for DHEA.[16,18]

About 60% of serum DHEA originates from adrenal and ovarian secretions and about 40% comes from complex peripheral interconversions.[35] It appears to be a less important substrate for both aromatase and 5α-reductase activities than for androstenedione. The serum levels and blood production rate are approximately twice as high for DHEA than for androstenedione before and after menopause,[35,56] but the conversion to testosterone or 3α-Adiol-G is one-fifth for DHEA than for androstenedione.[35,37]

In short, serum values of testosterone, SHBG, BT or DHEA have not been convincingly helpful for the diagnosis of potential androgen deficiency in postmenopausal women. Assuming that, in women, the most important part of active testosterone and DHT is synthesized directly within the target tissue and do not circulate, the most informative serum measurements already feasible are the levels of the major physiological DHT precursor, androstenedione, and DHT metabolite, 3α-Adiol-G. They have been documented in hyperandrogenic states and should be included in future androgen deficiency studies.

ANDROGEN DEFICIENCY IN POSTMENOPAUSAL WOMEN: CLINICAL DIAGNOSIS

Because the biological diagnosis of androgen deficiency has remained largely inadequate, clinical features may be used to identify candidates for AT.[15,34,56] A popular hypothesis is that physiological levels of androgens in women have strong influences on the brain, lean and fat mass, and bone. Some hormone-dependent dysfunctions in these tissues are expected to translate into clinical symptoms, which are helpful for the diagnosis of androgen deficiency. Because most women become symptomatic during the menopausal transition, it seems an appropriate time to identify the potential correlations between occurrences of symptoms and specific changes in sex steroid metabolism.[61]

LIBIDO

Sexual functioning is obviously multifactorial and involves the woman's sexual self and self-image, emotional intimacy, partner history, past relationships, mental health status and current medical problems;[19] more than 40% of women aged 18 to 59 complain of sexual dysfunction.[31] Hormonal status also plays a role, as in the largest longitudinal study it was observed that libido declined concurrently with the decline in serum oestradiol during the menopausal transition.[16] Similarly, in a cross-sectional study of perimenopausal women, the strong reverse correlation found between serum androstenedione and sexual desire in untreated postmenopausal women disappeared in postmenopausal women treated with oestrogens.[20] These studies strongly suggest that physiological levels of oestrogens have more influence than androgens on female sexual functioning, and that postmenopausal women complaining of low libido should first be treated with oestrogens. Because oral ET increases the liver synthesis of SHBG (also triglycerides, C-reactive protein and coagulation factors) and decreases BT (as well as LDL-cholesterol particle size), they might be treated by non-oral oestradiol.[34,49]

To investigate the potential benefits of adding androgens, surgically induced menopausal women with impaired sexual function (despite oral ET) were randomized to placebo or testosterone patch delivering either 150 or 300 µg per day.[48] At baseline, all women had a low BT, in comparison with premenopausal women. There was a strong placebo effect, and a further improvement in the scores for frequency of sexual activity and pleasure but only when the higher testosterone dose increased mean BT to the upper normal limit for premenopausal women, and beyond in an unspecified number of users. The lower dose, increasing BT to the midnormal range, was not different from a placebo. If pharmacological doses of testosterone clearly influence sexual functioning in postmenopausal women, then there is still no evidence that changes in BT within the physiological range have more than a placebo effect.[19,34,39]

These studies may have missed important information about actual androgen activities in tissues. They may also have missed serum variation from baseline, which may be important for optimal physiological adaptation to behavior and environment, such as physical exercise and sexual arousal. For example, physical exercise normally coincides with an acute increase in testosterone levels, but the maximal increase appears to be lower in post- than premenopausal women.[14] Similarly, sexual arousal in men also normally coincides with a rapid increase in testosterone levels[53] but this information is missing in women. On the other hand, an acute increase in libido seems to follow the i.m. injection of oestradiol plus testosterone immediately in postmenopausal women suggesting that rapid fluctuations of sex hormone secretion, and not only stable baseline levels, may play an important role.[47] Therefore baseline resting levels of serum androgens may not detect a defect of androgens in reacting to sexual stimulation or physical exercise, and a continuous slow-release delivery of androgens may not provide a fully effective AT.

However, clinical symptoms of sexual dysfunction, and specifically loss of libido, cannot be easily used for the diagnosis of androgen deficiency, and, knowing the large placebo effect, for monitoring AT in current postmenopausal users of oestrogens.

LEAN AND FAT MASS

Changes in body composition have multiple causes but the menopause transition coincides with a weight gain in most women in parallel with the oestradiol drop.[1] Normal premenopausal women have enlarged fat cells with high lipoprotein lipase activity in the subcutaneous gluteofemoral adipose tissue, while hyperandrogenic women tend to have most of their adipose tissue in the central and visceral part of the body. Lean body mass tends to increase with androgen levels, as does BMI, percentage of body fat and weight.[1,6,52] In postmenopausal women BT levels correlate positively with lean body mass but also with central abdominal fat.[1,21,23] The effects of various androgen supplements and differences between physiological replacement and pharmacology remain unclear without an appropriate monitoring of the doses.[43] Therefore BMI, or even body composition, may follow changes in androgen levels in populations but they are not reliable markers of androgen deficiency in a current postmenopausal user of oestrogen.

BONE MINERAL DENSITY

The menopause transition coincides with an accelerated decrease in BMD in parallel with the oestradiol drop. Androgens also influence bone mass partly through their aromatization to oestrogens but also as DHT via 5α-reductases in both osteoclasts and osteoblasts.[24,25] Therefore, if ET after menopause is expected to replace both the drop in endogenous oestradiol and a potential deficiency in aromatized androgens, a deficit in DHT precursors may translate into impaired BMD. Women with complete androgen insensitivity syndrome and current users of oestrogens show only moderate deficits in spine BMD, which suggests that severe osteopenia reflects an inadequate ET rather than androgen lack alone.[36] Accordingly, adequate ET maintains or increases BMD in the lumbar spine and hip of postmenopausal women, but several studies show a further increase when AT is added.[3,34]

In short, typical candidates for AT complain of loss of libido and have a relatively low BMI and BMD, despite careful individual adjustment of a non-oral ET HRT.[34]

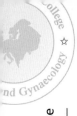

ANDROGEN REPLACEMENT THERAPY FORMULATIONS

Endogenous androgen excess in women is associated with side-effects such as anger, aggressiveness, seborrhoea, acne, hirsutism, baldness, central and visceral obesity, insulin resistance, an increase in LDL particle density, and increases in cardiovascular and breast cancer risks, the latter through an increased aromatization.[2,6,9,11–13,26,33,40,44,55,57] Conversely, androgen deficiency may also have more serious consequences than those previously cited, such as endothelial dysfunction, arrhythmias[10,41,59] and breast cancer,[29,42,54] through a relative deficit in DHT synthesis via the arterial walls, myocardium and breast. Therefore, with too much hype and not enough data at present,[43] AT in postmenopausal women should be a carefully monitored replacement for what seems to be lacking in comparison with normal premenopausal women. Because sexual dysfunction and osteopenia are largely oestrogen dependent, AT should be prescribed to current users of a non-oral ET HRT aiming to normalize androgen transportation and metabolism.[34,49]

TESTOSTERONE THERAPY

Testosterone can be administered in various injectable and transdermal formulations, theoretically able to mimic the endogenous secretion. However, identifying a testosterone deficit and simply replacing it is quite impossible in most AT candidates. The physiological way for female androgen target cells to receive their appropriate load of testosterone and DHT is *in-situ* synthesis, mostly from circulating precursors but only marginally from serum BT or DHT.

Serum total testosterone or BT levels do not correlate with symptoms of androgen deficiency before testosterone therapy, and, when reaching the physiological premenopausal range during treatment, do not provide any benefit beyond a placebo effect in most users.[39,48] Therefore testosterone therapy cannot be carefully monitored following physiological thresholds in most women and should not be recommended at the moment as a first choice for treating remaining sexual dysfunction or osteopenia in postmenopausal oestrogen users.[19,39,43]

DHEA THERAPY

DHEA can be administered in oral and non-oral formulations, theoretically able to mimic the endogenous secretion.[4,28] Serum DHEA clearly decreases with age but there is no obvious inverse relationship with symptoms or diseases expected to be related to androgen deficiency, specifically with libido.[16,18] Conversely, the higher DHEA serum levels coincide with the higher risks of cardiovascular disease and breast cancer.[26,33,40,44,55] DHEA appears to be a less important substrate for 5α-reductase activities than androstenedione with a conversion rate to testosterone or 3α-Adiol-G of approximately one-fifth.[35,37] It may be a better oestrogen than androgen precursor.[40] Most clinical trials with DHEA therapy involving postmenopausal women show limited or no benefits on libido and muscle mass and bone effects similar to low-dose oestrogen treatment.[4,39,45,58] DHEA associated with an anti-oestrogen may become a more attractive therapy[28] but it is no substitute for a physiological replacement.

ANDROSTENEDIONE THERAPY

Androstenedione can be administered in oral and non-oral formulations, theoretically able to mimic the endogenous secretion[20,32] but no one is available as a controlled pharmaceutical product. Serum androstenedione is the main physiological substrate for the tissular synthesis of DHT. Its levels clearly decrease with age and the onset of menopause,[34,56] with a limited influence of oral ET[49] and hysterectomy.[30] One cross-sectional study shows an inverse relationship with libido.[18] Breast cancer risk increases with the serum levels of androstenedione and DHEA in untreated postmenopausal women through metabolization to oestradiol.[27] However, the *in-vivo* conversion rate to 3α-Adiol-G is four or five times higher from androstenedione than DHEA,[35,37] and exogenous androstenedione administered to women (by contrast with men) uses the pathways to DHT more than those to oestradiol.[20,32] Since DHT is also highly protective for the breast,[29,42,54] androstenedione therapy is likely to be more effective and less risky than DHEA. Unfortunately androstenedione is only on the non-pharmaceutical market and, for obvious sponsoring reasons, no large clinical trial can be expected in the near future.

'FLASH' THERAPY

The fluctuations observed in serum androgens during the day in normal premenopausal women may not just be random but may reflect an important part of physiology by improving adaptations to physical activity or even, as in men, to sexual arousal.[14,53] Accordingly, the i.m. administration of androgen (plus oestradiol) seems to have an almost immediate effect on the sexual behavior of postmenopausal women. Formulations able to create a peak of serum androgen within a few minutes, followed by a return to baseline within a few hours,[60] may have a favourable efficacy/safety ratio when used just before physical exercise or sexual intercourse.

CONCLUSION

While the strategy to detect androgen excess seems adequate after many years' research, there is still no consensus on the way to diagnose women with androgen deficiency. Nevertheless, none of the anticipated important data regarding the potential consequences of this deficiency can be obtained from epidemiological investigations or clinical trials, as long as the populations studied cannot be classified and compared on the basis of sufficiently precise, informative and consensual biological measurements. Compared to total testosterone, the measurement of BT is an important improvement in laboratory tests for the identification of androgen deficiency in men over 50 but not in women. Biochemical investigations are not seeking evidence of simple hypogonadism decreasing blood production and serum levels, but they must deal with a complex situation involving multiple metabolic changes in target tissues, poorly reflected by current serum analysis. Only substantial progress in the biochemical investigations of aromatase and 5α-reductase activities, such as the analysis of serum androstenedione and 3α-Adiol-G, may improve the screening and the treatment of postmenopausal women suspected of being androgen deficient. Treatments with several formulations of testosterone or DHEA, often associated with oral ET, remain largely empirical and should not be recommended in current practice.

References

1. Bancroft J, Cawood E H H 1996 Androgens and the menopause; a study of 40–60-year-old women. Clinical Endocrinology 45:577–587
2. Barrett-Connor E, Khaw K T 1987 Absence of an inverse relation of dehydroepiandrosterone sulfate with cardiovascular mortality in postmenopausal women. The New England Journal of Medicine 317:711
3. Barrett-Connor E, Young R, Notelovitz M et al 1999 A two-year, double-blind comparison of oestrogen–androgen and conjugated oestrogens in surgically menopausal women. Effects on bone mineral density, symptoms and lipid profiles. The Journal of Reproductive Medicine 44:1012–1020
4. Baulieu E E, Thomas G, Legrain S et al 2000 Dehydroepiandrosterone (DHEA), DHEA sulfate, and aging. Contribution of the DHEAge study to a sociobiomedical issue. Proceedings of the National Academy of Sciences of the USA 97:4279–4284
5. Berman J R, Almeida F G, Jolin J et al 2003 Correlation of androgen receptors, aromatase, and 5α-reductase in the human vagina with menopausal status. Fertility and Sterility 79:925–931
6. Björntorp P 1996 The android woman – a risky condition. Journal of Internal Medicine 239:105–110
7. Breitkopf D M, Rosen M P, Young S L et al 2003 Efficacy of second versus third generation oral contraceptives in the treatment of hirsutism. Contraception 67:349–353
8. Burger H G, Dudley E C, Cui J et al 2000 A prospective longitudinal study of serum testosterone, dehydroepiandrosterone sulfate, and sex hormone-binding globulin levels through the menopause transition.

The Journal of Clinical Endocrinology and Metabolism 85:2832–2838
9. Carmina E, Ferin M, Gonzalez F et al 1999 Evidence that insulin and androgens may participate in the regulation of serum leptin levels in women. Fertility and Sterility 72:926–931
10. Carnes C A, Dech S J 2002 Effects of dihydrotestosterone on cardiac inward rectifier K(+) current. International Journal of Andrology 25:210–214
11. Cashdan E 2003 Hormones and competitive aggression in women. Aggressive Behavior 29:107–115
12. Cauley J A, Lucas F L, Kuller L H et al 1999 Elevated serum estradiol and testosterone concentrations are associated with a high risk of breast cancer. Study of Osteoporotic Fractures Research Group. Annals of Internal Medicine 130:270–277
13. Chen W, Thiboutot D, Zouboulis C C 2002 Cutaneous androgen metabolism: basic research and clinical perspectives. The Journal of Investigative Dermatology 119:992–1007
14. Copeland J L, Consitt L A, Tremblay M S 2002 Hormonal responses to endurance and resistance exercise in females aged 19–69 years. The Journals of Gerontology 57A:B158–B165
15. Davis S R, Burger H G 2003 The role of androgen therapy. Best Practice & Research. Clinical Obstetrics & Gynaecology 17:165–175
16. Dennerstein L, Randolph J, Taffe J et al 2002 Hormones, mood, sexuality and the menopausal transition. Fertility and Sterility 77:S42–S48
17. Fassnacht M, Schlenz N, Schneider S B et al 2003 Beyond adrenal and ovarian

androgen generation: increased peripheral 5 alpha-reductase activity in women with polycystic ovary syndrome. The Journal of Clinical Endocrinology and Metabolism 88:2760–2766

18. Floter A, Nathorst-Böös J, Carlström K et al 1997 Androgen status and sexual life in perimenopausal women. Menopause 4:95–100

19. Fourcroy J L 2003 Female sexual dysfunction. Potential for pharmacotherapy. Drugs 63:1445–1457

20. Gompel A, Wright F, Kuttenn F et al 1986 Contribution of plasma androstenedione to 5α-androstanediol glucuronide in women with idiopathic hirsutism. The Journal of Clinical Endocrinology and Metabolism 62:441–444

21. Gower B A, Nyman L 2000 Associations among oral oestrogen use, free testosterone concentration, and lean body mass among postmenopausal women. The Journal of Clinical Endocrinology and Metabolism 85:4476–4480

22. Gruber D M, Sator M O, Kirchengast S et al 1998 Effect of percutaneous androgen replacement therapy on body composition and body weight in postmenopausal women. Maturitas 29:253–259

23. Guthrie J R, Dennerstein L, Taffe J R et al 2003 Central abdominal fat and endogenous hormones during the menopausal transition. Fertility and Sterility 79:1335–1340

24. Huber D M, Bendixen A C, Pathrose P et al 2001 Androgens suppress osteoclast formation induced by RANKI and macrophage-colony stimulating factor. Endocrinology 142:3800–3808

25. Isaa S, Schnadel D, Feix M et al 2002 Human osteoblast-like cells express predominantly steroid 5alpha-reductase type 1. The Journal of Clinical Endocrinology and Metabolism 87:5401–5407

26. Johannes C B, Stellato R K, Feldman H A et al 1999 Relation of dehydroepiandrosterone and dehydroepiandrosterone sulfate with cardiovascular disease risk factors in women. Longitudinal results from the Massachusetts Women's Health Study. Journal of Clinical Epidemiology 52:95–103

27. Key T J, Appleby P N, Reeves G K et al 2003 Body mass index, serum sex hormones, and breast cancer risks in postmenopausal women. Journal of the National Cancer Institute 95:1218–1226

28. Labrie F 2003 Extragonadal synthesis of sex steroids: intracrinology. Annales d'endocrinologie (Paris) 64:95–107

29. Lapointe J, Labrie C 2001 Role of the cyclin-dependent kinase inhibitor p27 in androgen-induced inhibition of CAMA-1 breast cancer cell proliferation. Endocrinology 142:4331–4338

30. Laughlin G A, Barrett-Connor E, Kritz-Silverstein D et al 2000 Hysterectomy, oophorectomy, and endogenous sex hormone levels in older women. The Rancho Bernardo Study. The Journal of Clinical Endocrinology and Metabolism 85:645–651

31. Laumann E O, Paik A, Rosen R C 1999 Sexual dysfunction in the United States. Prevalence and predictors. The Journal of the American Medical Association 281:537–544

32. Leder B Z, Leblanc K M, Longcope C et al 2002 Effects of oral androstenedione administration on serum testosterone and estradiol levels in postmenopausal women. The Journal of Clinical Endocrinology and Metabolism 87:5449–5454

33. Liu Y, Ding J, Bush TL et al 2001 Relative androgen excess and increased cardiovascular risk after menopause: a hypothesized relation. American Journal of Epidemiology 154:489–494

34. Lobo R A 2001 Androgens in postmenopausal women: production, possible role, and replacement options. Obstetrical & Gynecological Survey 56:361–376

35. Longcope C 1998 Androgen metabolism and the menopause. Seminars in Reproductive Endocrinology 16:111–115

36. Marcus R, Leary D, Schneider D L et al 2000 The contribution of testosterone to skeletal development and maintenance: lessons from the androgen insensitivity syndrome. The Journal of Clinical Endocrinology and Metabolism 85:1032–1037

37. Mauvais-Jarvis P, Kuttenn F, Mowszowicz I (eds) 1981 Hirsutism. Springer-Verlag, Berlin

38. Miller K K 2001 Androgen deficiency in women. The Journal of Clinical Endocrinology and Metabolism 86:2395–2401

39. Modelska K, Cummings S 2003 Female sexual dysfunction in postmenopausal women: systematic review of placebo-controlled trials. American Journal of Obstetrics and Gynecology 188:286–293

40. Morris K T, Toth-Fejel S, Schmidt J et al 2001 High dehydroepiandrosterone sulfate predicts breast cancer progression during new aromatase inhibitor therapy and stimulates breast cancer cell growth in

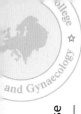

tissue culture: a renewed role for adrenalectomy. Surgery 130:947–953

41. Nowinski K, Pripp U, Carlstrom K et al 2002 Repolarization measures and their relation to sex hormones in postmenopausal women with cardiovascular disease receiving hormone replacement therapy. The American Journal of Cardiology 90:1050–1055

42. Ortmann J, Prifiti S, Bohlmann M K et al 2002 Testosterone and 5-alpha-dihydrotestosterone inhibit in vitro growth of human breast cancer cell lines. Gynecological Endocrinology 16:113–120

43. Padero M C M, Bhasin S, Friedman T C 2002 Androgen supplementation in older women: too much hype, not enough data. Journal of the American Geriatrics Society 50:1131–1140

44. Paridisi G, Steinberg H O, Hempfling A et al 2001 Polycystic ovary syndrome is associated with endothelial dysfunction. Circulation 103:1410–1415

45. Percheron G, Hogrel J Y, Denot-Ledunois S et al 2003 Effect of 1-year oral administration of dehydroepiandrosterone to 60- to 80-year-old individuals on muscle function and cross-sectional area. Archives of Internal Medicine 163:720–727

46. Puche C, Jose M, Cabero A et al 2002 Expression and enzymatic activity of the P450c17 gene in human adipose tissue. European Journal of Endocrinology 146:223–229

47. Sherwin B B 1985 Changes in sexual behavior as a function of plasma sex steroid levels in post-menopausal women. Maturitas 7:225–233

48. Shifren J L, Braunstein G D, Simon J A et al 2000 Transdermal testosterone treatment in women with impaired sexual function after oophorectomy. The New England Journal of Medicine 343:682–688

49. Simon J A 2002 Estrogen replacement therapy: effects on the endogenous androgen milieu. Fertility and Sterility 4:S77–S82

50. Simpson E R 2002 Aromatization of androgens in women: current concepts and findings. Fertility and Sterility 77 (Suppl 4):6–10

51. Slater C C, Chang L, Stanczyk F Z et al 2001 Altered balance between the 5 alpha-reductase and aromatase pathways of androgen metabolism during controlled ovarian hyperstimulation with human menopausal gonadrotropins. Journal of Assisted Reproduction and Genetics 18:527–533

52. Sowers M F, Beebe J L, McConnell D et al 2001 Testosterone concentrations in women aged 25–50 years: association with lifestyle, body composition, and ovarian status. American Journal of Epidemiology 153:256–264

53. Stoleru S G, Ennaji A, Cournot A et al 1993 LH pulsatile secretion and testosterone blood levels are influenced by sexual arousal in human males. Psychoneuroendocrinology 18:205–218

54. Suzuki T, Darnel A D, Akahira J I et al 2001 5-alpha-reductases in human breast carcinoma: possible modulator of in situ androgenic actions. The Journal of Clinical Endocrinology and Metabolism 86:2250–2257

55. Trivedi D P, Khaw K T 2001 Dehydroepiandrosterone sulfate and mortality in elderly men and women. The Journal of Clinical Endocrinology and Metabolism 86:4171–4177

56. Vermeulen A 1998 Plasma androgens in women. The Journal of Reproductive Medicine 43:725–733

57. Von der Pahlen B, Lindman R, Sarkola T et al 2002 An exploratory study on self-evaluated aggression and androgens in women. Aggressive Behavior 28:273–280

58. Wolf O T, Neumann O, Hellhammer D H et al 1997 Effects of a two-week physiological dehydroepiandrosterone substitution on cognitive performance and well-being in healthy elderly women and men. The Journal of Clinical Endocrinology and Metabolism 82:2363–2367

59. Worboys S, Kotsopoulos D, Teed H et al 2001 Evidence that parenteral testosterone therapy may improve endothelium-dependent and -independent vasodilation in postmenopausal women already receiving estrogen. The Journal of Clinical Endocrinology and Metabolism 86:158–161

60. Wren B G, Day R O, McLachlan A J et al 2003 Pharmacokinetics of estradiol, progesterone, testosterone and dehydroepiandrosterone after transbuccal administration to postmenopausal women. Climacteric 6:104–111

61. Zapantis G, Santoro N 2003 The menopausal transition: characteristics and management. Best Practice & Research. Clinical Endocrinology & Metabolism 17:33–52

Addendum

Recent reports suggest that when testosterone is added to HRT, the risk of breast cancer might be lowered. In Australia, women receiving implants containing 50–150 mg of testosterone every 5 months, with the mean follow-up time of 5.8 years, had a breast cancer rate of 238 per 100 000 woman-years, while those having HRT without testosterone had a cancer rate of 293 per 100 000 woman-years (a difference of –18.8%).[1] In animal studies, artificially induced breast cancer has either disappeared or reduced in size when DHT has been added to HRT.[3] This is biologically plausible since, in Rhesus monkeys, testosterone has been shown to inhibit the mitogenic effects of oestrogen.[2] This is an extremely interesting optional possibility for reducing the suggested risk of breast cancer in women who receive a combined oestrogen–progestin HRT.

Risto Erkkola

References

1. Dimitrakakis C, Jones R A, Liu A et al 2004 Breast cancer incidence in postmenopausal women using testosterone in addition to usual hormone therapy. Menopause 11:531–535
2. Gelfand M M 2004 It might be wise to consider adding androgen to the estrogen or estrogen–progestin regimens in the appropriate patients. Menopause 11:505–507
3. Somboonporn W, Davis S R 2004 Postmenopausal testosterone therapy and breast cancer risk. Maturitas 49:267–275

20

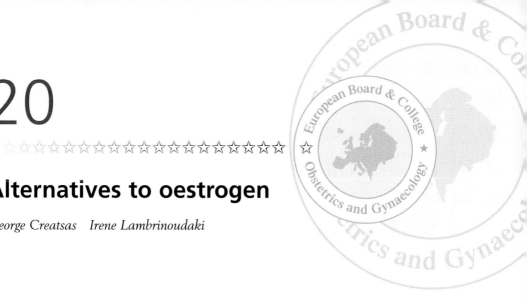

☆☆☆☆☆☆☆☆☆☆☆☆☆☆☆☆☆☆ ☆

Alternatives to oestrogen

George Creatsas   Irene Lambrinoudaki

ABSTRACT

Tibolone is a synthetic steroid with oestrogenic, progestogenic and androgenic activity. It is effective in alleviating climacteric symptoms and sexual dysfunction and in increasing bone mineral density (BMD) at the lumbar spine and hip. It does not promote endometrial growth and it appears to be less stimulative to the breast than conventional oestrogen or oestrogen–progestogen hormone replacement therapy (HRT), although data on breast cancer risk is still missing. Tibolone lowers triglyceride and HDL cholesterol and has subtle effects on LDL cholesterol.

Raloxifene is a SERM (selective oestrogen receptor modulator) with partial oestrogenic and anti-oestrogenic activity. It does not affect – and it may in some cases aggravate – climacteric symptoms. Raloxifene increases BMD at the lumbar spine and hip and decreases the risk for vertebral fractures. It has no effect on the endometrium and it decreases the risk for invasive breast cancer, at least in postmenopausal women with osteoporosis. Raloxifene lowers total and LDL cholesterol, while it does not modulate HDL cholesterol and triglyceride levels.

KEYWORDS

Bone mineral density (BMD), breast, endometrium, hormone replacement therapy (HRT), lipids, osteoporosis, raloxifene, tibolone

INTRODUCTION

Hormone replacement therapy (HRT) is the treatment of choice for the alleviation of climacteric symptoms and the prevention of postmenopausal osteoporosis. Prolonged treatment, however, may be associated with slight increases in the occurrence of breast cancer. However, the effect of prolonged HRT on the incidence of cardiovascular disease still remains a matter of debate. The need for long-term medical support of postmenopausal women regarding quality of life and the prevention of bone loss has led physicians to seek alternatives to conventional HRT. Currently the two most widely employed alternative regimens to HRT are tibolone and raloxifene.

Tibolone is a synthetic steroid with tissue-selective activity, which has been available in Europe for over 15 years, for the treatment of climacteric symptoms and postmenopausal osteoporosis.

Raloxifene is a SERM, which was launched for the prevention and treatment for postmenopausal osteoporosis but appears to exert oestrogenic or anti-oestrogenic activity on other tissues as well, depending on the target cell type.

This chapter deals with the available data on the efficacy and safety of these two compounds with regard to the climacteric symptoms, the skeleton, the reproductive tract, the breast and the cardiovascular system in postmenopausal women.

TIBOLONE

Tibolone is a synthetic steroid with a tissue-specific action. It is available as a 2.5 mg oral preparation and is absorbed rapidly and irrespectively of meals, peaking in the blood after 4 hours. It is metabolized in the liver and excreted in the urine, with a plasma half-life of 45 hours.[59] Tibolone itself is devoid of steroid activity. Its main actions are exerted through its metabolites 3α-hydroxytibolone (3αOH-tibolone), 3β-hydroxytibolone and the Δ4 isomer. After oral intake tibolone is rapidly converted to these metabolites, which appear in the circulation predominantly as sulphate forms.[79] The 3α- and 3β-OH metabolites possess oestrogenic activity and mainly stimulate the oestrogen receptor α (ERα), while the Δ4 isomer stimulates both the progesterone and androgen receptors, with relative binding and agonistic activity similar to that of progesterone and testosterone, respectively.[26] Tibolone is devoid of glucocorticoid activity.[26] In addition to its actions on steroid receptors, tibolone locally inhibits sulphatase activity, resulting in lower levels of active unbound oestrogenic compounds in tissues expressing these enzymes, such as the human breast and endometrium.[25]

TIBOLONE AND CLIMACTERIC SYMPTOMS

Climacteric symptoms are divided into three categories: vasomotor symptoms (e.g. hot flushes and night sweats); mood instability (e.g. mood swings, fatigue, loss of interest, insomnia and headaches); and sexual disorders (vaginal dryness, dyspareunia and diminished sexual desire, arousability and frequency of orgasms).

Tiblone lowers the frequency of hot flushes and night sweats significantly more than to placebo.[24,52] Compared to HRT, tibolone appears to be equally effective in reducing vasomotor symptoms.[1,47] Moreover, it improves mood parameters, such as sleep, emotional reactions, general well-being and psychological instability.[24,57] The alleviation of vasomotor symptoms, however, is related to improvements in sleep and fatigue and thus it may be difficult to assess the direct effect of tibolone on mood parameters. Beyond the short-term influence of tibolone on mood, its long-term administration may be associated with positive effects on cognitive functions in postmenopausal women.[36]

Sexuality is a complex issue requiring adequacy of both oestrogen and androgen activity in the brain and reproductive system. Physical symptoms such as vaginal dryness, recurrent urogenital infections and dyspareunia mainly result from oestrogen deprivation and are effectively treated by either tibolone or HRT. Psychological symptoms, however, such as low sexual desire and arousability are dependent on androgen deprivation. Tibolone exerts androgenic activity directly (through its Δ4 metabolite) and indirectly (by reducing SHBG serum levels and increasing free testosterone).[29] In this context, tibolone appears to be superior to HRT in improving sexual dysfunction in postmenopausal women. Compared to placebo and HRT, tibolone significantly increases sexual desire, sexual fantasies, arousability, frequency of intercourse and orgasm.[47,50,51,84] Tibolone's efficacy on sexual dysfunction is reported to be equivalent to combined replacement therapy with oestrogen and androgen, though its adverse androgenic effects with respect to other parameters, such as liver toxicity and lipid profile, are considerably less than with pure androgenic compounds.[10]

TIBOLONE AND OSTEOPOROSIS

Tibolone exerts its protective effect on bone through the ER.[30] In prospective randomized clinical trials tibolone therapy is associated with increases in BMD in the lumbar spine and hip.[5,38] Ten years' therapy with tibolone is reported to result in 12% greater BMD in the lumbar spine and hip when compared to non-users;[69] tibolone also appears to be effective in elderly women.[6] Moreover, 1.25 mg of tibolone (half of the usual dose) is also capable of reducing post-menopausal decreases in BMD.[6,38,68] Compared to HRT, two studies have demonstrated the superior efficacy of tibolone when compared with either transdermal or oral oestrogen,[64,75] while, in another trial, 17β-oestradiol combined with norethisterone acetate resulted in greater increases in BMD compared with tibolone.[68] However, no data currently exist with respect to the efficacy of tibolone in reducing fracture incidence. A placebo-controlled trial is underway to investigate the effect of tibolone on fracture risk and other important safety parameters – Long-term Intervention of Fractures with Tibolone: LIFT.

TIBOLONE AND THE ENDOMETRIUM

Tibolone is converted locally in endometrial tissue into its Δ4-metabolite, which exerts progestogenic activity, so there is no stimulation of the endometrium by tibolone.[26] Histologically, tibolone produces an atrophic endometrium in 90% of

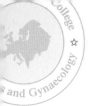
The menopause

cases and a clinically insignificant and mildly proliferative endometrium in the remainder. Compared to placebo, tibolone doubles the rate of vaginal bleeding during the first months of treatment,[4] but compared to continuous combined HRT (17β-oestradiol/norethisterone) tibolone is associated with approximately half the rate of vaginal bleeding.[44,83] Clinically, this effect is translated to 10–15% vaginal bleeding during the first 6 months, which is later reduced to 4%. Women having a recent menopause are more prone to vaginal bleeding although endometrial biopsies from women who bled showed no evidence of endometrial hyperplasia.[4] Tibolone does not appear to have any effect on the size of uterine fibroids.[74] A prospective study concerning the effects of tibolone on the endometrium and breast with 3200 participants (THEBES: Tibolone History of the Endometrium and Breast Endpoints Study) is due to end in 2005.

TIBOLONE AND BREAST

There are numerous studies evaluating, *in vitro*, the effects of tibolone on normal breast and breast cancer cell lines. Tibolone and its 3-OH metabolites inhibit sulphatase activity and to a lesser extent 17β-hydroxysteroid dehydrogenase activity, thus diminishing active steroid concentrations.[13,65,76] Tibolone and its Δ4 isomer have antiproliferative and pro-apoptotic actions and promote differentiation in normal breast cells. Tibolone is also pro-apoptotic in breast cancer cell lines.[41,42] On clinical grounds, tibolone does not affect mammographic breast density in the majority of cases.[15,22] Compared to oestrogen/progestin regimens, tibolone increases breast density to a much lesser degree[23,32,55] and causes substantially less breast discomfort.[44] Moreover, tibolone alleviates mastopathic complaints and reduces breast density in selected patients with benign mastopathy.[31] In this context, tibolone appears to be safe with respect to the risk of breast cancer although controlled randomized trials with breast cancer risk as the primary end-point are still missing. A 5-year prospective placebo-controlled study on 2600 breast cancer patients (LIBERATE: Livial Intervention following Breast cancer – Efficacy, Recurrence And Tolerability Endpoints) will end in 2009.

TIBOLONE, LIPIDS AND THE CARDIOVASCULAR SYSTEM

Tibolone's effect on lipid parameters appears to be a consequence of both oestrogenic and androgenic activity. In contrast to HRT, tibolone reduces plasma high-density lipoprotein (HDL) cholesterol by approximately 30% and plasma triglycerides by 20–30%. Total and low-density lipoprotein (LDL) cholesterol are not significantly influenced by tibolone.[2,7,40,53] Despite the decrease in HDL cholesterol, tibolone does not affect serum cholesterol efflux potential, implying that tibolone has no effect on the anti-atherogenic activity of HDL cholesterol.[58,77,78] Data with respect to other cardiovascular risk parameters are limited. Tibolone may increase nitric oxide (NO) and decrease endothelin-1 plasma levels.[19,43] Similarly to oestrogens, tibolone is reported to reduce fibrinogen, factor VIIc, antithrombin and plasminogen activator inhibitor-1 (PAI-1) antigen and to increase fibrin degradation products, indicating an increased fibrin turnover state.[63,83] Furthermore, tibolone increases C-reactive protein (CRP) [39] and has no effect on plasma homocysteine levels.[12,17] Beyond the effect on lipids, however, tibolone's effect on other cardiovascular parameters remains to be documented in large placebo-controlled trials. Recently it has been demonstrated that in cholesterol-fed ovariectomized monkeys tibolone had a strong dose-dependent anti-atherosclerotic effect.[85] In healthy postmenopausal women, tibolone treatment is reported to decrease the intimal–medial thickness and the resistance indices of the common carotid artery.[33] The long-term effect of tibolone, however, on the incidence and evolution of cardiovascular disease in postmenopausal women remains to be elucidated in randomized controlled trials.

CONCLUSION ON TIBOLONE

Tibolone is an effective alternative to HRT in the treatment of climacteric symptoms, namely hot flushes, urogenital symptoms and mood swings, and may be more effective than HRT in improving sexuality. Tibolone increases BMD in the lumbar spine and hip and has no stimulatory activity on the endometrium. The effect on the breast appears to be favourable, although long-term data on the incidence of breast cancer are still missing. The overall effect of tibolone on surrogate markers of cardiovascular disease is considered to be positive. The influence, however, on cardiovascular events in postmenopausal women remains to be clarified.

RALOXIFENE

Raloxifene is a major representative of SERMs. Tamoxifen, the first available SERM, is widely used for the prevention and treatment of breast cancer. Raloxifene is also approved for the prevention and treatment of osteoporosis but appears to have a wide range of action in other oestrogen-responsive tissues.

SERMs are compounds structurally related but chemically distinct from oestrogen and which have the ability to bind to ER and exert differential activity, depending on the target tissue. This unique characteristic of SERMs depends on three inherent properties of the ER activation system:

1. There are two identified ERs: ERα and ERβ. The activation of ERα almost always results in oestrogen agonist activity, while ERβ may inhibit the activation of ERα by forming ERα-β heterodimers or by inhibiting the transcription of oestrogen responsive genes. Therefore raloxifene is an oestrogen agonist through the ERα while being an oestrogen antagonist through the ERβ in tissues containing oestrogen response elements.
2. Oestrogen receptors sustain a unique conformational change depending on the ligand. SERMs may induce a spectrum of conformational changes ranging from that induced by oestrogens to that induced by pure anti-oestrogens.

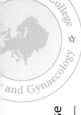

3. The final genomic action of the activated ER depends on the activity of co-regulatory proteins, some of them stimulating (coactivators) and others inhibiting (co-repressors) gene transcription. SERMs can induce different sets of co-regulatory proteins, depending on the receptor conformational changes induced in each target tissue.

These three parameters enable SERMs selectively to exert oestrogenic or anti-oestrogenic activities depending on the target cell type.[67]

RALOXIFENE AND CLIMACTERIC SYMPTOMS

Raloxifene functions as an anti-oestrogen in hypothalamic centres regulating gonadotrophin production. Therefore raloxifene is not indicated for the treatment of hot flushes or other climacteric complaints related to low endogenous oestrogen levels. In recently menopausal women, raloxifene increases hot flushes by up to 7% (compared to placebo) while tamoxifen increases hot flushes by 17%.[48] In late postmenopausal women, raloxifene does not affect the incidence of hot flushes,[34] enabling clinicians to prescribe this drug for indications other than the treatment of climacteric symptoms.

RALOXIFENE AND OSTEOPOROSIS

Raloxifene's effect in preventing and treating postmenopausal osteoporosis is well documented. In randomized placebo-controlled trials raloxifene is reported to induce a 2–3% increase in BMD in the lumbar spine and hip after the second year of treatment in postmenopausal women with osteoporosis.[34,54] Furthermore, raloxifene was associated with a 40% reduction of vertebral fractures in postmenopausal women with osteoporosis after 3 years' treatment in the MORE trial, a large-scale placebo-controlled trial aimed to evaluate the effect of raloxifene on fracture risk in osteoporotic postmenopausal women.[34] This effect was consistent across age groups and independent of the severity of bone loss or of prevalent vertebral fractures. The fact that raloxifene has almost equal efficacy in reducing vertebral fracture risk compared to bisphosphonates, while increasing BMD to a lesser extent, has been attributed to the bone micro-architechture preserving properties of raloxifene.[66] The MORE trial, however, failed to show an effect of raloxifene in reducing hip fracture risk. Raloxifene is also effective in the prevention of osteoporosis, increasing BMD by 2–3% in the lumbar spine and hip in healthy postmenopausal women after the second year of treatment.[27,48]

RALOXIFENE AND THE ENDOMETRIUM

In contrast to oestrogen, raloxifene has no stimulatory effect on the endometrium. Long-term treatment with raloxifene does not increase endometrial thickness and is not associated with endometrial hyperplasia or polyp formation,[34,61] in contrast to tamoxifen, which induces endometrial hyperplasia and polyp formation in 18% and 25–30% of cases, respectively[60] and increases endometrial cancer risk 2.5-fold.[35] Thus raloxifene is not associated with uterine bleeding, which is one of the main reasons for early drop-outs in women receiving oestrogen–progestin therapy.[1,21]

RALOXIFENE AND THE BREAST

Raloxifene acts as an anti-oestrogen on the breast. It has recently been shown that this action is mediated by the recruitment of co-repressors to inhibit activated ER action on target gene promoters.[72] This action is also shared by tamoxifen. On the contrary, while tamoxifen recruits coactivators for oestrogen responsive gene expression in the endometrium, this does not happen with raloxifene, which has no effect on that tissue. The anti-oestrogenic effect of raloxifene on the breast has been documented in the MORE trial.[11] This trial – originally designed to assess the effect of raloxifene on fracture risk in 7705 postmenopausal women with osteoporosis assigned either to raloxifene or placebo – evaluated as a secondary end-point the incidence of invasive breast cancer. After a median of 40 months raloxifene reduced the incidence of invasive breast cancer by 76% (RR 0.24; 95% CI; range 0.13–0.44). This effect was confined to ER-positive tumours, where the reduction in incidence was 90% (RR 0.10; 95% CI; range 0.04–0.24). Recent results from 8-year follow-up of the MORE participants[56] documented a persistent effect in the reduction of the incidence of ER-positive tumours (RR 0.24; 95% CI; range 0.15–0.40). It must be remembered, however, that the population studied was not at a high risk for developing breast cancer and we cannot therefore extrapolate these results to high-risk women. Currently, there is a large-scale trial under way which aims to assess the efficacy of raloxifene compared to tamoxifen in the primary prevention of breast cancer in 22 000 postmenopausal women at high risk for breast cancer (Study of Tamoxifen and Raloxifene: STAR). The results of this study are expected to answer the question of the long-term use of raloxifene in healthy postmenopausal women at increased risk for breast cancer.

In contrast to HRT, which increases breast density in mammography by 10–34%,[18] raloxifene has no effect on breast density[15] or it may even induce involution of breast parenchyma, similar to the regression in fibroglandular tissue seen in healthy postmenopausal women under no therapy.[37] This is particularly important for screening purposes as it does not diminish the sensitivity of mammography to diagnose breast cancer and thus there is no need to discontinue the drug temporarily before mammography.

RALOXIFENE, LIPIDS AND THE CARDIOVASCULAR SYSTEM

Raloxifene's effect on lipids is considered as favourable. Similarly to oestrogens, raloxifene decreases LDL cholesterol by up to 12% in postmenopausal

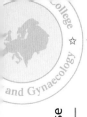
The menopause

women;[2,48,62,80] this effect is apparent across the whole age spectrum of post-menopausal women.[45] In contrast to oestrogens, which increase HDL cholesterol and triglyceride levels, raloxifene has no effect on either parameter.[2,27,80] There is some evidence, however, that raloxifene might actually increase the HDL_2 cholesterol subfraction, although to a lesser extent than oestrogens.[80] Moreover raloxifene reduces Lp(a) levels by approximately 7%, compared to a 19% decrease induced by oestrogen.[80]

The effect of raloxifene on other cardiovascular risk factors is less well defined. Raloxifene probably decreases serum homocysteine and fibrinogen, while it has no effect on PAI-1.[16,28,80,81] In contrast to HRT, which increases CRP, an independent risk factor for cardiovascular events, raloxifene has no effect on this parameter.[81] This is particularly important for the safety profile of this drug, given the long-term intake of raloxifene in postmenopausal women. Also, raloxifene is reported to increase serum NO, to decrease serum endothelin-1 and to augment NO-dependent vasodilatation.[14,70,71,73]

In animal models raloxifene is reported to inhibit evolution of atherosclerosis. In ovariectomized rabbits fed with atherogenic diet raloxifene retarded the development of atherosclerotic plaques[7] and inhibited the progression in already formed plaques.[9] This effect was not confirmed, however, in ovariectomized monkeys, where raloxifene had no effect on the progression of atherosclerosis.[20]

Data on the effect of raloxifene on cardiovascular events come mainly from the MORE study. After 3 years of follow-up there was no difference concerning the total number of coronary and cerebrovascular events between the raloxifene and the placebo group in 7705 enrolled postmenopausal women with osteoporosis.[46] No excess risk for cardiovascular events was identified, either during the first or subsequent years of the trial. No excess risk was documented in the subgroup of women with pre-existing coronary artery disease. The 4-year results of the MORE trial have subsequently shown that although no effect of raloxifene on cardiovascular risk was apparent in the whole cohort, women at high cardiovascular risk exhibited a significant reduction in the incidence of cardiovascular events.[3] An increased risk for thromboembolic events was identified in the MORE trial similar to those associated with HRT.[34] A large trial currently under way evaluating the effect of raloxifene on the incidence of coronary events in high cardiovascular risk postmenopausal women will elucidate the efficacy of raloxifene in the prevention of cardiovascular disease (Raloxifene Use for the Heart: RUTH).[81]

CONCLUSION ON RALOXIFENE

Raloxifene is a very good therapeutic option for the prevention and treatment of postmenopausal osteoporosis, especially for the prevention of vertebral fractures in women not recently menopausal. Raloxifene has no effect on the endometrium, it does not increase breast density and it may also reduce the incidence of ER-positive invasive breast cancer. The drug has lipid-lowering properties and its safety profile with respect to the cardiovascular system may prove superior to that of HRT in the long term. The results of the two large trials currently under way (STAR and RUTH) are awaited to validate the effect of raloxifene on the breast and heart.

References

1. Al-Azzawi F, Wahab M, Habiba M et al 1999 Continuous combined hormone replacement therapy compared with tibolone. Obstetrics and Gynecology 93:258–264

2. Barnes J F, Farish E, Rankin M et al 2002 A comparison of the effects of two continuous HRT regimens on cardio-vascular risk factors. Atherosclerosis 160:185–193

3. Barrett-Connor E, Grady D, Sashegyi A et al 2002 Raloxifene and cardiovascular events in osteoporotic postmenopausal women. Four-year results from the MORE trial. The Journal of the American Medical Association 287:847–857

4. Berning B, van Kuijk J W, Fauser B C 2000 Absent correlation between vaginal bleeding and oestradiol levels or endome-trial morphology during tibolone use in early postmenopausal women. Maturitas 35:81–88

5. Berning B, Bennink H J, Fauser B C 2001 Tibolone and its effects on bone: a review. Climacteric 4:120–136

6. Bjarnason N H, Bjarnason K, Haarbo J et al 1996 Tibolone: prevention of bone loss in late postmenopausal women. The Journal of Clinical Endocrinology and Metabolism 81:2419–2422

7. Bjarnason N, Bjarnason K H, Bennink H J et al 1997 Tibolone: influence on markers of cardiovascular disease. The Journal of Clinical Endocrinology and Metabolism 82:1752–1756

8. Bjarnason N H, Haarbo J, Byrjalsen I et al 1997 Raloxifene inhibits aortic accumu-lation of cholesterol in ovariectomized, cholesterol-fed rabbits. Circulation 96:1964–1969

9. Bjarnason N H, Haarbo J, Byrjalsen I et al 2001 Raloxifene and estrogen reduces progression of advanced atherosclerosis: a study in ovariectomized, cholesterol-fed rabbits. Atherosclerosis 154:97–102

10. Castelo-Branco C, Vicente J J, Figueras F et al 2000 Comparative effects of estrogens plus androgens and tibolone on bone, lipid pattern and sexuality in postmenopausal women. Maturitas 34:161–168

11. Cauley J A, Nortol L, Lippman M E et al 2001 Continued breast cancer risk reduction in postmenopausal women treated with raloxifene: 4-year results from the MORE randomized trial. Multiple Outcomes of Raloxifene Evaluation. Breast Cancer Research and Treatment 65:125–134

12. Celic H, Ayar A, Tug N et al 2002 Effects of tibolone on plasma homocysteine levels in postmenopausal women. Fertility and Sterility 78:347–350

13. Chetrite G, Kloosterboer H J, Pasqualini J R 1997 Effect of tibolone (Org OD14) and its metabolites on estrone sulphatase activity in MCF-7 and T-47D mammary cancer cells. Anticancer Research 17:135–140

14. Christodoulakos G, Panoulis C, Kouskouni E et al 2002 Effects of estrogen–progestin and raloxifene therapy on nitric oxide, prostacyclin and endothelin-1 synthesis. Gynecological Endocrinology 16:9–17

15. Christodoulakos G, Lambrinoudaki I, Vourtsi A et al 2002 Mammographic changes associated with raloxifene and tibolone therapy in postmenopausal women. A prospective study. Menopause 9:110–116

16. Christodoulakos G, Lambrinoudaki I, Panoulis C et al 2003 Effect of raloxifene, estrogen, and hormone replacement therapy on serum homocysteine levels in postmenopausal women. Fertility and Sterility 79:455–456

17. Christodoulakos G, Panoulis C, Lambrinoudaki I et al 2004 Effect of hormone replacement therapy and tibolone on serum total homocysteine levels. European Journal of Obstetrics, Gynecology, and Reproductive Biology 112:74–79

18. Christodoulakos G, Lambrinoudaki I, Panoulis C et al 2003 The effect of oestrogen and hormone replacement therapy on mammography. Maturitas 45:109–118

19. Cicinelli E, Ignarro L J, Galantino P et al 2002 Effects of tibolone on plasma levels of nitric oxide in postmenopausal women. Fertility and Sterility 78:464–468

20. Clarkson T B, Anthony M S, Jerome C P 1998 Lack of effect of raloxifene on coronary artery atherosclerosis of post-menopausal monkeys. The Journal of Clinical Endocrinology and Metabolism 83:721–726

21. Cohen F, Watts S, Shah A et al 2000 Uterine effects of 3-year raloxifene therapy in postmenopausal women younger than age 60. Obstetrics and Gynecology 95:104–110

22. Colacurci N, Mele D, De Franciscis P et al 1998 Effects of tibolone on the breast. European Journal of Obstetrics, Gyne-cology, and Reproductive Biology 80:235–238

23. Colacurci N, Fornaro F, De Franciscis P et al 2001 Effects of different types of hormone replacement therapy on mammographic density. Maturitas 40:159–164

24. Davis S R 2002 The effects of tibolone on mood and libido. Menopause 9:162–170

25. De Gooyer M E, Kleyn G T, Smits K C et al 2001 Tibolone: a compound with tissue-specific inhibitory effects on sulfatase. Molecular and Cellular Endocri-nology 183:55–62

26. De Gooyer M, Deckers G, Schoonen W et al 2003 Receptor profiling and endocrine interactions of tibolone. Steroids 68:21–30

27. Delmas P D, Bjarnason N H, Mitlak B H et al 1997 Effects of raloxifene on bone mineral density, serum cholesterol concentrations and uterine endometrium in postmenopausal women. The New England Journal of Medicine 337:1641–1647

28. De Valk-de Roo G W, Stehouwer C D A, Meijer P et al 1999 Both raloxifene and estrogen reduce major cardiovascular risk factors in healthy postmenopausal women. A 2-year, placebo-controlled study. Arterio-sclerosis, Thrombosis, and Vascular Biology 19:2993–3000

29. Doren M, Rubig A, Coelingh Bennink H J et al 2001 Differential effects on the androgen status of postmenopausal women treated with tibolone and continuous combined estradiol and norethindrone acetate replacement therapy. Fertility and Sterility 75:554–559

30. Ederveen A G, Kloosterboer H J 2001 Tibolone exerts its protective effect on trabecular bone loss through the estrogen receptor. Journal of Bone and Mineral Research 16:1651–1657

31. Egarter C, Eppel W, Vogel S et al 2001 A pilot study of hormone replacement therapy with tibolone in women with mastopathic breasts. Maturitas 40:165–171

32. Erel C T, Esen G, Seyisoglu H et al 2001 Mammographic density increase in women receiving different hormone replacement regimens. Maturitas 40:151–157

33. Erenus M, Ilhan H, Elter K 2003 Effect of tibolone treatment on intima-media thickness and the resistive indices of the carotid arteries. Fertility and Sterility 79:268–273

34. Ettinger B, Black D M, Mitlak B H et al 1999 Reduction of vertebral fracture risk in postmenopausal women with osteoporosis treated with raloxifene: results from a 3-year randomized clinical trial. The Journal of the American Medical Association 282:637–645

35. Fisher B, Constantino J P, Wickerham D L et al 1998 Tamoxifen for the prevention of breast cancer. Report of the National Surgical Adjuvant Breast and Bowel Project P-1 study. Journal of the National Cancer Institute 90:1371–1388

36. Fluck E, File S E, Rymer J 2002 Cognitive effects of 10 years of hormone replacement therapy with tibolone. Journal of Clinical Psychopharmacology 22:62–67

37. Freedman M, Martin J S, O'Gorman J et al 2001 Digitized mammography: a clinical trial of postmenopausal women randomly assigned to receive raloxifene, estrogen or placebo. Journal of the National Cancer Institute 93:51–56

38. Gallagher J C, Baylink D J, Freeman R et al 2001 Prevention of bone loss with tibolone in postmenopausal women. Results of two randomized, double-blind, placebo-controlled, dose-finding studies. The Journal of Clinical Endocrinology and Metabolism 86:4717–4726

39. Garnero P, Jamin C, Benhamou C L et al 2002 Effects of tibolone and combined 17beta-estradiol and norethisterone acetate on serum C-reactive protein in healthy post-menopausal women: a randomized trial. Human Reproduction 17:2748–2753

40. Godsland I F 2001 Effects of postmen-opausal hormone replacement therapy on lipid, lipoprotein and lipoprotein(a) concentrations: analysis of studies pub-lished from 1974–2000. Fertility and Sterility 75:898–915

41. Gompel A, Siromachkova M, Lombet A et al 2000 Tibolone actions on normal and breast cancer cells. European Journal of Cancer 36:S76–S77

42. Gompel A, Chaouat M, Jacob D et al 2002 In vitro studies of tibolone in breast cells. Fertility and Sterility 78:351–359

43. Haenggi W, Bersinger N A, Mueller M D et al 1999 Decrease of serum endothelin levels with postmenopausal hormone replacement therapy or tibolone. Gynecological Endocrinology 13:202–205

44. Hammar M, Christau J, Rud T et al 1998 A double-blind randomized trial comparing the effects of tibolone and continuous combined hormone replacement therapy in postmenopausal women with menopausal symptoms. British Journal of Obstetrics and Gynaecology 105:904–911

45. Harper K, Sarkar S, Cox D et al 2000 Raloxifene improves serum lipids and lowers fibrinogen in older postmenopausal women. Journal of the American Geriatrics Society 48 (Suppl):S51

46. Harper K D, Barrett-Connor E, Sashegyi A et al 2001 The effect of raloxifene on cardiovascular risk in osteoporotic postmenopausal women: 3-year results from the MORE (Multiple Outcomes of Raloxifene Evaluation) trial. Journal of the American Geriatrics Society 49:S5–S6

47. Huber J, Palacios S, Berglund L et al 2002 Effects of tibolone and continuous combined hormone replacement therapy on bleeding rates, quality of life and tolerability in postmenopausal women. British Journal of Obstetrics and Gynaecology 109:886–893

48. Johnston C C, Bjarnanson N H, Cohen F J et al 2000 Long-term effects of raloxifene on bone mineral density, bone turnover and serum lipid levels in early postmenopausal women: three year data from 2 double-blind randomized placebo-controlled trials. Archives of Internal Medicine 160:3444–3450

49. Kloosterboer H J, Ederveen A G 2002 Pros and cons of existing treatment modalities in osteoporosis: a comparison between tibolone, SERMs and estrogen (+/−progestogen) treatments. The Journal of Steroid Biochemistry and Molecular Biology 83:157–165

50. Kokcu A, Cetinkaya M B, Yanik F et al 2000 The comparison of effects of tibolone and conjugated estrogen–medroxyprogesterone acetate therapy on sexual performance in postmenopausal women. Maturitas 36:75–80

51. Laan E, van Lunsen R H, Everaerd W 2001 The effects of tibolone on vaginal blood flow, sexual desire and arousability in postmenopausal women. Climacteric 4:28–41

52. Landgren B M, Bennink H J, Helmond F A et al 2002 Dose-response analysis of effects of tibolone on climacteric symptoms. British Journal of Obstetrics and Gynaecology 109:1109–1114

53. Lloyd G, McGing A, Patel N et al 2000 A randomized placebo-controlled trial of the effects of tibolone on blood pressure and lipids in hypertensive women. Journal of Human Hypertension 14:99–104

54. Lufkin E G, Whitaker M D, Nickelsen T et al 1998 Treatment of established postmenopausal osteoporosis with raloxifene: a randomized trial. Journal of Bone and Mineral Research 13:1747–1754

55. Lundström E, Christow A, Kersemaekers W et al 2002 Effects of tibolone and continuous combined hormone replacement therapy on mammographic breast density. American Journal of Obstetrics and Gynecology 186:717–722

56. Martino S, Cauley J A, Barrett-Connor E et al 2004 Continuing outcomes relevant to Evista. Breast cancer incidence in postmenopausal osteoporotic women in a randomized trial of raloxifene. Journal of the National Cancer Institute 96:1751–1761

57. Meeuwsen I B, Samson M M, Duursma S A et al 2002 The influence of tibolone on quality of life in postmenopausal women. Maturitas 41:35–43

58. Mikkola T S, Anthony M S, Clarkson T B et al 2002 Serum cholesterol efflux potential in postmenopausal monkeys treated with tibolone or conjugated estrogens. Metabolism 51:523–530

59. Modelska K, Cummings S 2002 Tibolone for postmenopausal women: systematic review of randomized trials. The Journal of Clinical Endocrinology and Metabolism 87:16–23

60. Neven P, Vernaeve H 2000 Guidelines for monitoring patients taking tamoxifen treatment. Drug Safety 22:1–11

61. Neven P, Lunde T, Benedetti-Panici P et al 2003 A multicentric randomized trial to compare uterine safety of raloxifene with continuous combined hormone replacement therapy containing oestradiol and norethisterone acetate. British Journal of Obstetrics and Gynaecology 110:157–167

62. Nickelsen T, Creatsas G, Rechberger T et al 2001 Differential effects of raloxifene and continuous combined hormone replacement therapy on biochemical markers of

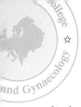

cardiovascular risk. Results from the Euralox 1 study. Climacteric 4:320–331

63. Norris L A, Joyce M, O'Keefe N et al 2002 Haemostatic risk factors in healthy postmenopausal women taking hormone replacement therapy. Maturitas 43:125–133

64. Prelevic G M, Bartram C, Wood J et al 1996 Comparative effects on bone mineral density of tibolone, transdermal estrogen and oral estrogen/progestogen therapy in postmenopausal women. Gynecological Endocrinology 10:413–420

65. Purohit A, Malini B, Hooymans C et al 2002 Inhibition of oestrone sulphatase activity by tibolone and its metabolites. Hormone and Metabolic Research 34:1–6

66. Riggs B L, Melton L J III 2002 Bone turnover matters: the raloxifene treatment paradox of dramatic decreases in vertebral fractures without commensurate increases in bone density. Journal of Bone and Mineral Research 17:11–14

67. Riggs B L, Hartmann L C 2003 Selective estrogen-receptor modulators. Mechanisms of action and application to clinical practice. The New England Journal of Medicine 348:618–629

68. Roux C, Pelissier C, Fechtenbaum J et al 2002 Randomized, double-masked, 2-year comparison of tibolone with 17beta-estradiol and norethindrone acetate in preventing postmenopausal bone loss. Osteoporos International 13:241–248

69. Rymer J, Robinson J, Fogelman I 2002 Ten years of treatment with tibolone 2.5 mg daily: effects on bone loss in postmenopausal women. Climacteric 5:390–398

70. Saitta A, Morabito N, Frisina N et al 2001 Cardiovascular effects of raloxifene hydrochloride. Cardiovascular Drug Reviews 19:57–74

71. Sarrel P M, Nawaz H, Chan W et al 2003 Raloxifene and endothelial function in healthy postmenopausal women. American Journal of Obstetrics and Gynecology 188:304–309

72. Shang Y, Brown M 2002 Molecular determinants for the tissue specificity of SERMs. Science 295:2465–2468

73. Simoncini T, Genazzani A R, Liao J K 2002 Nongenomic mechanisms of endothelial nitric oxide synthase activation by the selective estrogen receptor modulator raloxifene. Circulation 105:1368–1373

74. Simsek T, Karakus C, Trak B 2002 Impact of different hormone replacement therapy regimens on the size of myoma uteri in postmenopausal period. Tibolone versus transdermal hormonal replacement system. Maturitas 42:243–246

75. Thiebaud D, Bigler J M, Renteria S et al 1998 A 3-year study of prevention of postmenopausal bone loss: conjugated equine estrogens plus medroxyprogesterone acetate versus tibolone. Climacteric 1:202–210

76. Van de Ven J, Donker G H, Sprong M et al 2002 Effect of tibolone (Org OD14) and its metabolites on aromatase and estrone sulfatase activity in human breast adipose stromal cells and in MCF-7 and T47D breast cancer cells. The Journal of Steroid Biochemistry and Molecular Biology 81:237–247

77. Von Eckardstein A, Schmiddem K, Hovels A et al 2001 Lowering of HDL cholesterol in post-menopausal women by tibolone is not associated with changes in cholesterol efflux capacity or paraoxonase activity. Atherosclerosis 159:433–439

78. Von Eckardstein A, Crook D, Elbers J et al 2003 Tibolone lowers high-density lipoprotein cholesterol by increasing hepatic lipase activity but does not impair cholesterol efflux. Clinical Endocrinology 58:49–58

79. Vos R M, Krebbers S F, Verhoeven C H et al 2002 The in vivo human metabolism of tibolone. Drug Metabolism and Disposition 30:106–112

80. Walsh B W, Kuller L H, Wild R A et al 1998 Effects of raloxifene on serum lipids and coagulation factors in healthy postmenopausal women. The Journal of the American Medical Association 279:1445–1451

81. Walsh B W, Paul S, Wild R A et al 2000 The effects of hormone replacement therapy and raloxifene on C-reactive protein and homocysteine in healthy postmenopausal women: a randomized controlled trial. The Journal of Clinical Endocrinology and Metabolism 85:214–218

82. Wenger N K, Barrett-Connor E, Collins P et al 2002 Baseline characteristics of participants in the Raloxifene Use for The Heart (RUTH) trial. American Journal of Cardiology 90:1204–1210

83. Winkler U, Altkemper B, Helmond F A et al 2000 Effects of tibolone and continuous combined hormone replacement therapy on parameters in the clotting cascade: a multicenter, double-

blind, randomized study. Fertility and
Sterility 74:10–19

84. Wu M H, Pan H A, Wang S T et al 2001
Quality of life and sexuality changes in
postmenopausal women receiving tibolone
therapy. Climacteric 4:314–319

85. Zandberg P, Peters J L M, Demacker P N
et al 2001 Comparison of the
antiatherosclerotic effect of tibolone with
that of estradiol and ethinyl estradiol in
cholesterol-fed, ovariectomized rabbits.
Menopause 8:96–105

21

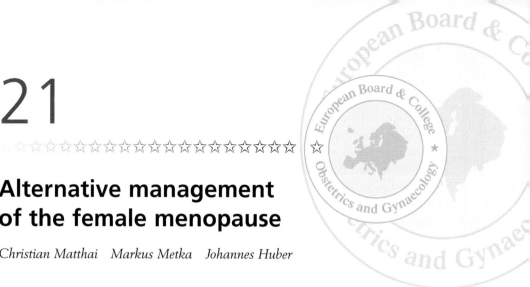

☆☆☆☆☆☆☆☆☆☆☆☆☆☆☆☆☆☆☆☆☆☆ ☆

Alternative management of the female menopause

Christian Matthai   Markus Metka   Johannes Huber

ABSTRACT

The oestrogenic properties of the polyphenolic non-steroidal phyto-oestrogens may provide a range of health benefits. These natural plant compounds particularly occur in soya products and red clover and could be a helpful alternative to the conventional hormone replacement therapy (HRT) in special cases. Three major chemical types of phyto-oestrogens have been identified. One of them comprises the well known isoflavones (including genistein or 4′,5,7-trihydroxyisoflavone), which has been investigated and described the most. Isoflavones appear to possess tissue selectivity in their agonist and antagonist effects. Because of a significantly higher binding affinity to oestrogen receptor β (ER-β)[29] isoflavones can be regarded as selective oestrogen-receptor modulators (SERMs). The latest developments and their controversial results concerning the role of phyto-oestrogens in diseases such as breast and prostate cancer, osteoporosis, menopausal symptoms or cardiovascular diseases are discussed here.

KEYWORDS

Genistein (4′,5,7-trihydroxyisoflavone), isoflavones, menopause, phyto-oestrogens

INTRODUCTION

The public interest in complementary and alternative therapies for the treatment of medical conditions is expanding and will continue to increase in the years ahead. In 1997, about 40% of Americans reported using alternative therapies for the relief of complaints.[12] The number of women aged 45–60, who reported using non-prescription therapies for the management of menopausal symptoms

225

was 80%.[25] Over 23% of women older than 65 years suffer from osteoporosis caused by an endogenous oestrogen deficiency.[38]

Hormone replacement therapy and bisphosphonates are currently accepted as the best pharmaceutical methods for maintaining bone mineral density (BMD) in postmenopausal women,[56] although some women are not candidates for hormone treatment because of a clotting disorder (thromboembolism) or a history of breast cancer. Reasons such as discomfort, decline in cardiovascular function or loss of BMD induce patients to look for something else.

Red clover (*Trifolium pratense*) and soya products are valuable sources of phyto-oestrogens. The three major chemical types that have been identified are isoflavones, lignans and coumestans. The most important of these are the four isoflavones: genistein; daidzein; biochanin A; and formononetin (a precursor of genistein and daidzein). Red clover contains all four. Isoflavones are natural plant compounds with a striking similarity to the chemical structure of mammalian oestrogens. Clinical data are now accumulating suggesting that isoflavones (which have the most potent oestrogenic activity of these natural compounds) may provide a range of health benefits with few side-effects and could be a natural alternative to conventional HRT. Among the isoflavones, genistein is the most active oestrogen with the highest binding affinity for oestrogen receptors (ERs)[47] and the highest bioavailability.[45]

Isoflavones are attached to a sugar molecule; they are also referred to as glucones and, after conversion, they become the biologically active aglycone form. The conjugates (glucones) are split by microbial enzymes in the intestine and are commonly taken up, in the unconjugated form, as aglycones. The precursors and metabolites all exert oestrogenic activity.[50] After absorption, isoflavones are transported to the liver and then eliminated via the kidneys.

Basically, isoflavones act as weak oestrogens on ERs, and are strong enough to promote bone formation and reduce the risk of cardiovascular disease but not strong enough to induce hormone-related cancer.[32,54]

Isoflavones appear to possess tissue selectivity (ER-α, ER-β) in their agonist and antagonist effects. Because of a significantly higher affinity to ER-β,[29] isoflavones can be regarded as SERMs. Isoflavones also compete with endogenous oestrogen for receptor sites. If the endogenous oestrogen level is high, they may exhibit anti-oestrogenic properties but oestrogenic properties if the level is low. Genistein is supposed to be effective in many medical conditions. Questions regarding the therapeutic benefits of isoflavones have been raised and many studies have been carried out. However, further investigations are necessary to explore the potential of this alternative therapeutic agent.

EFFECTS ON MENOPAUSAL SYMPTOMS

HOT FLUSHES AND NIGHT SWEATS

By studying the literature on the effects of genistein on vasomotor symptoms, one will find numerous controversial opinions. For example, the examinations of

Nachtigall et al[36] and Faure et al[11] concerning the effects of isoflavones on vaso-motor symptoms are cited. Their investigations resulted in a decrease of hot flushes and night sweats. Thus the use of genistein was proclaimed as an attractive addition to the choices available. Contradictory results were reported by Baber et al[3] who found no significant difference between active and placebo groups in the reduction of hot flushes.

OSTEOPOROSIS

Morabito et al[35] investigated (in a randomized, double-blind, placebo-controlled study) that genistein reduces bone resorption markers and enhances new bone formation markers. They also confirmed the suppressive effect on osteoclasts and their induction of apoptosis through the pathway intracellular Ca^{2+} signalling. There was significant enhancement in B-ALP (alkaline phosphatase) and osteocalcin (both of which are markers of osteoblast activity), which differs from the HRT effect.

BLOOD LEVELS

Recent animal studies also demonstrated the benefits of isoflavones on total and LDL cholesterol[7] although various cross-sectional analyses demonstrated the opposite result.[21] By occupying the receptor and stimulating the steroid hormone-binding globulin production in the liver, isoflavones are able to reduce the amount of free oestradiol (E_2) in the plasma.[42]

ISOFLAVONES AND CANCER

Genistein may also have potential for the prevention of cancer (breast, colon, prostate). It may inhibit cancer cell growth by various mechanisms including the stimulation of apoptosis, inducing changes in signalling pathways of transforming growth factors, inhibition of angiogenesis and the differentiation of some malignant cells into benign cells.[8,16,26,28] Genistein also works as an antioxidant, particularly in the skin and intestine, preventing cell damage from free radicals.[4,44,55]

The increased phyto-oestrogen intake in premenopausal women is also useful for preventing several hormone-related cancers through the suppression of gonadotrophin output, which leads to a lengthening of the menstrual cycle and, consequently, a lower lifetime exposure to E_2 levels.[5]

Genistein is able to influence signal transduction mechanisms through the inhibition of the enzymes protein tyrosine kinase (PTK) and DNA topoisomerase (I, II). By inhibiting PTK, genistein activates natural killer cells.[59] It also modulates many nuclear events including the G_2/M cell cycle. Genistein interferes with the passage through the G_2 phase to the M phase checkpoint by altering the level of phosphorylation of the cyclon B-Cdc2 complex, which is required for transition from the G_2 phase to the M phase.[17] In a recent case-control study, McCann et al support a protective effect on ovarian cancer of phyto-oestrogen intake and the hypothesis that a plant-based diet may be important in reducing the risks of hormone-related neoplasms.[34]

In 1997 Adlercreutz[2] reported that genistein inhibits the proliferation of human prostate cancer cells (LNCaP) and decreases the intracellular and extra-cellular prostate-specific antigen concentration.

ISOFLAVONES AND BREAST CANCER

Oestrogens are likely to be involved in the initiation and particularly the promotion of breast cancer. Therefore, it seems to be surprising that phyto-oestrogens may play a preventive role. There are many epidemiological studies on isoflavones and breast cancer showing the benefits of eastern nutritional behaviour (median intake of isoflavones 12 mg per day) and their protective role, which may be accepted as potential evidence.[30,31,58] Zheng et al reported on the urinary excretion of isoflavonoids and the risk of breast cancer. In a case-control study they estimated a lower urinary excretion of isoflavonoids in breast cancer patients (50–65%) than in controls. The adjusted odds ratio for breast cancer was 0.14 (95% CI) for women whose urinary excretion of phenol and total isoflavonoids was in the upper 50% compared with those in the lower 50%.[60]

Alternative studies have shown that genistein stimulates breast cancer cell growth in culture; this occurs in lower concentrations. At higher, mostly non-physiological, concentrations genistein inhibits oestrogen and growth factor-stimulated growth; this is independent of the presence of ER.[40] Ju et al reported that dietary treatment with genistein at physiological concentrations produces blood levels of genistein sufficient to stimulate oestrogenic effects, such as breast tumour growth, in athymic mice.[22]

ER-α AND ER-β RECEPTORS

Interpretations and conclusions concerning the regulation of ER-α- and ER-β receptors have been contradictory. However, the results of Pettersson et al demonstrated that ER-β can act as a negative or positive dominant regulator of ER activity, which is manifested through reduced transcriptional activity at low concentrations of E_2.[41] They found that in certain cellular backgrounds ER-β has the ability to regulate the activity of the α/β heterodimer dominantly, both positively through genistein and negatively through low levels of E_2 or tamoxifen, perhaps through modification of the activity of ER-α AF-1.

ER-β functionally suppresses ER-α transcriptional activity,[39,41,57] and changes in the ER-α/ER-β ratio are associated with different types of cancer.[39,40]

Transcriptional activity in response to genistein is enhanced when ER-α and ER-β are coexpressed to levels that could not be obtained with either receptor alone. ER-β expression may also amplify the agonistic effect of genistein in tissues that also express ER-α.[41] Chen and Anderson reported that genistein and daidzein independently modify cytokine production and reduce ovarian cancer cell proliferation via, at least in part, an oestrogen receptor-dependent pathway.[6]

E$_2$ METABOLISM AND DETOXIFICATION

Girrbach et al investigated the influence of genistein on E$_2$ metabolism.[18] The carcinogenic effect of E$_2$ is, among other things, caused by the oxidative metabolites catechol oestrogens and the lack of detoxification through methylation and conjugation. Girrbach et al reported an inhibition of E$_2$-oxidative metabolism of 30% through genistein and daidzein.[18] Phyto-oestrogens are metabolized in the same way as E$_2$ but only at a minor level. In conclusion, there was a strong inhibition of hydroxylation and conjugation of E$_2$ through isoflavones, whereas O-methylation was unchanged.

Aromatic hydroxycarbon receptor (AHR) is a suspected carcinogen and a non-genotoxic liver tumour promotor in animal models.[27,37,43,52] The prototype AHR agonist is 2,3,7,8-tetrachlorodibenzo-p-dioxin (i.e. dioxin), which induces CYP1A1 enzyme activity. CYP1A1 catalyses the hydroxylation of β-oestradiol, forming the 2,3-catechol and 3,4-catechol forms.[19] Shertzer et al found that genistein inhibits CYP1A1 directly in a metabolic process requiring NADPH, to prevent CYP1A1-mediated covalent binding of benzo[a]pyrene (BaP) metabolites to DNA.[46]

VITAMIN D

The serum 1,25-dihydroxyvitamin D$_3$ level is inversely related to the incidence of some cancers. *In-vitro* studies have shown that 1,25-D$_3$ inhibits proliferation, promotes differentiation and induces apoptosis in many cancer cells.[53] 1,25-D$_3$ levels are determined by the cytochrome P450 hydroxylases CYP27A1 (responsible for the conversion of the precursor vitamin D to the active hormone), CYP27B1 (for synthesis) and CYP24 (responsible for catabolism in the liver and kidneys). Genistein elevates the CYP27B1 level and decreases the CYP24 level. Previous *in-vitro*[9,51] and *in-vivo*[24] studies demonstrated that 1,25-D$_3$ may act as antimitotic and prodifferentiating agents, for example in colon cancer cells. Cross et al were the first to demonstrate that colon cancer cells in culture can synthesize 1,25-D$_3$ from the precursor 25-D$_3$.[10] Thus genistein could affect the vitamin D-related inhibition of tumour growth. Interactions between vitamin D and oestrogen have been observed in breast cancer cells[49] and in murine colon cancer.[48]

Killay et al demonstrated that the administration of genistein resulted in consistent downregulation of CYP24 in the mouse colon, which again would lead to optimal autocrine/paracrine production of the antimitotic secosteroid 1,25-D$_3$.[23] High levels of CYP24 were found in prostate cancer cells. This indicates a specific role for genistein in maintaining the antineoplastic activity of 1,25-D$_3$ in the human prostate. Farahan et al identified genistein as a potent inhibitor of 24-hydroxylation in the prostatic cancer cell line DU-145 and suggest a new mechanism for the tumour-preventive action of isoflavone compounds.[13]

CONCLUSION

Less than 25% of Japanese women report experiencing hot flushes.[33] It is estimated that the Japanese consume 200 mg of phyto-oestrogens per day, 50 mg of which are isoflavones.[1] It is unlikely that foods can offer an adequate alternative for oestrogens full and well-documented benefits.

A new aspect has to be taken into consideration if postmenopausal women with coronary disease have a sequence variant in the gene encoding ER-α. Herrington et al examined the effect of various ER-α polymorphisms on the response to HRT.[20] They found that women with the ER-α polymorphism have an augmented response of HDL cholesterol to HRT.

Phyto-oestrogens bind weakly to the ER-α receptor and more strongly to the ER-β receptor. They possess organ-specific oestrogenic and anti-oestrogenic effects working as partial agonists in some tissues and antagonists in others. ER-β receptors are located in vascular walls and bone cells and ER-α are found in the endometrium and breast tissue.

Women with the ER-α polymorphism receiving HRT in combination with phyto-oestrogens could benefit in two ways. On the one hand HRT increases the HDL cholesterol, and on the other hand the α-receptor would be downregulated by phyto-oestrogens binding to the β-receptor. This would have a protective effect for the endometrium where ERαs are located.

The huge range of contrary results from studies and trials makes a conclusion difficult. It is very difficult to carry out case-control studies because, for example, many vegetables contain isoflavones. So many kinds of food must not be eaten by the control group to achieve clear results – that is hardly practicable.

Nevertheless, isoflavones should be welcomed as a safe and effective form of treatment in addition to HRT or even alone (if there are any contraindications for the HRT). Phyto-oestrogens offer benefits but future studies and controlled clinical trials are needed to achieve definitive conclusions.

References

1. Adlercreutz H, Hämäläinen E, Gorbach S et al 1992 Dietary phytoestrogens and menopause in Japan. The Lancet 339:1233
2. Adlercreutz H 1999 Phytoestrogens. State of the art. Environmental Toxicology and Pharmacology 7:201–207
3. Baber R J, Templeman C, Morton T et al 1999 Randomized placebo-controlled trial of an isoflavone supplement and menopausal symptoms in women. Climacteric 2:85–92
4. Cai Q, Wei H 1996 Effect of dietary genistein on antioxidant enzyme activities in SENCAR mice. Nutrition and Cancer 25:1–7
5. Cassidy A, Bingham S, Setchell K 1995 Biological effects of isoflavones in young women: importance of the chemical composition of soybean products. The British Journal of Nutrition 74:587–601
6. Chen X, Anderson J J 2001 Isoflavones inhibit proliferation of ovarian cancer cells in vitro via an estrogen receptor-dependent pathway. Nutrition and Cancer 41(1–2):165–171
7. Clarkson R, Anthony M, Williams J et al 1998 The potential of soybean phyto-estrogens for postmenopausal hormone replacement therapy. Proceedings of the Society for Experimental Biology and Medicine 217:365–368
8. Constantinou A I, Krygier A E, Mehta R R 1998 Genistein induces maturation of cultured human breast cancer cells and prevents tumor growth in nude mice. The American Journal of Clinical Nutrition 68:1426–1430
9. Cross H S, Pavelka M, Slavik J et al 1992 Growth control of human colon cancer cells by vitamin D and calcium in vitro. Journal of the National Cancer Institute 84:1355–1357
10. Cross H S, Peterlik M, Reddy G S et al 1997 Vitamin D metabolism in human

colon adenocarcinoma-derived Caco-2 cells: expression of 25-hydroxyvitamin D3-1α hydroxylase activity and regulation of sidechain metabolism. The Journal of Steroid Biochemistry and Molecular Biology 62:21–28

11. Drapier Faure E, Chantre P, Mares P 2002 Effects of a standardized soy extract on hot flushes: a multicenter, double-blind, randomized, placebo-controlled study. Menopause 9:329–334

12. Eisenberg D M, Davis R B, Ettner S L et al 1998 Trends in alternative medicine in the US. Results of a follow-up national survey. The Journal of the American Medical Association 16:2377–2381

13. Farhan H, Wähälä K, Adlercreutz H et al 2002 Isoflavonoids inhibit catabolism of vitamin D in prostate cancer cells. Journal of Chromatography B 777:261–268

14. Filardo E J, Quinn J A, Bland K I et al 2000 Estrogen-induced activation of Erk-1 and Erk-2 requires the G protein-coupled receptor homolog, GPR 30, and occurs via transactivation of the epidermal growth factor receptor through release of HB-EGF. Molecular Endocrinology 14:1649–1660

15. Foley E F, Jazaeri A A, Shupnik M A et al 2000 Selective loss of estrogen receptor beta in malignant human colon. Cancer Research 60:245–248

16. Fotsis T, Pepper M, Adlercreutz H et al 1993 Genistein, a dietary-derived inhibitor of in vitro angiogenesis. Proceedings of the National Academy of Sciences of the USA 90:2690–2694

17. Frey S, Singletary K W 2003 Genistein activates p38 mitogen-activated protein kinase, inactivates ERK1/ERK2 and decreases Cdc25C expression in immortalized human mammary epithelial cells. The Journal of Nutrition 133:226–231

18. Girrbach S, Pfeiffer E, Metzler M 2003 Einfluss der Isoflavone Daidzein und Genistein auf den Metabolismus von 17β-Estradiol in Präzisionsschnitten aus Rattenleber. Lebensmittelchemie 57:1–16

19. Hayes C L, Spink D C, Spink B C et al 1996 17β-Estradiol hydroxylation catalyzed by human cytochrome P450 1B1. Proceedings of the National Academy of Sciences of the USA 33:9776–9781

20. Herrington D M, Howard T D, Hawkins G A et al 2002 Estrogen-receptor polymorphisms and effects of estrogen replacement on high-density lipoprotein cholesterol in women with coronary disease. The New England Journal of Medicine 3346:967–974

21. Howes J B, Sullivan D, Lai N et al 2000 The effects of dietary supplementation with isoflavones from red clover on lipoprotein profiles of post menopausal women with mild to moderate hypercholesterolemia. Atherosclerosis 152:143–147

22. Ju Y, Allred C D, Allred K F et al 2001 Physiological concentrations of dietary genistein dose-dependently stimulate growth of estrogen-dependent human breast cancer (MCF-7) tumors implanted in athymic nude mice. The Journal of Nutrition 131:2957–2962

23. Kállay E, Adlercreutz H, Farhan H et al 2002 Phytoestrogens regulate vitamin D metabolism in the mouse colon: relevance for colon tumor prevention and therapy. The Journal of Nutrition 132:3490–3493

24. Kállay E, Pietschmann P, Toyokuni S et al 2001 Characterization of a vitamin D receptor knockout mouse as a model of colorectal hyperproliferation and DNA damage. Carcinogenesis 22:1429–1435

25. Kaufert P, Boggs P, Ettinger B et al 1998 Women and menopause: beliefs, attitudes and behaviors. The North American Menopause Society 1997 survey. Menopause 54:197–202

26. Kim H, Peterson T G, Barnes S 1998 Mechanisms of action of the soy isoflavone genistein: emerging role for its effects via transforming growth factor beta signaling pathways. The American Journal of Clinical Nutrition 68:1418–1425

27. Kociba R J, Keyes D G, Beyer J E et al 1978 Results of a two-year chronic toxicity and oncogenity study of 2,3,7,8-tetrachlorodibenzo-p-dioxin in rats. Toxicology and Applied Pharmacology 46:279–303

28. Koroma B M, de Juan E Jr 1994 Phosphotyrosine inhibition and control of vascular endothelial cell proliferation by genistein. Biochemical Pharmacology 48:809–818

29. Kuiper G G J M, Lemmen J G, Carlsson B et al 1998 Interaction of estrogenic chemicals and phytoestrogens with the estrogen receptor β. Endocrinology 139:4252–4263

30. Lee H P, Gourley L, Duffy S W et al 1999 Dietary effects on breast cancer risk in Singapore. The Lancet 331:1197–1200

31. Lee H P, Gourley L, Duffy S W et al 1992 Risk factor for breast cancer by age and menopausal status: a case-control study in Singapore. Cancer Causes & Control 3:313–322

32. Lichtenstein A H 1998 Soy protein, isoflavones and cardiovascular disease risk. The Journal of Nutrition 128:1589–1592

33. Lock M 1993 Encounters in Aging: Mythologies of menopause in Japan and North America. University of California Press, Berkeley and Los Angeles

34. McCann S E, Freudenheim J L, Marshall J R et al 2003 Risk of human ovarian cancer is related to dietary intake of selective nutrients, phytochemicals and food groups. The Journal of Nutrition 133:1937–1942

35. Morabito N, Crisafulli A, Vergara C et al 2002 Effects of genistein and hormone-replacement therapy on bone loss in early postmenopausal women: a randomized double-blind placebo-controlled study. Journal of Bone and Mineral Research 17:1904–1912

36. Nachtigall L E 2001 Isoflavones in the management of menopause. The Journal of the British Menopause Society 7 (Suppl 1):8–12

37. National Toxicology Program 1982 Carcinogenesis bioassay of 2,3,7,8-tetrachlorodibenzo-*p*-dioxin in Osborne–Mendel rats and B6C3F1 mice (gavage study). NTP Technical Report, p 209

38. Osteoporosis among estrogen-deficient women – United States, 1988–1994. Morbidity and Mortality Weekly Report 1998;47:969–973

39. Paech K, Webb P, Kuiper G G et al 1997 Differential ligand activation of estrogen receptors Eralpha and Erbeta at AP1 sites. Science 277:1508–1510

40. Peterson G, Barnes S 1996 Genistein inhibits both estrogen and growth factor-stimulated proliferation of human breast cancer cells. Cell Growth & Differentiation 7:1345–1351

41. Pettersson K, Delaunay F, Gustaffson J A 2000 Estrogen receptor beta acts as a dominant regulator of estrogen signaling. Oncogene 19:4970–4978

42. Pino A M, Valladares L E, Palma M A et al 2000 Dietary isoflavones affect sex hormone-binding globulin levels in postmenopausal women. The Journal of Clinical Endocrinology and Metabolism 88:450–458

43. Pitot H C, Goldsworthy T, Campbell H A et al 1980 Quantitative evaluation of the promotion by 2,3,7,8-tetrachlorodibenzo-*p*-dioxin of hepatocarcinogenesis from diethylnitrosamine. Cancer Research 40:3616–3620

44. Riuz-Larrea M B, Mohan A R, Paganga G et al 1997 Antioxidant activity of phytoestrogenic isoflavones. Free Radical Research 26:63–70

45. Setchell K D R, Brown N M, Desai P et al 2001 Bioavailability of pure isoflavones in healthy humans and analysis of commercial soy isoflavone supplements. The Journal of Nutrition 131:1362–1375

46. Shertzer H G, Puga A, Chang C et al 1999 Inhibition of CYP1A1 enzyme activity in mouse hepatoma cell culture by soybean isoflavones. Chemico-Biological Interactions 123:31–49

47. Shutt D A, Cox R 1972 Steroid and phyto-estrogen binding to sheep uterine receptors in vitro. The Journal of Endocrinology 52:299–310

48. Smirnoff P, Liel Y, Gnainsky J et al 1999 The protective effect of estrogen against chemically induced murine colon carcinogenesis is associated with decreased CpG island methylation and increased mRNA and protein expression of the colonic vitamin D receptor. Oncology Research 11:255–264

49. Swami S, Krishnan A V, Feldman D 2000 1-alpha 25 Dihydroxyvitamin D3 down regulates estrogen receptor abundance and suppresses estrogen actions in MCF-7 human breast cancer cells. Clinical Cancer Research 6:3371–3379

50. Tham D M, Gardner C D, Haskell W L 1998 Clinical review 97. Potential health benefits of dietary phytoestrogens: a review of the clinical, epidemiological, and mechanistic evidence. The Journal of Clinical Endocrinology and Metabolism 83:-2223–2235

51. Tong W M, Bises G, Sheinin Y et al 1998 Establishment of primary cultures from human colonic tissue during tumor progression. Vitamin D responses and vitamin D receptor expression. International Journal of Cancer 75:467–472

52. Toth K, Somfai-Relle S, Sugar J et al 1979 Carcinogenicity testing of herbizide 2,4,5-trichlorophenoxyethanol containing dioxin and of pure dioxin in Swiss mice. Nature 27:548–549

53. Van den Bemd G J, Pols H A, van Leewen J P 2000 Anti-tumor effects of 1,25-dihydroxyvitamin D3 and vitamin D analogues. Current Pharmaceutical Design 6:717

54. Verma S P, Goldin B R, Lin P S 1998 The inhibition of the estrogenic effects of pesticides and environmental chemical by curcumin and isoflavonoids, Environmental Health Perspectives 106:807–812

55. Wei H, Bowen R, Cai Q et al 1995 Anti oxidant and antipromotional effects of the soybean isoflavone genistein. Proceedings of the Society for Experimental Biology and Medicine 208:124–130

56. Who are candidates for prevention and treatment for osteoporosis? Osteoporosis International 1997;7:1–6

57. Windahl S H, Vidal O, Andersson G et al 1994 Increased cortical bone mineral content but unchanged trabecular bone mineral density in female ER beta mice. The Journal of Clinical Investigation 104:895–901

58. Wu A H, Wan P, Hankin J et al 2002 Adolescent and adult soy intake and risk of breast cancer in Asian-Americans. Carcinogenesis 23:1491–1496

59. Zhang Y, Song T T, Cunnick J E et al 1999 Daidzein and genistein glucuronides in vitro are weakly estrogenic and active human natural killer cells at nutritionally relevant concentrations. The Journal of Nutrition 129:399–405

60. Zheng W, Dai Q, Custer L J et al 1999 Urinary excretion of isoflavonoids and the risk of breast cancer. Cancer Epidemiology, Biomarkers and Prevention 8:35–4

22

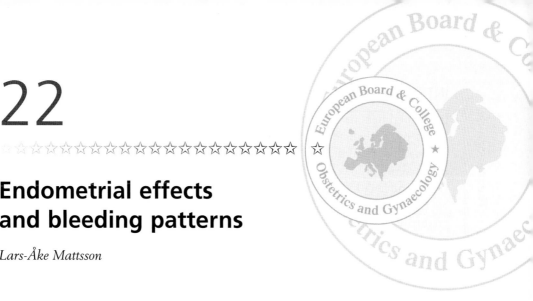

Endometrial effects and bleeding patterns

Lars-Åke Mattsson

ABSTRACT

In the perimenopausal period a number of endocrine changes take place in the ovary which influence the production of oestrogens and progestogens. The most common reason for bleeding disturbances in the perimenopausal period is anovulation. Bleeding problems associated with anovulation should preferably be treated with the addition of progestogens cyclically. Irregular bleedings in the postmenopausal period in women not taking hormone replacement therapy (HRT) are, in 10% of cases, associated with endometrial cancer. Epidemiological studies have reported an increased risk of adenocarcinoma of the endometrium in women taking HRT. Relative risks of 1.4 for less than 1 year of use and of 9.5 for more than 10 years of use have been reported.. The risk of endometrial cancer is low in women on continuous combined oestrogen–progestogen therapy (CCEPT). Bleeding patterns do not predict endometrial histopathology.

Over 90% of women on sequential oestrogen–progestogen therapy (CSEPT) will experience withdrawal bleedings. Median blood loss is around 20–30 ml per month although a large interindividual variability has been reported. A majority of women prefer HRT that does not induce uterine bleedings. In women on CCEPT, especially those containing low doses of oestrogens and progestogens, a high frequency of amenorrhoea is reached after a few months of treatment. Continuous combined formulations have been proposed for women in the postmenopausal period. Bleeding in the postmenopausal period may be a presenting sign of endometrial cancer and should always be investigated. A number of methods such as transvaginal sonography, endometrial biopsies, hydrosonography and hysteroscopy have been proposed for detecting benign and malignant lesions of the endometrium.

KEYWORDS

Bleeding disturbances, endometrial cancer, hormone replacement therapy (HRT), hysteroscopy, transvaginal sonography

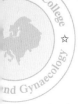
INTRODUCTION

In the perimenopausal period of a woman's life a number of changes take place in the ovaries which influence the production of oestrogens and progestogens. During this phase there is a gradual decrease in oestradiol and inhibin levels and a concomitant increase in circulating levels of follicle-stimulating hormone (FSH) and later luteinizing hormone. During the menopausal transition, FSH levels fluctuate markedly as do the levels oestradiol and progesterone. The ovaries gradually become less responsive to FSH several years before menstruation ceases. Menopause occurs when ovarian failure becomes pronounced and the production of oestradiol has reached such a low level that the endometrial lining is no longer stimulated.[23,26]

The most common reason for bleeding disturbances in the perimenopausal period is anovulation. When the endometrium is stimulated by oestrogens (but without a concomitant secretion of progesterone) the endometrium will often develop hyperplasia. The target cells in the endometrium are extremely responsive to even low concentrations of oestrogens and the endometrium might respond by the profileration of glandular and stromal cells. The glandular epithelium becomes more vascularized with poor stromal support and, accordingly, the fragility of the mucosa will increase, which may lead to uncontrolled bleeding. It is typical with tall and pseudostratified or stratified glands. The cell nuclei are elongated, the chromatin is dense with frequent mitosis and the cytoplasm contains abundant RNA. The content of oestrogen receptors is greatly increased. With prolonged oestrogen stimulation the endometrium responds with glandular cystic and adenomatous hyperplasia in which the stroma becomes compressed and less prominent.[6]

When the origin of bleeding disturbances is anovulation it may be sufficient to add progestogens cyclically, e.g. medroxyprogesterone acetate (MPA) 5–10 mg per day or norethisterone acetate (NETA) 2.5–5 mg per day from Day 16 to Day 25 in the cycle. This treatment can be repeated for three or four cycles or even longer. The risk of progression of simple hyperplasia to endometrial cancer in the perimenopausal period is low.

In postmenopausal women the endometrium is normally thin due to low oestrogen stimulation. However, in some women endogenous oestrogen production is fairly high due to the peripheral conversion of androstenedione. If there is a simultaneous lack of progestogen secretion, the endometrium can proliferate and develop a variety of hyperplastic conditions. There is normally a continuum in the progression of different stages in the endometrium due to oestrogenic stimulation as shown in Figure 22.1.

Risk factors for the development of endometrial cancer (apart from exogenous oestrogen exposure) are obesity, nulliparity, diabetes and hypertension. In postmenopausal women the frequency of irregular bleeding decreases with age. In about 10% of irregular bleedings in postmenopausal women who are not on HRT, the underlying reason is endometrial cancer and about 50% of such bleedings are associated with atrophic mucosa.[11]

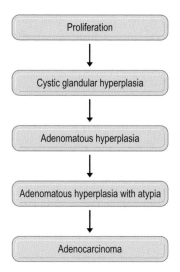

Fig 22.1 Progression of the endometrial histopathology during long-term estrogen stimulation.

The risk of developing endometrial malignancies in women with cystic hyperplasia is low and has been reported to be less than 2%. In women with atypical adenomatous hyperplasia, the risk has been reported to vary between 20 and 80%.[25,34] In this context it should be stressed that significant disagreement exists among pathologists with regard to the classification of different states of hyperplasia. It is therefore critical that physicians are familiar with how their pathologist reads and reports the results from endometrial biopsies since this may have a major impact on the management of individual patients.

A number of epidemiological studies have reported associations between long-term oestrogen therapy (ET) and the development of adenocarcinoma of the endometrium.[3,10] The size of this risk depends on the dose of oestrogens given and the duration of treatment. The association between ET only and endometrial malignancy was demonstrated in 1975 by Ziel and Finkle[36] and Smith et al.[28] Numerous studies later confirmed their results. In a meta-analysis by Grady et al it was found that the relative risk (RR) increased from 1.4 (95% CI; range 1.0–1.8) for less than 1 year of use to 9.5 (95% CI; range 7.4–12.3) for more than 10 years of use.[10] It was also reported by them that the increased incidence of endometrial cancer persisted for 5 years or more following the discontinuation of unopposed oestrogen use (RR 2.3; 95% CI; range 1.8–3.1).[10]

In women with an intact uterus HRT with oestrogens and progestogens in combination is recommended. There are two main reasons to recommend combined therapy:

1. To avoid the risk of developing atypical hyperplasia and its possible progression to endometrial cancer in women given unopposed oestrogens.
2. To create regular and predictable withdrawal bleedings.

When progestogens are added to oestrogens, the endometrium will change into a secretory condition normally creating predictable withdrawal bleedings. It is probably not necessary with a fully secretory transformation of the endometrium to protect against hyperplasia since a number of effects (besides shedding) are involved. It has been demonstrated that progestogens exert antiproliferative effects and modulate the endometrium by different mechanisms as shown in Box 22.1.

The duration of the progestogen supplement is more important than the dose for protection of the endometrium. In one early study the frequency of hyperplasia was reported to be 3–4% with 7 days, 2% with 10 days and 0% after 12–13 days of progestogen supplement each month. Lower doses are needed for the protection of the development of atypical hyperplasia compared to the doses needed for induction of regular bleedings or amenorrhoea. In one study with CCEPT, 0.1 mg NETA daily in combination with 1 mg oestradiol was found to protect atypical mucosa, while 0.5 mg was needed to secure acceptable bleeding patterns.[18] The progestogen dose can be reduced if the oestrogenic potency is decreased.

In CSEPT, progestogens should be added for at least 10–14 days per cycle. Hence higher does are recommended in CSEPT as compared to those needed in CCEPT. Doses of a selected number of progestogens needed for endometrial transformation are shown in Table 22.1.[24]

BLEEDING PATTERNS

COMBINED SEQUENTIAL OESTROGEN–PROGESTOGEN THERAPY

The sequential addition of progestogens to ET has been proposed at a duration of 10–14 days on a monthly basis. This regimen will inevitably lead to withdrawal bleeding in over 90% of women; this therapy should be advocated in women in the perimenopausal period. There are no studies to show how the duration or dosage of the progestogen supplement will influence the duration or amount of the monthly withdrawal bleed. A few studies have reported a median blood loss of around 20–30 ml each month but with a large interindividual variability.[22,29] This blood loss should be compared with about 35 ml during normal menstruation.[15] No difference in the amount of bleeding could be detected when women were given 10 mg MPA or 250 mg levonorgestrel added to 2 mg oestradiol valerate administered orally.[29] The mean duration of the withdrawal bleed each

---

Box 22.1 Progestogenic effects in the endometrium

- Reduction of DNA synthesis in the endometrium and decreased number of oestrogen receptors;

- Stimulation of oestradiol conversion into less active oestrogens (oestrone, oestrone sulphate) by an increase in, for example, 17α-hydroxysteroid dehydrogenase;

- Secretory transformation, decidualization and shedding of the endometrium;

- Reduction of insulin-like growth factor (IGF-I) action.

Table 22.1 Progestogen doses needed for endometrial transformation.

Progestogen	Transformation dose (mg per cycle)
Progesterone	4200
Dydrogesterone	140
Medroxyprogesterone acetate	80
Drospirenone	50
Norethisterone acetate	30–60
Dienogest	6
Desogestrel	2

month was 3.8 ± 2.1 days (mean ± standard deviation). It has been proposed that the amount of bleeding decreases with increasing age but there are little data to support this statement.

One study on the variability in cycle length during a 6-month period in 103 women given 2 mg oestradiol valerate daily with the addition of 1 mg NETA from Day 17 to 28 each cycle was conducted. Of 275 completed cycles, bleeding was found to begin before the last day of progestogen supplement (Day 29) in 36% and after Day 29 in 64%. If the onset of bleeding occurred later than Day 29 this was associated with less intra-individual cycle-to-cycle variability. Women with early bleeding (before Day 29) exhibited a significantly longer duration of bleeding.[14] There is some evidence that bleeding could be delayed with an increase in the potency of progestogen supplement.

Padwick et al[21] proposed that the characteristics of the withdrawal bleed could give some indication of the status of the endometrium. They found that bleedings that occurred on Day 11 or later of the progestogen supplement were associated with a predominantly secretory endometrium. However, their study was not supported by data presented later by Sturdee et al.[31] In their study on 413 women, no association between the day of onset of bleeding and endometrial histopathology could be found. In that study, 50 out of 105 women with a fully secretory transformation of the endometrium reported bleeding before the 11th day. Furthermore, seven women with complex hyperplasia had regular bleeds after Day 11.

In a large multicenter study two different sequential regimens with conjugated oestrogens (0.625 mg) in combination with 5 or 10 mg MPA for the last 14 days of a 28-day cycle were compared. Bleedings were considered to be regular if they occurred within Days 20–28 of one cycle and Days 1–5 of the next cycle. It was stated that most cycles (81.3 and 77%, respectively) were considered to be regular in patients taking 5 and 10 mg MPA. Obviously the frequency of 'regular' bleeding depends on how this is defined, and this differs between various studies.[2]

CONTINUOUS COMBINED OESTROGEN–PROGESTOGEN THERAPY

As mentioned above, the majority of women on CSHRT will experience withdrawal bleeding. Many women are reluctant to start HRT due to the induction of

Endometrial effects and bleeding patterns

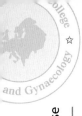

uterine bleedings and few discontinue because of bleeding disturbances. In epidemiological studies it has been found that around 80% of postmenopausal women prefer HRT regimens that do not induce bleeding periods.[32] It may be important to be aware of women's attitudes to and knowledge of treatment to increase adherence to and satisfaction with therapy.

CCHRT was developed in an attempt to reduce bleeding disturbances;[20] some studies have shown excellent compliance with different formulations of CCHRT.[7] Most studies of CCHRT have shown that bleedings occur early in the therapy and that the number of bleeding episodes gradually decreases with increasing duration of treatment. Higher rates of amenorrhoea have been demonstrated with low-dose combinations compared to conventional dose formulations.[16] It has been proposed that these types of formulation are best suited for postmenopausal women.[20] In one large study, two different formulations of CCHRT were tested, namely conjugated oestrogens (0.625 mg) in combination with either 2.5 or 5 mg MPA as a daily tablet.[2] In that study it was concluded that the two regimens produced amenorrhoea in 61.4 and 72.8%, respectively, of all available cycles and that no cases of atypical hyperplasia were detected.[1]

Efforts have been made to reduce the doses of oestrogens and progestogens in CCEPT. In one small study, 1 mg oestradiol was combined with various doses of NETA; a high frequency of amenorrhoea was reported.[30] Few women reported bleeding and they were often characterized as spottings.

With regard to climacteric complaints, low HRT has been reported to be almost as effective as conventional-dose HRT, especially in elderly women. In a large study, the highest frequency of amenorrhoea was reported in women taking 1 mg oestradiol valerate and 5 mg MPA on a daily basis.[1] In a comparative study of orally given and transdermally applied oestradiol, the best bleeding profile was obtained with a patch delivering 25 µg oestradiol per day.[19] High frequencies of amenorrhoea were also reported in a large study with different combinations of low doses of oestradiol valerate and MPA.[16] After a few months of treatment, an amenorrhoea frequency of almost 90% was found in women given 1 mg oestradiol valerate in combination with 2.5 mg MPA. Few women discontinue treatment due to bleeding problems when given low-dose CCHRT. It has also been shown that further bleeding is uncommon in women on CCHRT once amenorrhoea has been established. If irregular bleedings occur in women on CCHRT after 6 months, it is important to exclude other underlying reasons such as polyps and fibromas.

LONG-CYCLE THERAPY

A number of women do not accept monthly withdrawal bleeds or do not tolerate the addition of progestogens each month. In order to reduce such progestogen side-effects, long-cycle treatment with the addition of progestogens for 10–14 days every second or third month were introduced as a possible alternative to standard therapy. In this type of therapy, endometrial safety has been less extensively evaluated compared to other regimens. In a Scandinavian long-cycle study, the regimen consisted of cycles of 2 mg oestradiol daily for 68 days followed by 2 mg oestradiol and 1 mg NETA for 10 days, and then 1 mg oestradiol was given alone for 6 days.[5] This study was discontinued after 3 years when 15 out of 243 patients had developed simple or complex hyperplasia. One case with endometrial cancer was detected. However, the addition of 20 mg MPA for 14 days every third month in combination with one week without therapy has shown no increased risk of hyperplasia.[9] However, breakthrough bleedings may be more frequent with long-cycle therapy.

In a comparative study, breakthrough bleedings were reported to occur at a frequency of 15.5% in long-cycle versus 6.8% in monthly CSHRT regimens. Also, withdrawal bleedings were found to be longer in the long-cycle therapy. It has also been found that the blood loss is doubled if the progestogen supplement is given every third month compared to monthly.

INDIVIDUALIZATION OF THERAPY

It may be wise to individualize HRT to suit a particular woman's needs if adherence to HRT is to be ensured. Women in the perimenopausal period should be offered CSEPT regimens. Since there is a gradual decrease in ovarian activity, and probably also in receptor sensitivity in the uterus, HRT must be adapted to the woman's menopausal status. In the perimenopausal period many women are willing to accept withdrawal bleedings, and accordingly CSHRT should be the first-line choice at this time. Later, in the postmenopausal period, many women prefer treatment that does not induce bleeding irregularities. At this time CCHRT or long-cycle CSHRT may be preferable. The dose should be reduced by age and a large number of studies have produced evidence to show that a majority of women cope well with low-dose HRT regimens. It may be prudent to choose the lowest effective dose for women in need of short- or long-term HRT.

THE MANAGEMENT OF BLEEDING DISORDERS

In the postmenopausal period, vaginal bleeding is an important and common problem; it is often the presenting problem of endometrial cancer. Even though endometrial atropy is a common feature associated with postmenopausal bleeding,[11] several studies have indicated other anatomical causes, such as polyps, fibromas and adenomatous hyperplasia, may be combined in postmenopausal bleeding.[8,17,27] Previously, a conventional dilatation and curettage was the method of choice but the accuracy of that for detecting benign and malignant lesions has been questioned.[8,12]

The measurement of endometrial thickness by transvaginal sonography (TVS) has become a useful tool for evaluating the endometria of postmenopausal women.[13] If TVS is combined with saline infusion sonography, the diagnostic accuracy can be increased. This technique has been extensively described and is performed by inserting a catheter into the endometrial cavity and injecting sterile saline solution while scanning transvaginally.[4,35] Another procedure that can

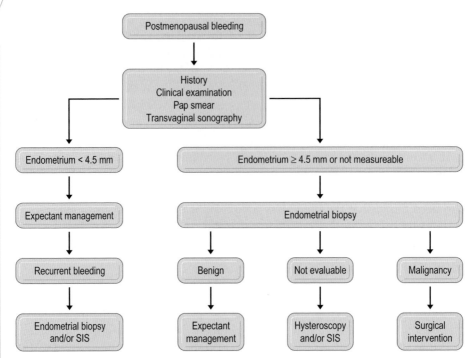

Fig 22.2 A simplified algorithm for the management of postmenopausal bleeding.
SIS, Saline Infusion Sonography.

enable the physician to detect focal anatomical aberrations is hysteroscopy, which can also be used as an outpatient procedure for diagnosis and therapy.[33]

It may be important to be familiar with different diagnostic procedures to optimize the diagnostic efforts. In Figure 22.2 an algorithm for the management of postmenopausal bleeding is proposed. It should also be emphasized that many pathological changes in the uterus are small and localized to a minor area. Biopsies of focal lesions under hysteroscopic guidance might be an attractive option in such cases.[12,33]

References

1. Archer D, Dorin M, Heine W et al 1999 Uterine bleeding in postmenopausal women on continuous therapy with estradiol and norethindrone acetate. Obstetrics and Gynecology 94:323–329
2. Archer D F, Picker J H, Bottiglioni F 1994 Bleeding patterns in postmenopausal women taking continuous combined or sequential regimens of conjugated estrogens with medroxyprogesterone acetate. Obstetrics and Gynecology 83:686–692
3. Biglia N, Gadduchi A, Ponzone R et al 2004 Hormone replacement therapy in cancer survivors. Maturitas 48:333–346
4. Bree R L 1997 Ultrasound of the endometrium: facts, controversies, and future trends. Abdominal Imaging 22:557–569
5. Cern A, Heldaas K, Moeller B for the Scandinavian Long-Cycle Study Group 1996 Adverse endometrial effects of long-cycle estrogen and progestogen replacement therapy (letter). The New England Journal of Medicine 334:668–669
6. Dallenbach-Hellweg G 1987 Histopathology of the Endometrium. Springer Verlag, Berlin

7. Dören M, Reuther G, Minne H et al 1995 Superior compliance and efficacy of continuous combined oral estrogen–progestogen replacement therapy in postmenopausal women. American Journal of Obstetrics and Gynecology 173:1446–1451

8. Epstein E, Ramirez A, Skoog L et al 2001 Dilatation and curettage fails to detect most focal lesions in the uterine cavity in women with postmenopausal bleeding. Acta Obstetricia et Gynecologica Scandinavica 80:1488–1494

9. Erkkola R, Kumento U, Lehmuskoski S et al 2002 No increased risk of endometrial hyperplasia with fixed long-hormone replacement therapy after two years. The Journal of the British Menopause Society 8:155–156

10. Grady D, Gebresadik T, Kerlikowske K et al 1995 Hormone replacement therapy and endometrial cancer risk. A meta-analysis. Obstetrics and Gynecology 85:304–313

11. Gredmark T, Kvint S, Havel G et al 1995 Histopathological findings in women with postmenopausal bleeding. British Journal of Obstetrics and Gynaecology 102:133–136

12. Grimes D A 1982 Diagnostic dilation and curettage: a reappraisal. American Journal of Obstetrics and Gynecology 142:1–6

13. Gull B, Karlsson B, Milsom I et al 2003 Can ultrasound replace dilatation and curettage? A longitudinal evaluation of postmenopausal bleeding and transvaginal sonographic measurement of the endometrium as predictors of endometrial cancer. American Journal of Obstetrics and Gynecology 188:401–408

14. Habiba M A, Bell S C, Abrams K et al 1996 Endometrial responses to hormone replacement therapy: the bleeding pattern. Human Reproduction 11:503–508

15. Hallberg L, Högdahl A M, Nilsson I et al 1966 Menstrual blood loss: a population study. Variation at different ages and attempts to define normality. Acta Obstetricia et Gynecologica Scandinavica 45:25–56

16. Heikkinen J E, Vaheri R T, Ahomäki S M et al 2000 Optimizing continuous-combined hormone replacement therapy for postmenopausal women: a comparison of six different treatment regimens. American Journal of Obstetrics and Gynecology 182:560–567

17. Karlsson B, Granberg S, Wikland M et al 1995 Transvaginal ultrasonography of the endometrium in women with postmenopausal bleeding. A Nordic multicenter study. American Journal of Obstetrics and Gynecology 172(5):1488–1494

18. Kurman R J, Felix J C, Archer D F et al 2000 Norethindrone acetate and estradiol-induced endometrial hyperplasia. Obstetrics and Gynecology 96:373–379

19. Mattsson L-Å, Bohnet H G, Gredmark T et al 1999 Continuous combined hormone replacement. Randomized comparison of transdermal and oral preparations. Obstetrics and Gynecology 94:61–65

20. Mattsson L-Å, Cullberg G, Samsioe G 1982 Evaluation of a continuous estrogen–progestogen regimen for climacteric complaints. Maturitas 4:95–102

21. Padwick M L, Pryse-Davies J, Whitehead M I 1986 A simple method for determining the optimal dosage of progestin in postmenopausal women receiving estrogens. The New England Journal of Medicine 315:930–934

22. Rees M C P, Barlow D H 1991 Quantification of hormone replacement-induced withdrawal bleeds. British Journal of Obstetrics and Gynaecology 98:106–107

23. Richardson S J 1993 The biological basis of the menopause. Baillière's Clinical Endocrinology & Metabolism 7:1–16

24. Schindler A E, Campaglioni C, Druckmann R et al 2003 Classification and pharmacology of progestins. Maturitas 46 (Suppl 1): S7–S16

25. Sherman A I, Brown S 1979 The precursors of endometrial carcinoma. American Journal of Obstetrics and Gynecology 135:947–956

26. Sherman B M, West J, Korenman S G 1976 The menopausal transition. Analysis of LH, FSH, estradiol, and progesterone concentrations during menstrual cycles of older women. The Journal of Clinical Endocrinology and Metabolism 42:629–636

27. Smith Bindman R, Kerlikowske K, Feldstein V A et al 1998 Endovaginal ultrasound to exclude endometrial cancer and other endometrial abnormalities. The Journal of the American Medical Association 280:1510–1517

28. Smith D C, Prentice R, Thompson D J et al 1975 Association of exogenous estrogen and endometrial carcinoma. The New England Journal of Medicine 293:1164–1167

29. Sporrong T, Rybo G, Mattsson L-Å et al 1992 An objective and subjective assessment of uterine blood loss in postmenopausal women on hormone replacement therapy. British Journal of Obstetrics and Gynaecology 99:399–401

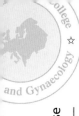

30. Stadberg E, Mattson L-Å, Uvebrant M 1996 17β-estradiol and norethisterone acetate in low doses as continuous combined hormone replacement therapy. Maturitas 23:31–39

31. Sturdee D W, Barlow D H, Ulrich L G et al 1994 Is the timing of withdrawal bleeding a guide to endometrial safety during different sequential combined HRT regimens in current use? The Lancet 343:979–982

32. Thunell L, Stadberg E, Mattsson L-Å et al 2000 Treatment of climacteric symptoms. A longitudinal study. Maturitas 35 (Suppl 1):51

33. Timmerman D, Deprest J, Bourne T et al 1999 A randomized trial on the use of ultrasonography or hysteroscopy for endometrial assessment in postmenopausal patients with breast cancer who were treated with tamoxifen. American Journal of Obstetrics and Gynecology 179:62–70

34. Wentz W B 1974 Progestin therapy in endometrial cancer. Gynecologic Oncology 2:362–367

35. Williams C D, Marshburn P B 1998 A prospective study of transvaginal hydrosonography in the evaluation of abnormal uterine bleeding. American Journal of Obstetrics and Gynecology 179:292–298

36. Ziel H K, Finkle W D 1975 Increased risk of endometrial carcinoma among users of conjugated estrogens. The New England Journal of Medicine 293:1167–1170

23

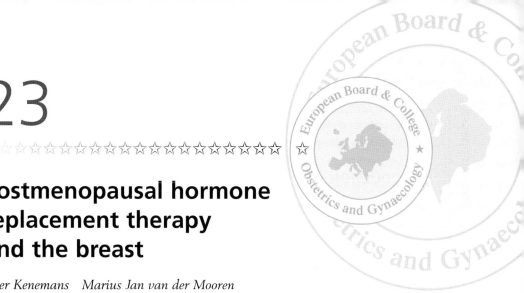

Postmenopausal hormone replacement therapy and the breast

Peter Kenemans   Marius Jan van der Mooren

ABSTRACT

The human breast is an organ that is highly sensitive to sex hormones. Clinical signs of this are mastalgia and mammographic breast density. Prolonged exposure to endogenous or exogenous oestrogens increases the risk of breast cancer. Oestrogens act as tumour promoters as they induce mitosis, leading to the proliferation and therefore the accelerated growth of clinically occult, pre-existing tumours. Oestrogens are also genotoxic mutagenic carcinogens, although very weak as such. In addition, oestrogens could induce tumours by the accumulation of incessant DNA replication damage mechanisms.

Opinions differ as to the influence of a progestogen when added to an oestrogen. Theoretically, the action of a progestogen on the cellular mitotic activity induced by oestrogen could be antagonistic – by different pathways: oestrogen receptor (ER) downregulation; the activation of metabolic pathways within the breast; or stimulation of apoptosis – but it is probably synergistic.

Over 60 observational studies and two randomized controlled trials provide evidence that a small but significant increase in the risk of breast cancer appears with long-term current postmenopausal combined oestrogen-plus-progestogen (EPT) use. Compared to non-hormone replacement therapy (HRT) users, the relative risk (RR) would be around 1.25 for current use for, on average, 6 years. One recent randomized controlled trial confirmed earlier observational studies that unopposed oestrogen therapy (ET) does not increase breast cancer risk in the first 6.8 years of use.

There are still many questions to be answered. Is the risk increase limited to lean women only? Are tumours detected under HRT less aggressive? Is there a better prognosis and a lower mortality? What about risk-modifying factors such as alcohol use, obesity and a positive family history of breast cancer? And is mammographic breast density a biomarker for breast cancer?

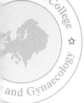

☆ | ☆☆☆☆☆☆☆☆☆☆☆☆☆☆☆☆☆☆☆☆

KEYWORDS

Apoptosis, breast, breast cancer, breast cancer mortality, breast cancer risk, breast density, hormone replacement therapy (HRT), incessant replication damage, mammography, proliferation

INTRODUCTION

Breast cancer is a major challenge to modern western society. In addition to lifestyle factors such as alcohol use and obesity, the use of exogenous sex hormones has been found to increase the risk of breast cancer.[14] As breast cancer is a hormone-dependent disease, medical inventions such as postmenopausal HRT should ideally result in hormonal prevention of a hormone-dependent tumour like breast cancer.[11, 24] However, on the basis of observational studies[8],[17, 20] as well as randomized clinical trials[6,13] there is a great concern that this is not the case. These studies indicate an increase in breast cancer risk in HRT users and a lack of an overall benefit.

HRT consists of a wide variety of natural and synthetic substances, with many possible routes of administration. The risk for breast cancer might differ with the regimen used, the route of administration, and the type of oestrogen and progestogen used. Breast density on the mammogram is observed to increase in HRT users, especially in women on combined EPT, with a decreased accuracy in diagnosing breast cancer.[4] Other HRT substances such as tibolone and raloxifene, which are increasingly used in postmenopausal HRT, might influence breast cancer risk and mammographic density in a way different from EPT.

OESTROGENS AND THE BREAST

Oestrogens bind to the intranuclear ERs α and β. Subsequent binding of the ligand receptor complex to oestrogen-response elements within DNA ultimately results in mitotic activity and, therefore, tissue proliferation. Occult breast tumours will start to grow and become clinically evident. This is the so-called late stage tumour promotion. Carcinogenesis is a multistep process involving some 5–7 mutations in important regulatory genes.

Oestrogens are only weak mutagenic carcinogens[18] but there is a second carcinogenic pathway, according to the Incessant DNA Replication Damage Hypothesis.[11,14] During DNA replication at the time of oestrogen-driven mitosis, damage to the DNA is likely to occur but this is commonly corrected by intrinsic repair mechanisms. Any abnormal cells that have escaped DNA repair mechanisms go into programmed cell death (apoptosis). Several of these apoptotic pathways are modulated by sex hormones. Oestradiol is known to induce an anti-apoptotic pathway via Bcl-2.

Theoretically, continuous oestrogen stimulation should result in incessant mitotic cellular activity, with a steadily growing accumulation of unrepaired DNA replication damage. The ensuing inactivation of important regulatory genes, such as tumour suppressor genes, would ultimately lead to impairment of the above-mentioned DNA repair and apoptotic destruction mechanisms, and therefore cancer.

In conclusion, induction or initiation of tumours by oestrogens is a possibility, via two different pathways, in addition to the late-stage promoter effect of oestrogens, which lead to accelerated growth of clinically occult, pre-existing tumours (Fig. 23.1).

In addition to these cell biological, preclinical data, epidemiological studies also suggest that prolonged exposure to oestrogens plays an important role in

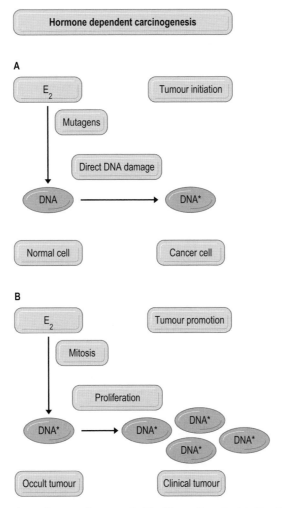

Fig 23.1 Hormone dependent carcinogenesis. The illustration depicts the three possible hypothetical roles oestrogens play in the carcinogenesis of breast tumours. (a) Oestrogen acts here as a genotoxic mutagenic carcinogen. The International Agency for Research on Cancer (Lyon, France) has classified oestradiol as a weak carcinogen, as oestradiol (E_2) via its catechol metabolites can cause free radical-mediated DNA damage to epithelial breast cells.[18] (b) This depicts oestrogen as a late-stage tumour promoter via oestrogen receptor-mediated proto-oncogene activation and subsequent mitotic activity and proliferation, leading to the acceler-ated growth of pre-existing occult tumours which are clinically less aggressive.

Continued

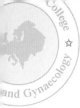
The menopause

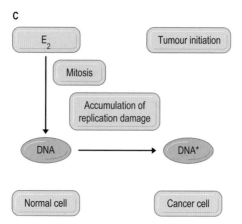

c

Fig 23.1 cont'd (c) This depicts oestrogen as a tumour initiator, resulting from incessant mitotic activity, leading to the accumulation of unrepaired replication DNA damage with subsequent damage to the tumour suppressor genes and the impairment of mismatch repair and apoptosis mechanisms.
Reproduced with permission from reference 14.

relation to breast cancer risk. Established risk factors for breast cancer are hormone exposure related: early age at menarche, late onset of menopause and postmenopausal obesity.

Postmenopausal women with a relatively high blood concentration of endogenous oestrogens have been shown to have a substantially increased risk for breast cancer, compared to those with low levels.[9] However, local tissue concentrations of oestrogens are not directly related to blood oestradiol concentrations, probably due to differences in local metabolism.

Many observational studies have provided evidence that a small but significant risk increase exists with current postmenopausal oestrogen use. Data from 51 epidemiological studies, including 52 705 women with breast cancer and 108 411 controls, have been re-analysed by the Collaborative Group for hormonal effects on breast cancer.[8] About 80% of the users were on unopposed ET. For long-term users, the RR of developing breast cancer was 1.35 (95% CI; range 1.21–1.49). The absolute increase in breast cancer cases attributable to postmenopausal hormone use is relatively low. After a period of 25 years, in a group of 1000 women (all having used HRT for 5 years) there would be only two extra cases of breast cancer (Fig. 23.2).

The increase in risk was present from the start of use and was roughly equivalent to the RR increase that was associated with each year that menopause came later (beyond 50 years of age) in non-HRT users within the same population. Within 5 years after cessation of HRT the effect on breast cancer risk had largely disappeared.[8]

Following the publication of the re-analysis in 1997,[8] 12 observational studies have been published, of which the Million Women Study is the largest.[20] Most of these studies confirm the existence of a small but consistent increase in breast cancer risk with long-term use of unopposed oestrogen. In the Million Women

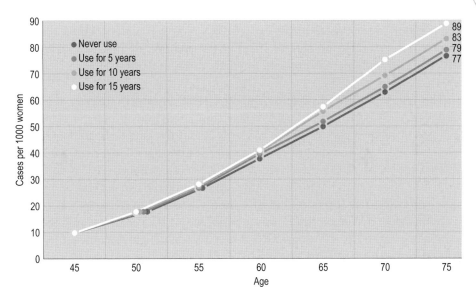

Fig 23.2 Estimate of the increase in the cumulative number of breast cancers per 1000 postmenopausal women using HRT for 0, 5, 10 and 15 years, respectively, all having started at age 50 years.
Reproduced with permission from reference 8.

Study current users of oestrogen-only had their RR for breast cancer increased to 1.32 (range 1.20–1.46) after 5–9 years of use.[20]

Until now, besides observational studies, results on unopposed oestrogen use are only available from the recently published randomized clinical trial from the Women's Health Initiative (WHI). After an average of 6.8 years of ET, this trial found no increased breast cancer risk (RR 0.77; 95% CI; range 0.59–1.01).[2]

PROGESTOGENS AND THE BREAST

The two known progesterone receptor isoforms (PR-A, PR-B) have different physiological functions via differential gene regulation. Four genes are uniquely regulated via PR-A, 65 genes uniquely by PR-B and only 25 by both receptors.[22]

Various preclinical studies show that the action of a progestogen on the oestrogen-induced cellular mitotic activity is antagonistic by downregulation of the ER, activation of certain metabolic pathways or by the stimulation of apoptosis. Other studies show synergism.[14]

Moreover, the action of progestogens in combination with oestrogens on mitotic epithelial activity is tissue-specific. Proliferation in the endometrium is observed in the follicular phase, while proliferation in the breast is typically observed in the luteal phase, when progesterone levels are high.

However, in the breast in the luteal phase, not only does the mitotic rate peak, so does the rate of apoptosis. It is probable that the ultimate effect of sex hormones on the breast should not be understood solely in terms of mitosis but rather in terms of the balance between mitotic and apoptotic rates.[10]

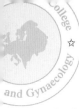
While the influence of the addition of a progestogen to an oestrogen on breast proliferation in relation to breast cancer risk is not well understood on the basis of preclinical studies, the clinical effect of the addition of a progestogen to ET, necessary for endometrial protection, seems to be undoubtedly adverse for the breast.

The effect of EPT on mammographic breast density is stronger than that observed with oestrogens alone.[4] When compared to non-users, a significant increase in relative risk for breast cancer is found for long-term combined EPT users.[6,8,13,14,17,20] A number of observational studies have looked specifically at the risk for breast cancer associated with the use of combined EPT, as compared to that of ET users and non-users in the same population. In general, an increase in breast cancer risk is reported in EPT users compared to ET users.[14]

In the Million Women Study, this increase with EPT versus ET only was substantially greater: RR 2.0 versus RR 1.3, a statistically highly significant increase. It is estimated that 10 years' use of HRT will result in five additional breast cancers per 1000 oestrogen-only users, and 19 additional cancers per 1000 combined EPT users.[20] The Million Women Study found little variation in results between transdermal and oral, and between sequentially and continuously combined, regimens.

Two recent, prospective, placebo-controlled, clinical trials reported that continuously combined EPT induced a higher risk than that which existed among women in the control group.[6,13] In the Heart and Estrogen/progestin Replacement Study[13] long-term use (average 6.8 years) of continuously combined EPT (CCEPT) resulted in a RR of 1.27 (95% CI; range 0.84–1.94). In the WHI study, CCEPT use led to a RR of 1.24 (95% CI; range 1.01–1.54) after an average follow-up of 5.6 years, with an adjusted 95% CI of 0.97–1.59.[6] In view of the large population of women on CCEPT (N = 8506) and the lack of overall benefit in this group, the CCEPT study of the WHI was stopped prematurely in 2002. In 2004, the ET-only WHI study was also stopped prematurely because of an increased risk of stroke; however, this study found no increased breast cancer risk.[2]

TUMOUR CHARACTERISTICS OF BREAST CANCER UNDER HORMONE REPLACEMENT THERAPY

The large Collaborative Group reanalysis reported breast cancer tumours found in women on HRT to be more localized in nature.[8] The majority of studies have reported that tumours in HRT users are more often well-differentiated, more often receptor positive, significantly smaller and less likely to spread to the axillary lymph nodes. However, not all studies found this. For example, the WHI trial reported that tumours in the HRT group were less localized, slightly larger and with more positive nodes.[6] It could be that HRT users developed an increased risk for relatively mild breast tumours while probably not reducing their baseline risk for aggressive tumours, which have a poorer prognosis. A point that deserves further investigation is the suggestion that HRT only elevates the risk of lobular carcinoma.[17]

In conclusion, there is no clear evidence to show that breast cancers arising in HRT users have better prognostic characteristics than those found in non-users. For a long time the general opinion was that mortality in breast cancer patients, diagnosed when on HRT, was not increased.[21] The Million Women Study has now reported an increase in fatal breast cancer in current users.[20]

It is possible that the phenomenon of a better prognosis of breast cancer in HRT users is due to confounding factors. This could be the case when HRT users have easier access to medical care, have more mammograms, have tumours diagnosed earlier and adhere more frequently to a healthier lifestyle, thereby favourably influencing their prognosis.

RISK-MODIFYING FACTORS

Obesity, more than moderate alcohol use, and a positive family history of breast cancer are factors that might modify the risk of breast cancer when using HRT. Obese, postmenopausal non-HRT users have an increased risk of breast cancer. Conversely, lean, non-HRT users have lower concentrations of sex hormones compared to more obese women. Interestingly, various studies found a higher excess risk of breast cancer in lean women, when using HRT, than in obese HRT users.[8,14]

Postmenopausal alcohol intake of two drinks or more increases the risk of developing breast cancer. In the Collaborative Group re-analysis[8] breast cancer risk among long-term HRT users was modified by alcohol intake but this was not so in the Million Women Study.[20]

Surprisingly, women with a family history of breast cancer, using HRT after a natural or surgical menopause, have not been shown to have an increased risk of breast cancer.[8,20,23] This is especially important for women with a BRCA-1 or -2 gene mutation, who are frequently offered bilateral oophorectomy during the premenopause as a prophylactic measure against ovarian cancer. For these particular groups of women, HRT is very important, both in relation to climacteric complaints and for protection against osteoporosis.

In women with a history of breast cancer, the use of oestrogen-containing replacement regimens is highly controversial and HRT has generally been considered to be contraindicated.[14] As ovarian ablation in premenopausal women with breast cancer leads to a significantly longer disease-free survival and a reduced mortality, it is felt that dormant residual breast cancer cells could be activated by oestrogens, and therefore might precipitate the recurrence of clinical breast cancer. Also, oestrogens could induce a new tumour in the contralateral breast in these women.

Quality of life is an important issue in these breast cancer patients, especially in young premenopausal women who enter menopause prematurely and artificially due to surgery or chemotherapy. After treatment a substantial portion of these women will survive without tumours but they will suffer from hot flushes and vaginal dryness, and an impaired quality of life, while osteoporosis and cardiovascular disease are long-term health concerns in women with an induced, premature menopause. Therefore, a history of breast cancer should not be an absolute contraindication for oestrogen-containing HRT. Recently, a review of 11 studies found no adverse impact on recurrence and mortality in cancer survivors using HRT.[7] Although these data are reassuring, they might be confounded to a significant extent. The HABITS (HRT after breast cancer – is it safe?), an open, randomized, clinical trial in women treated with HRT after a diagnosis of breast cancer, was stopped prematurely in 2003 and reported an adjusted RR of 3.5 (95% CI; range 1.5–8.1) for a new breast cancer event in HRT users after a median follow-up of 2.1 years.[12] The LIBERATE trial (Livial intervention following breast cancer: efficacy, recurrence and tolerability) is an ongoing, randomized, clinical trial in women after breast cancer treated with either tibolone or placebo.[16]

ALTERNATIVES TO OESTROGEN-CONTAINING HORMONE REPLACEMENT THERAPY

Tibolone[15] and raloxifene3 are options for women seeking alternatives to oestrogen-containing HRT. In preclinical and mammographic studies, breast stimulation was low or absent.[4]

Tibolone is effective in reducing hot flushes and other climacteric complaints, while raloxifene is not. However, while raloxifene has been shown to reduce breast cancer risk (in women with osteoporosis),[5] tibolone has been reported in one study to increase breast cancer risk to the same degree as unopposed ET but not as much as combined EPT.[20] Both are useful in protection for osteoporosis.

Phyto-oestrogens are a complex group of plant-derived substances of which soya foods and black cohosh (*Cimicifuga racemosa*) are the best known. It is claimed that they reduce the number of hot flushes, and also LDL cholesterol, but the effect on the breast is not well-documented and the effects on the nervous system are controversial.[1]

Progestogens such as megestrol acetate, when given continuously, reduce hot flushes in most patients. In severe cases, a selective serotonin reuptake inhibitor (e.g. fluoxetine,[19] venlafaxine or paroxetine), or cardiovascular drugs such as clonidine, can be considered.

For vaginal dryness and dyspareunia, a limited intravaginal dose of oestradiol or oestriol is an option. A nonhormonal vaginal lubricant may offer an acceptable alternative.

Women with climacteric complaints in the perimenopause (or directly afterwards) should be advised not to smoke, to eat a healthy diet, to get adequate exercise, reduce stress, and attain or keep to a healthy weight. Women with hot flushes should reduce their intake of alcohol and hot beverages, and limit their consumption of spicy foods. So-called paced respiration (deep breathing) might be effective in some patients.

To reduce the risk of osteoporosis, daily exercise and an adequate dose of calcium and vitamin D are advised. In women with osteopenia or osteoporosis, raloxifene and bisphosphonates have been proven to be very effective. To reduce the risk of cardiovascular disease, the control of blood pressure and cholesterol level are important. Appropriate preventive treatment options are now available, e.g. aspirin and statins.

CONCLUSION

To summarize, long-term, current combined EPT increases breast cancer risk slightly and probably more than unopposed oestrogen use. Mammographic breast density and breast tenderness also differ between regimens. It is not clear if breast density and breast pain can be considered as biomarkers for breast cancer risk.

The idea that the excess breast cancers found under EPT tend to be more localized and less aggressive has recently been challenged, and the effect on breast cancer mortality is not clear. Our knowledge of other routes of administration (than the oral route) is very limited. Lean women have a higher RR for breast cancer with HRT use than obese women. A family history of breast cancer does not increase the HRT-induced risk further. In women with a history of breast cancer, HRT for climacteric symptoms, vaginal dryness and feelings of well-being is highly controversial. In addition to HRT, effective alternative options exist for treating hot flushes and vaginal dryness, or to prevent osteoporosis.

References

1. Albertazzi P, Purdie D W 2002 The nature and utility of the phytoestrogens: a review of the evidence. Maturitas 42:173–185
2. Anderson G L, Limacher M, Assaf A R et al for the Women's Health Initiative Steering Committee 2004 Effects of conjugated equine estrogen in postmenopausal women with hysterectomy. The Women's Health Initiative randomized controlled trial. The Journal of the American Medical Association 291:1701–1712
3. Barrett-Connor E 2001 Raloxifene: risks and benefits. Annals of the New York Academy of Science 949:295–303
4. Bosman A, van der Mooren M J, Kenemans P Postmenopausal hormone therapy and mammographic breast density (in press)
5. Cauley J A, Norton L, Lippman M E 2001 Continued breast cancer risk reduction in postmenopausal women treated with raloxifene: 4-year results from the MORE trial. Multiple Outcomes of Raloxifene Evaluation. Breast Cancer Research and Treatment 65:125–134
6. Chlebowski R T, Hendrix S L, Langer R D et al 2003 Influence of estrogen plus progestin on breast cancer and mammography in healthy postmenopausal women. The Journal of the American Medical Association 289:3243–3253
7. Col N F, Hirota L K, Orr R K et al 2001 Hormone replacement therapy after breast cancer: a systematic review and quantitative assessment of risk. Journal of Clinical Oncology 19:2357–2363
8. Collaborative Group on Hormonal Factors in Breast Cancer 1997 Breast cancer and hormone replacement therapy. Collaborative reanalysis of data from 51 epidemiological studies of 52,705 women with breast cancer and 108,411 women without breast cancer. The Lancet 350:1047–1059
9. Endogenous Hormones and Breast Cancer Collaborative Group 2002 Endogenous sex hormones and breast cancer in postmenopausal women: reanalysis of nine prospective studies. Journal of the National Cancer Institute 94:606–616
10. Franke H R, Vermes I 2003 Differential effects of progestogens on breast cancer cell lines. Maturitas 46 (Suppl 1):S55–S58
11. Hesch R-D, Kenemans P 1999 Hormonal prevention of breast cancer: proposal for a

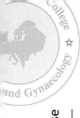
change in paradigm. British Journal of Obstetrics and Gynaecology 106:1006–1008

12. Holmberg L, Anderson H for the HABITS steering and data monitoring committees 2004 HABITS (hormonal replacement therapy after breast cancer – is it safe?). A randomised comparison: trial stopped. The Lancet 363:453–455

13. Hulley S, Furberg C, Barret-Connor E et al 2002 Noncardiovascular disease outcomes during 6.8 years of hormone therapy. The Journal of the American Medical Association 288:58–66

14. Kenemans P, Bosman A 2003 Breast cancer and post-menopausal hormone therapy. Best Practice & Research. Clinical Endocrinology & Metabolism 17:123–137

15. Kloosterboer H J 2001 Tibolone: a steroid with a tissue-specific mode of action. The Journal of Steroid Biochemistry and Molecular Biology 76:231–238

16. Kubista E 2003 Behandlung klimakterischer Symptome nach Brustkrebs mit Livial® – Die LIBERATE-Studie. Journal für Menopause 10 (Sonderheft/Special Edition 3):16–19

17. Li C I, Malone K E, Porter P L et al 2003 Relationship between long durations and different regimens of hormone therapy and risk of breast cancer. The Journal of the American Medical Association 289:3254–3263

18. Liehr J G 2000 Is estradiol a genotoxic mutagenic carcinogen? Endocrine Reviews 21:40–54

19. Loprinzi C L, Sloan J A, Perez E A et al 2002 Phase III evaluation of fluoxetine for treatment of hot flushes. Journal of Clinical Oncology 20:1578–1583

20. Million Women Study Collaborators 2003 Breast cancer and hormone replacement therapy in the Million Women Study. The Lancet 362:419–427

21. Nanda K, Bastian L A, Schulz K 2002 Hormone replacement therapy and the risk of death from breast cancer. A systematic review. American Journal of Obstetrics and Gynecology 186:325–334

22. Richer J K, Jacobsen B M, Manning N G et al 2002 Differential gene regulation by the two progesterone receptor isoforms in human breast cancer cells. The Journal of Biological Chemistry 277:5209–5218

23. Scheele F, Burger C W, Kenemans P 1999 Postmenopausal hormone replacement in the woman with a reproductive risk factor for breast cancer. Maturitas 33:191–196

24. Spicer D V, Pike M C 1992 The prevention of breast cancer through reduced ovarian steroid exposure. Acta Oncologica 31:167–174

24

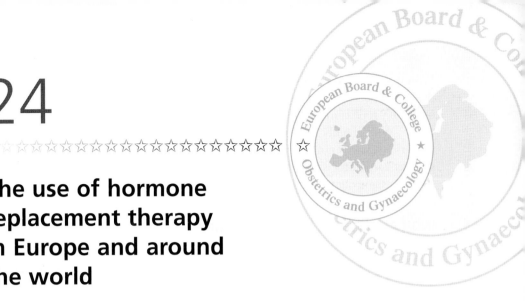

☆☆☆☆☆☆☆☆☆☆☆☆☆☆☆☆☆☆   ☆

The use of hormone replacement therapy in Europe and around the world

Margaret Rees

ABSTRACT

The main reason for taking hormone replacement therapy (HRT) is to relieve vasomotor symptoms such as hot flushes and night sweats. Compliance with HRT is low and over 50% of women will have stopped therapy after one year. Women receive much of their information from the media, resulting in an incomplete understanding of the issues. The quality of information is variable. Scares about the risks and side-effects of HRT will receive more publicity than any studies showing benefits. It is therefore not surprising that compliance is greater in health professionals. Publication of the Women's Health Initiative (WHI) and the Million Women Study (MWS) has led to the publication of new guidelines regarding HRT prescribing. This has led to a reduction in systemic HRT use with a tendency to use lower doses and more vaginal preparations.

KEYWORDS

Breast cancer, cardiovascular disease, hormone replacement therapy (HRT), menopause, osteoporosis

INTRODUCTION

The concept of oestrogen replacement was first explored in the late 19th century. In 1896, ovarian therapy was first tried in a Berlin clinic by the gynaecologist Ludwig Fraenkel.[6] The patient was a 23-year-old woman who had undergone oophorectomy; other cases were reported three weeks later in Germany and five weeks later in Vienna. The 1930s saw the isolation and manufacture of sex steroids, which shortly afterwards became commercially available. In 1966 Robert

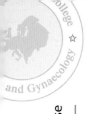

Wilson published a best-selling book, *Feminine Forever*, in which he maintained that menopause was an oestrogen-deficiency disease that should be treated with oestrogen replacement therapy (ET) to prevent the otherwise inevitable 'living decay'. While highly debated, this gave rise to the idea that oestrogen could be a universal panacea not only dealing with the consequences of oestrogen deficiency such as vasomotor symptoms but also delaying ageing. The past few years have shown a significant reversal of this initial optimism.[23]

INDICATIONS FOR TAKING HORMONE REPLACEMENT THERAPY

The main reason for taking HRT is to relieve vasomotor symptoms such as hot flushes and night sweats. While it has been shown to reduce the risk of vertebral and hip fractures, continuation of its use is poor even in a targeted population such as those having undergone oophorectomy. Menopause symptomatology is not distributed equally, either between or among populations of peri- and post-menopausal women.[11] For example, there is lower reporting of vasomotor symptoms in India, Indonesia, Japan, China and rural Mayans living in Yucatan, Mexico, than in their North American or European counterparts. Thus HRT use varies widely from less than 5% to 45%.[9,11]

Since use is related to menopause symptomatology, it is not surprising that most women will use it between the ages of 50 and 54 and for 5 years or less.[14] The greater use in oophorectomized women (66%) versus women who had not undergone hysterectomy or oophorectomy (27%) as demonstrated in the MWS in the UK and a survey in Sweden, is a reflection of use to control menopausal symptoms.[14,19]

Studies that have examined the reasons as to why women stop therapy emphasize the dislike of continued menstruation, side-effects, lack of efficacy and concerns about long-term risks such as breast cancer.[9,20,21] There is also the opinion that the menopause is a natural process, which should not be interfered with.

CHARACTERISTICS OF HORMONE REPLACEMENT THERAPY USERS

HRT users differ from nonusers in ways that are known or believed to alter risk. While this has been described as a healthy user effect, there are also characteristics that may increase the risk of developing certain diseases. For example, HRT users tend to be more affluent, leaner and more educated, and they exercise more often and drink alcohol more frequently.[5,13,17] These factors are associated with an increased risk of breast cancer and decreased risk for cardiovascular disease. Further, women who have undergone hysterectomy and oophorectomy, which are associated with decreased risk of breast cancer and increased risk of osteoporosis, use HRT more often. Also, by definition, women who take HRT have access to healthcare and have a greater likelihood of being treated for other medical conditions that may also decrease their risks for certain clinical outcomes.

THE DECISION-MAKING PROCESS FOR THE USE OF HORMONE REPLACEMENT THERAPY

Compliance with HRT is low and over 50% of women will have stopped therapy after one year.[9] Women receive much of their information from the media, resulting in an incomplete understanding of the issues. Scares about the risks and side-effects of HRT, such as that following the initial publication of the WHI, will obtain more publicity than any studies showing benefits.[23] It is therefore not surprising that compliance is greater in female gynaecologists, general practitioners or the spouses of their male counterparts suggesting that good information and a positive attitude to therapy are important.[1]

A number of studies have reported that a major reason for taking HRT was a positive attitude of, and recommendation by, the physician. The gender of the doctor is also an important factor. For example, a study by Newton et al in the USA showed that controlling for age and practice type, HRT prescribing frequency was lower among men than women providers (odds ratio, OR, 0.38; 95% confidence interval, CI; range 0.21–0.65) and higher among the upper tertile versus the lower tertiles of an HRT encouragement scale (OR 2.50; 95% CI; range 1.29–4.85).[16] Clark et al in Canada also found that the most significant factor associated with the decision to take HRT, after the physician visit, was the physician preference (OR 62; 95% CI; range 13.3–289.7).[4]

Further, physician speciality is significantly associated with HRT use.[10] For example, current HRT use among women receiving care from gynaecologists has been found to be more than double that among women receiving care from family physicians.[10]

Women are turning to the Internet for information regarding the menopause and HRT. The quality of web-based information was recently assessed.[18] A sample of 25 sites (of varied ownership) was generated. Using a specific scoring tool, each site was assessed on factual information provided and quality of site. Certain types of ownership were associated with higher quality sites, including the pharmaceutical industry, community pharmacies, governments and charities. However, commercial sites could be biased towards particular products. The authors concluded that information about menopause and HRT on the Internet is often dubious with incomplete information being commonly provided.

THE WOMEN'S HEALTH INITIATIVE

The publication of the ending of the oestrogen–progestogen arm of the WHI in July 2002 (and further recent papers) has led to emotion in the media and considerable uncertainties about the role of HRT among health professionals and women.[23] Using a global index, the WHI investigators concluded that risks exceeded benefits of the combined regimen. The WHI was a randomized controlled trial designed in the early 1990s to examine various strategies for the primary prevention and control of some of the most common causes of morbidity and mortality among postmenopausal women aged 50–79 examining not only

HRT but also calcium and vitamin D supplementation and low-fat eating patterns. Publication of the oestrogen-only arm has led to more reassurance, but confusion among women and health professionals still prevails.[22]

The study has led regulatory authorities to publish new recommendations. For example, the Committee on Safety of Medicines in the UK, following a European review of the evidence, recommended in December 2003 that 'the risk/benefit is favourable for the treatment of menopausal symptoms, the lowest effective dose should be used for the shortest duration and that it should not be considered a first-line therapy for the long-term prevention of osteoporosis in women who are over 50 years of age.' This advice has, so far, not been changed following publication of the oestrogen-only arm of the WHI.[22] In addition, based on a scientific review, the US government has added steroidal oestrogens, used in HRT and oral contraceptives, to its official list of known human carcinogens.[15]

IMPACT OF THE WOMEN'S HEALTH INITIATIVE ON HORMONE REPLACEMENT THERAPY PRESCRIBING

Various studies worldwide have assessed women's knowledge of, attitudes and use of HRT following the first WHI publication.[23] Between 26 July and 6 August 2002 a national random-digit-dialling telephone survey was conducted in the USA in a sample of households which included women aged 40 to 79.[3] Of the 819 women interviewed, 64% had heard something about the WHI study results from the media or from talking to others, and 74% were confused about HRT use. Another 57% were worried about how the findings might affect them, and 79% were interested in obtaining additional information about HRT. Only 24% of those who had heard something had actually sought additional information. Current HRT users were most likely to be aware and informed. They were also more likely to be confused, worried, or to need or seek additional information; older women were less likely to be confused or worried, or to need or seek additional information. More highly educated women were more likely to be aware and less likely to be confused or uninformed but were more likely to have sought additional information.

HRT use has declined since the first WHI paper, and prescriptions of alternative therapies, such as clonidine, for menopausal symptoms have been documented.[2] There has been a reduction in systemic HRT use, especially with the preparation used in the WHI trial, a tendency to use lower doses and an increase in vaginal oestrogens.[7,8] However, a return to using systemic HRT has also been documented, presumably due to a recurrence of hot flushes.[12]

References

1. Andersson K, Pedersen A T, Mattsson L A et al 1998 Swedish gynecologists' and general practitioners' views on the climacteric period: knowledge, attitudes and management strategies. Acta Obstetricia et Gynecologica Scandinavica 77:909–916

2. Austin P C, Mamdani M M, Tu K 2004 The impact of the Women's Health Initiative study on incident clonidine use in Ontario, Canada. The Canadian Journal of Clinical Pharmacology 11:E191–E194

3 Breslau E S, Davis W W, Doner L et al 2003 The hormone therapy dilemma: women respond. Journal of the American Medical Women's Association 58:33–43

4. Clark H D, O'Connor A M, Graham I D et al 2003 What factors are associated with a woman's decision to take hormone replacement therapy? Evaluated in the context of a decision aid. Health Expectations 6:110–117

5. Derby C A, Hume A L, McPhillips J B et al 1995 Prior and current health characteristics of postmenopausal estrogen replacement therapy users compared with nonusers. American Journal of Obstetrics and Gynecology 173:544–550

6. Gruhn J G, Kazer R R 1989 Hormonal Regulation of the Menstrual Cycle: The evolution concepts. Plenum Publishing Co, New York

7. Haas J S, Kaplan C P, Gerstenberger E P et al 2004 Changes in the use of postmenopausal hormone therapy after the publication of clinical trial results. Annals of Internal Medicine 140:184–188

8. Hersh A L, Stefanick M L, Stafford R S 2004 National use of postmenopausal hormone therapy: annual trends and response to recent evidence. The Journal of the American Medical Association 291:47–53

9. Hope S, Wager E, Rees M 1998 Survey of British women's views on the menopause and HRT. The Journal of the British Menopause Society 4:33–36

10. Levy B T, Ritchie J M, Smith E et al 2003 Physician specialty is significantly associated with hormone replacement therapy use. Obstetrics and Gynecology 101:114–122

11. Lock M 2002 Symptom reporting at menopause: a review of cross cultural findings. The Journal of the British Menopause Society 8:132–136

12. MacLennan A H, Taylor A W, Wilson D H 2004 Hormone therapy use after the Women's Health Initiative. Climacteric 7:138–142

13. Matthews K A, Kuller L H, Wing R R et al 1996 Prior to use of estrogen replacement therapy, are users healthier than nonusers? American Journal of Epidemiology 143:971–978

14. Million Women Study Collaborators. Patterns of use of hormone replacement therapy in one million women in Britain, 1996–2000. British Journal of Obstetrics and Gynaecology 109:1319–1330

15. Nelson R 2002 Steroidal oestrogens added to list of known human carcinogens. The Lancet 360:2053

16. Newton K M, LaCroix A Z, Buist D S et al 2001 What factors account for hormone replacement therapy prescribing frequency? Maturitas 39:1–10

17. Persson I, Bergkvist L, Lindgren C et al 1997 Hormone replacement therapy and major risk factors for reproductive cancers, osteoporosis, and cardiovascular diseases: evidence of confounding by exposure characteristics. Journal of Clinical Epidemiology 50:611–618

18. Reed M, Anderson C 2002 Evaluation of patient information Internet web sites about menopause and hormone replacement therapy. Maturitas 43:135–154

19. Stadberg E, Mattsson L A, Milsom I 2000 Factors associated with climacteric symptoms and the use of hormone replacement therapy. Acta Obstetricia et Gynecologica Scandinavica 79:286–292

20. Stadberg E, Mattsson L A, Milsom I 1997 Women's attitudes and knowledge about the climacteric period and its treatment. A Swedish population-based study. Maturitas 27:109–116

21. Vihtamaki T, Savilahti R, Tuimala R 1999 Why do postmenopausal women discontinue hormone replacement therapy? Maturitas 33:99–105

22. Women's Health Initiative Steering Committee 2004 Effects of conjugated equine estrogen in postmenopausal women with hysterectomy. The Women's Health Initiative randomized controlled trial. The Journal of the American Medical Association 291:1701–1712

23. Writing Group for the Women's Health Initiative Investigators 2002 Risks and benefits of estrogen plus progestin in healthy postmenopausal women. Principal results from the Women's Health Initiative randomized controlled trial. The Journal of the American Medical Association 288:321–333

25

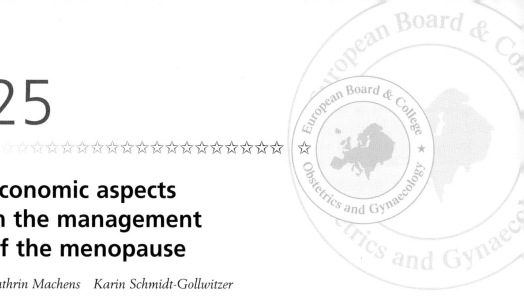

Economic aspects in the management of the menopause

Kathrin Machens   Karin Schmidt-Gollwitzer

ABSTRACT

Oestrogen deficiency in postmenopausal women is characterized by a variety of symptoms that involve different sites such as the nervous system, the urogenital tract, the skeleton and the cardiovascular system. In the industrialized world the number of people older than 65 years continues to rise, especially the subgroup of elderly women. Therefore the economic burden is likely to increase due to the rise in age-related chronic diseases. For single-target diseases special therapeutic agents exist that are effective, the actions of which are often limited to a single site or organ. Oestrogen with or without progestin is the only medication that exerts such broad effects, not only on immediate postmenopausal symptoms but also in the prevention of some age-related conditions. The results of the prematurely stopped Women's Health Initiative (WHI) study have shattered the confidence in postmenopausal hormone replacement therapy (HRT), especially long-term HRT. However, the extrapolation of the results from one specific HRT regimen (0.625 mg conjugated equine oestrogens, CEEs, alone or 0.625 mg CEEs plus 2.5 mg medroxyprogesterone acetate) on all HRT products apart from their doses, ingredients and administration routes, and on all postmenopausal women apart from their age and health status, is unjustifiable. A huge spectrum of different HRT products makes possible HRT adapted to the woman's individual needs. Furthermore, women usually start HRT around menopause and thus are 15 years younger and probably healthier than the WHI participants. Consequently, the failure of demonstrating some beneficial effects in these elderly postmenopausal women cannot be generalized to the general population of postmenopausal women. If HRT is given to appropriate women on an individualized basis this therapy combines cost-effectiveness and efficacy in a unique way.

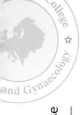

KEYWORDS

Chronic diseases, hormone replacement therapy (HRT), menopause, socioeconomy

INTRODUCTION: THE DEMOGRAPHIC SITUATION

In 1927 the world population reached 2 billion people, 5 billion in 1987, 6 billion in 1999 and is estimated to become 7 billion as early as 2011 or as late as 2015.[57] Because of historically low birth rates in Europe and Japan, the population continues to decline in these industrialized countries. The proportion of the younger relative to the older population is out of balance. Unlike the world population, where only 7% are 65 years of age or older, 15% of the European population and 18% of the Japanese belong to this age group. As a consequence of this demographic change, the health problems prevailing worldwide will increasingly be those of the elderly, the majority of whom will be women. In the developed countries, up to 70% of women, but only 40–50% of men, will reach the age of 80 years or more.

The economic burden of chronic diseases such as cardiovascular disease (CVD), osteoporosis or colorectal carcinoma that mainly affect elderly women is enormous. Early prevention, i.e. starting preventive measures around menopause at the latest, may decrease the severity of, and limit, some of these chronic conditions. Furthermore, these preventive measures may enhance quality of life in the elderly female due to the reduction or prevention of disability, pain or other complaints. This should help reduce the economic burden borne by society, mostly direct costs for hospitalization, ambulatory care and payments for drugs.

In the majority of observational and case-control studies, HRT prevented many of these chronic conditions. These promising findings – and the segment of menopausal women increasing as a result of demographic changes – account for the worldwide spread of HRT, especially during the past decade. While the use of HRT had attained a steady state in the 1980s, it has continued to surge steadily since the 1990s reaching, for example, 21.5% of women aged 40–64 years in the UK by 1994.[82] In the USA, a similar steady increase occurred, with an enormous leap in prescriptions mainly between 1999 and 2000. In 2000, 25% of menopausal women in the USA were on HRT, the same percentage as in Germany. With about 45% of menopausal women, France has the highest rate of HRT use in Europe. In most other European countries, the prevalence of HRT varies from 10% to 20%, with the exception of Mediterranean countries where HRT use is below 10%. In Japan, the prevalence of HRT is only 2%.[69]

It was the widely publicized premature termination of the WHI study[88,90] (because of a perceived higher risk of breast cancer and CVD) that stopped the continuous expansion of HRT. This randomized, double-blind, placebo-controlled multicentre trial sought to clarify the benefits and risks of HRT seen in observational and case-control studies. Herein, the protective effects of HRT against osteoporotic fractures and colorectal carcinoma were confirmed. Contrary to results from more than 50 observational and case-control studies, there was not only no evidence of cardiovascular prevention in the terminated WHI study but an increased risk for some cardiovascular events, e.g. stroke. This complex association cannot be handled here, therefore we will focus in the following on the treatment of menopausal complaints such as vasomotor and psychological symptoms, urogenital atrophy, and the proven preventive effects of HRT on age-related chronic diseases such as osteoporosis and colorectal carcinoma from a pharmacoeconomic point of view. Finally, the socioeconomic impact of prevention or delay of cognitive decline or Alzheimer's disease is explored, which is a major cost-driver of healthcare expenditure in the elderly.

MENOPAUSAL COMPLAINTS

The menopause and the sequelae of oestrogen/progestin loss have a socioeconomic dimension. In an investigation conducted in Germany in 1996, direct and indirect costs of diseases related to the women's decreased oestrogen production were estimated.[91] Combining direct costs such as outpatient care, hospitalization and rehabilitation, and indirect costs such as invalidity and death, the highest cost load was due to CVDs and cerebrovascular diseases. Second were the costs caused by diseases of the skeleton, and vasomotor and psychological disorders, each of around €450 million (US$600 million), followed by diseases of the urogenital tract.

VASOMOTOR AND PSYCHOLOGICAL SYMPTOMS

In the western hemisphere menopause is associated, for up to 80% of women, with a number of unpleasant vasomotor symptoms such as hot flushes and night sweats, which reduce their quality of life. Of those women experiencing vasomotor symptoms, 51% suffer severely, 33% moderately and 16% mildly.[39]

There are only a few studies that investigated the socioeconomic impact of vasomotor and psychological symptoms on women's quality of life. These pharmacoeconomic studies mostly focus on direct costs to healthcare systems,[81,82] and often compare the costs of different regimens with each another.[7,54,65] After the release of the WHI results,[88,90] an agreement seems to have emerged that HRT should primarily be used for the management of vasomotor and other menopausal symptoms. This treatment should be restricted to a short period. HRT has been demonstrated to be very cost-effective even for the short-term management of vasomotor symptoms, i.e. from 1 year to ≤3 years. This effect was more pronounced in women with more severe menopausal symptoms than in women with milder symptoms.[13] The onset of breakthrough bleeding or spotting, and the effectiveness of the individual HRT product in providing vasomotor symptom relief, also have an influence on the cost-effectiveness of short-term HRT.

There is wide range of HRT formulations; the monthly costs of therapy per patient for menopausal symptoms may differ according to the active ingredients, formulation (monotherapy or combination therapy) and route of administration

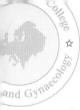
(costs of selected compounds in 2000; Tables 25.1 and 25.2). In general, oestrogen [mono]therapy (ET) is less expensive than oestrogen plus progestin combination therapy (EPT), and oral formulations are less expensive than patches. However, the woman's individual needs and preferences are the key determinants of which HRT product is chosen.

An alternative way of assessing the increments in quality of life with HRT is to evaluate the woman's willingness to pay. In an examination conducted in 1998, Swedish women with menopausal symptoms were willing to spend up to 12% of their annual pre-tax household income to continue HRT.[94] This was three times more than the 4% of the annual income they were willing to pay for continuing

Table 25.1 The cost of oestrogen replacement therapy per 28-day cycle (€) in the year 2000

Brand name	Hormone(s)	Formulation	Cost per 28-day cycle (€)
Elleste Solo® 1 mg	oestradiol 1 mg	Tablets	1.78
Hormonin®	oestriol 0.27 mg, oestrone 1.4 mg, oestradiol 0.6 mg	Tablets	2.20
Progynova® 1 mg	oestradiol 1 mg	Tablets	2.34
Zumenon 1 mg	oestradiol 1 mg	Tablets	2.55
Premarin® 0.625 mg	conjugated equine oestrogens 0.625 mg	Tablets	2.70
Harmogen®	estropipate 1.5 mg (equiv. oestrone 0.93 mg)	Tablets	3.00
Elleste Solo® MX 40	oestradiol 40 µg/24 h	Patches	5.19
FemSeven® 50	oestradiol 50 µg/24 h	Patches	5.20
Estraderm MX 50	oestradiol 50 µg/24 h	Patches	5.22
Fematrix® 40	oestradiol 40 µg/24 h	Patches	5.50
Progynova® TS	oestradiol 50 µg/24 h	Patches	5.96
Dermestril® 50	oestradiol 50 µg/24 h	Patches	6.06
Estraderm® TTS 50	oestradiol 50 µg/24 h	Patches	6.23
Menorest® 50	oestradiol 50 µg/24 h	Patches	6.44
Evorel® 50	oestradiol 50 µg/24 h	Patches	6.48
Sandrena® 0.5 mg	oestradiol 0.5 µg per 0.5 g single dose unit	Gel	5.68
Sandrena® 1 mg	oestradiol 1 mg per 1 g single dose unit	Gel	6.54
Oestrogel® CFC free pump	oestradiol 0.06% w/w; 1.5 mg oestradiol per 2 × 1.25 g measures	Gel	6.96
Duphaston® HRT	dydrogesterone 10 mg	Tablets	1.05
Micronor® HRT	norethisterone	Tablets	1.25
Crinone® 4%	progesterone 4% gel; progesterone 45 mg per 1.125 g gel	Vaginal gel	11.08

Adapted with permission from reference 8.

Table 25.2 The cost of HRT per 28-day cycle (€) in the year 2000

Brand name	Hormone(s)	Formulation	Cost per 28-day cycle (€)
Sequential preparations			
Elleste Duet® 1 mg	oestradiol, norethisterone	Tablets	3.24
Cyclo-Progynova® 1 mg	oestradiol, levonorgestrel	Tablets	3.34
Climagest® 1 mg	oestradiol, norethisterone	Tablets	4.38
Nuvelle®	oestradiol, levonorgestrel	Tablets	4.59
Trisequens®	oestradiol, norethisterone	Tablets	4.80
Prempak-C 0.625	conjugated oestrogens, norgestrel	Tablets	4.91
Femoston® 1/10	oestradiol, dydrogesterone	Tablets	4.99
Premique® Cycle	conjugated oestrogens, medroxyprogesterone	Tablets	7.54
Tridestra®	oestradiol, medroxyprogesterone	Tablets	7.66
Evorel-Pak®	oestradiol, norethisterone	Patches plus Tablets	8.45
Femapak® 80 μg	oestradiol, dydrogesterone	Patches plus Tablets	8.95
Estrapak®	oestradiol, norethisterone	Patches plus Tablets	9.48
Nuvelle® TS	oestradiol, levonorgestrel	Patches	10.51
Evorel® Sequi	oestradiol, norethisterone	Patches	11.00
Estracombi®	oestradiol, norethisterone	Patches	11.14
Continuous combined preparations			
Elleste Duet® Conti	oestradiol 2 mg, norethisterone 1 mg	Tablets	5.99
Nuvelle® Continuous	oestradiol 2 mg, norethisterone 1 mg	Tablets	6.01
Premique®	conjugated equine estrogens 0.625 mg, medroxyprogesterone 5 mg	Tablets	7.54
Climesse®	oestradiol 2 mg, norethisterone 0.7 mg	Tablets	7.90
Kliovance®	oestradiol 1 mg, norethisterone 0.5 mg	Tablets	8.65
Evorel® Conti	oestradiol 50 μg/24 h, norethisterone 170 μg/24 h	Patches	12.90
Livial®	tibolone 2.5 mg	Tablets	13.05

Adapted with permission from reference 8.

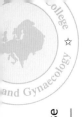

antihypertensive treatment.[36] This illustrates that the improvement in quality of life by HRT is far greater than the quality-of-life weightings applied in some studies.[28]

Psychological symptoms such as fatigue, headache, depressive mood, insomnia, muscular pain and palpitations have been considered to be associated with hot flushes, night sweats and consequent sleep disruption. HRT facilitates falling asleep and diminishes nocturnal restlessness and awakening, especially in women who experience a significant alleviation of their vasomotor symptoms.[16] ET also improves sleep in women without vasomotor symptoms, which may be due to a direct oestrogen effect on brain function.[56] Hence simple and reasonable HRT is a more cost-effective, comprehensive and interfering treatment than a therapy consisting of neuroleptics, antidepressants, analgesics or sleeping medicines (or a combination thereof).

UROGENITAL ATROPHY

In postmenopausal women, oestrogen deficiency results in a variety of symptoms as a consequence of urogenital atrophy such as vaginal dryness/irritation, vaginitis, itching and dyspareunia. All of these promptly respond to ET.[71] Additional urinary complaints include urinary incontinence, abacterial urethritis and cystitis. Changes in vaginal pH and flora may predispose older women to urinary tract infections.[50,66] Urinary incontinence is a common, debilitating and costly disease, involving more than one-third of community-dwelling women who are 65 years of age or older. Nearly half of the nursing home residents of the same age group suffer from this disorder. Incontinence causes substantial disability, social isolation, psychological stress and economic burden.[9,42,48,78]

The annual direct cost of urinary incontinence in the USA was estimated at US$16.2 billion (1995 value), including US$12.4 billion (76.5%) for women and US$3.8 billion (23.5%) for men. Costs for women over 65 years of age were US$7.6 billion. This is more than twice the cost for women under 65. These annual expenditures in women are similar to those of other chronic conditions.[84] Around 70% of the total cost of urinary incontinence is consumed by routine care such as laundry and supplies. Diagnostic measures only account for 1% of total costs. This observation may indicate that urinary incontinence is still a taboo subject that keeps many urogenital disorders from being diagnosed, allowing their chronic sequelae to evolve over time.

Oestrogen may be beneficial in treating urogenital atrophy and its related symptoms such as frequency, urgency, nocturia and dysuria.[5] The efficacy of oral and vaginal oestrogen formulations in the treatment of urinary urgency and incontinence was demonstrated in various studies,[12,18,43] but not in all studies.[19,30,34] Although the definite role of oestrogens in the management of urinary incontinence remains to be determined, these hormones – whether combined with α-adrenergic agonists or not – may be an efficient and cost-effective therapeutic option as compared to other treatment modalities for urinary incontinence in the elderly (Table 25.3).

Table 25.3 Cost estimates for the treatment of urinary incontinence in elderly people (€) in the year 2000

Therapy	Monthly cost estimates
Surgery	
Laparoscopic colposuspension	1315[a]
Tension-free vaginal tape procedure	1463–1671[a]
Burch procedure	4013[a]
Behavioral therapy	13.67–27.50
Pharmacological therapy	
Anticholinergics	6.54–43.74
Tricyclic antidepressants	5.08
α-Adrenergic agonist	1.67
Topical oestrogens	
Premarin® (intravaginal cream)	3.07
Ortho Dinoestrol® (cream)	3.66
Ortho Gynest® (vaginal cream)	3.81
Ortho Gynest® (pessaries)	7.41
Ovestin® (intravaginal cream)	7.30
Tampovagan® (pessaries)	9.80
Estring® (vaginal ring)	15.36[b]
Vagifem® (tablets)	20.47

[a] Total costs.
[b] Replacement every 3 months, costs €46.07 per 3 months.
Adapted with permission from references 27–31.

THE PREVENTION OF CHRONIC DISEASES

OSTEOPOROSIS

Osteoporosis is a systemic disease characterized by decreased bone mass and the microarchitectural deterioration of bone tissue leading to bone fragility and the increased risk of hip, spine and wrist fractures. These fractures may result in a life of dependency, immobility and limited autonomy. More than 200 million women worldwide have osteoporosis. Estimates suggest that the cost due to hip fractures in the USA may rise from around €4.5 billion per year to approximately €47 billion by the year 2020.[63] One in three women, who lives to the age of 80, will suffer a hip fracture, and more than 40% of elderly women will contract vertebral fractures.[33]

The economic burden caused by osteoporotic fractures is a societal charge. The direct and indirect cost estimates for osteoporotic fractures in Germany are approximately €3 billion per year.[53] In the USA, with more than 1.5 million osteoporotic fractures a year, expenditures for only direct medical care of osteoporotic fractures total around €6 billion per year.[49]

Worldwide costs of female hip fractures may reach around €45–50 billion in 2025. For men, the costs of hip fractures are estimated to total 'only' about €1 billion in the same year.[62] The remarkable disparity in the incidence of hip fractures between men and women is not only due to the differences in biology but also to the lower proportion of men reaching more than 80 years of age.

Controversy has been raging for some time about the efficacy of HRT on the reduction of osteoporotic fractures. A recent meta-analysis found that HRT reduces fractures by 30–60% at different sites (nonvertebral, hip, wrist and vertebral fractures)[46] as did the randomized WHI study.[13,88] In the MORE study, a 50% reduction of vertebral fractures with raloxifene in two different dosages relative to placebo was found.[72] While HRT and raloxifene are equally effective, they differ considerably in their annual costs. Relative to calcium or fluoride supplementation, conventional HRT is not only a cost-effective therapy in the prevention of osteoporosis but also addresses any additional needs of the elderly woman. Drugs that specifically combat osteoporosis such as bisphosphonates or calcitonin are much more expensive than preventive medicines (Table 25.4).

Closely related to bone health is dental health. Recently, the effect of HRT on dental outcomes was evaluated in postmenopausal women in a systematic review and economic analysis of clinical trials.[3] HRT was associated with a reduction in adverse dental outcomes and associated costs of dental care. HRT users less often needed full or partial dentures and have a higher chance of retaining more of their own teeth (Table 25.5). These data illustrate the health and economic benefits of HRT on dental care.

COLORECTAL CARCINOMA

Associated with a high mortality, colorectal carcinoma is one of the leading cancers in the western world. It is the third most common cause of cancer-related

Table 25.4 Annual cost estimates for the treatment of osteoporosis in elderly people: preventive and therapeutic drugs

Therapy	Annual cost estimates (€)
Calcium	44–94
HRT	37–291
Fluoride	58–116
Raloxifene	378
Bisphosphonates	153–487
Calcitonin s.c.	218–472
1,25-OH vitamin D	465
Strontium ranelate	548
Calcitonin nasal	1817

Adapted with permission from references 14, 46 and 47.

Table 25.5 Averages in dental outcome in women aged 50–75 years

	Studies (n)	Women (n)	Dentures (%)	Remaining teeth (n)
All women	10	5757	45.3	13.9
HRT	4	2881	27.6	14.4
No HRT	8	2073	55.6	11.4

Adapted with permission from reference 48.

death in women after breast and lung cancer. The risk of developing colorectal carcinoma starts to rise after the age of 50 years.[1] The evolution of colorectal carcinoma through the adenoma–carcinoma sequence is slow and may take decades.[58]

Due to its high incidence and often protracted diagnosis in old age, colorectal carcinoma poses a major health challenge, representing a great economic burden to western societies. In France, a cost-of-illness study revealed that the direct costs of colorectal carcinoma, such as hospital and ambulatory care, amounted to around €470 million in 1999, 98% of which went on hospitalization.[70] Indirect costs, such as short-term disability allowance, long-term disability allowance and production loss totalled approximately €87 million, 71% of which was due to disability allowances. From a societal point of view, indirect costs incurred through production losses were around €530 million. Altogether, the total cost of colorectal carcinoma in France amounted to more than €550 million for the social security system and almost €1 billion for the society in the year 1999.

Screening for adenomas, the precursors of most colorectal carcinomas,[20] and for early-stage colorectal carcinomas, decreases incidence and mortality associated with this disease.[10] Although screening for colorectal carcinoma has been shown to be cost-effective,[74] adherence to screening is rather poor.[14]

For women, oral contraceptive (OC) use and HRT may be an option for prevention. In 1969, a hormonal basis of colorectal carcinoma was recognized for the first time, based on the observation that nuns experience an excess rate of colorectal carcinoma.[22] This finding was further supported by the lower age-adjusted incidence rates for colorectal cancer in women compared with men.[87] In addition, populations with low parity have higher rates of colorectal carcinoma than populations with high parity.[59] Possible modes of action include a reduction of bile acid production, an exertion of direct preventive effects on the colorectal epithelium or a combination of these factors.[41,79] In several case-control studies,[47,60] cohort studies[11,25] and randomized controlled trials,[15,32] an inverse association was also identified between HRT and colorectal carcinoma. Three recent meta-analyses[26,29,45] found a reduction in the risk of colorectal carcinoma with HRT ranging from 10 to 30%, and a decrease in cancer related mortality of 30%. This effect was greater in current users and was more pronounced with increasing duration of use.

Another recent meta-analysis confirmed that OC use is inversely related to colorectal carcinoma risk.[21] OCs seem to prevent early precancerous lesions of the

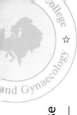
colorectal mucosa, and thus seem to protect against colorectal carcinoma in later life.

Aspirin and other nonsteroidal anti-inflammatory drugs are further agents used for the prevention of colorectal carcinoma. They inhibit both cyclooxygenase-1 (COX-1) and -2 (COX-2) by irreversible acetylation, and inhibit catalytic enzymes involved in prostaglandin synthesis by competitive inhibition,[77] the levels of which are elevated in colorectal adenoma and carcinoma.[17,92] The effectiveness of these compounds for the prevention of colorectal carcinoma, which, unlike HRT, can be used by men and women, has been intensively studied in case-control,[44,67] cohort[23,80] and randomized studies.[75] The results of these studies were conflicting. Despite its low cost, aspirin has not been adopted for chemoprevention because of its propensity to produce costly risks such as major gastrointestinal haemorrhage (Table 25.6). COX-2-specific inhibitors (i.e. COX-2 inhibitors) are associated with substantially higher costs than currently recommended screening strategies, and are suggested only as an adjunct to screening.[38] Furthermore, COX-2 inhibitors have come under scrutiny because of reports about an increased cardiovascular risk when used in colorectal adenoma prevention,[8,73] prompting an immediate withdrawal of Vioxx® (rofecoxib) from the market in 2005.

Recent reports suggest that supplemental folate, other vitamins, fibre and calcium have a preventive benefit but there are currently no prospective data to support these observations.[35]

COGNITION AND ALZHEIMER'S DISEASE

Cognitive and dementia disorders are a major burden for healthcare and social systems throughout the world. The worldwide number of people affected by

Table 25.6 Cost estimates for the screening and chemoprevention of colorectal carcinoma in elderly people

Method	Cost estimates per patient (€)
Faecal occult blood testing	6–17
Flexible sigmoidoscopy	86–384
Flexible sigmoidoscopy with biopsy	189–673
Colonoscopy	329–1095
Colonoscopy with biopsy	495–1565
Aspirin	2.30–6.90 per year
Aspirin plus management of aspirin-related complications	197 per year
Calcium	44–94 per year
HRT	37–291 per year
COX-2 inhibitor[a]	106–1679 per year

[a] COX-2 inhibitor, cyclooxygenase-2-specific inhibitor.
Adapted with permission from references 81, 82 and 88.

dementia in 2000 was estimated to vary between 25 million[86] and 38 million.[89] More women than men after the age of 75 years have dementia. Based on the United Nations prognosis for the demographic development of the world population until 2050 and the age-specific prevalence of dementia, it was estimated that the number of demented people in the world will increase to 63 million in 2030 and to 114 million in 2050.[85]

The most common form of dementia is Alzheimer's disease (AD). It is a progressive, degenerative disease of the brain and currently not curable. It is estimated that 10% of people over 65 and nearly half of those over 85 have AD; nearly half of all nursing home residents suffer from AD or a related disorder. A person with AD will live for an average of 8 years and for as many as 20 years or more from the onset of symptoms.[4] Although 70% of people with AD live at home, and 75% of home care is provided by the patients' families or friends, the total economic cost for society is exorbitant. For example, in the Netherlands dementia in women over 65 years of age amounted to 18.2% of total disease-specific costs, reaching first ranking throughout all disease-specific costs in 1994.[55] It was estimated that the cost of basic care (without any treatment) amount to almost €10 000 per patient-year, 50% of which results from care in a nursing home.[40] With special care, e.g. by an ambulatory Alzheimer's Disease Centre, the mean annual Medicare costs per patient surge to approximately €14 000.[6] The need for medical treatment, e.g. with the cholinesterase inhibitor donepezil, additionally increases the total costs per patient-year to almost €20 000.[86]

HRT, especially the oestrogen component, is thought to prevent or delay the onset of dementia or AD. Although there are conflicting results from several studies, the findings of a recent large cohort study supported this hypothesis.[93] According to this study, the start of HRT shortly after menopause is of paramount importance in preserving the preventive effect of oestrogen.

The main mechanisms of oestrogenic action in the brain are well known with:[51]

- increase of cerebral blood flow;
- forming of new synapses (in adult mice);
- and an antioxidant and antiinflammatory action.

The oestrogenic activity in parallel with specific progestogens improves cognitive performance, emotional state and memory.

It is doubtful whether AD, once established, can be successfully treated with any current medication. In general, the prevention of a disease is usually more cost-effective than treatment – this is especially true for dementia and AD. It has been estimated that a 5-year delay in onset of AD yields, in cost savings, at least €55 billion in annual healthcare costs, and that a 1-month delay in nursing home placement results in cost-savings of €1.1 billion per year.[68] From a socioeconomic point of view, HRT is an inexpensive way to save healthcare costs due to its ability to prevent or delay dementia or AD in older women.

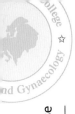
CONCLUSION

Even in the post-WHI era, the beneficial effects of HRT on menopausal complaints and some age-related chronic diseases remain unchallenged. These benefits include the treatment of vasomotor and psychological symptoms, and urogenital atrophy as well as preventive effects against osteoporosis and colorectal carcinoma. Compared to different screening, preventive or treatment measures, HRT has a favourable cost/benefit ratio. If HRT is given to appropriate women on an individualized basis this therapy combines cost-effectiveness and efficacy in a unique way.

References

1. Al-Azzawi F, Wahab M 2002 Oestrogen and colon cancer: current issues. Climacteric 5:3–14
2. Albertazzi P, Purdie D W 2001 Oestrogen and selective oestrogen receptor modulators (SERMs): current roles in the prevention and treatment of osteoporosis. Best Practice & Research. Clinical Rheumatology 15:451–468
3. Allen I E, Monroe M, Connelly J et al 2000 Effect of postmenopausal hormone replacement therapy on dental outcomes: systematic review of the literature and pharmacoeconomic analysis. Managed Care Interface 13:93–99
4. Alzheimer's Association. Statistics about Alzheimer's disease. http://www.alz.org/AboutAD/Statistics.asp (accessed 16 March 2005)
5. Azam U, Castleden M, Turner D 2001 Economics of lower urinary tract symptoms (LUTS) in older people. Drugs & Aging 18:213–223
6. Bloom B S, Chhatre S, Jayadevappa R 2004 Cost effects of a specialized care center for people with Alzheimer's disease. American Journal of Alzheimer's Disease and Other Dementias 19:226–232
7. Botteman M F, Shah N P, Lian J et al 2004 Cost-effectiveness evaluation of two continuous-combined hormone therapies for the management of moderate-to-severe vasomotor symptoms. Menopause 11:343–355
8. Bresalier R S, Sandler R S, Quan H et al 2005 Cardiovascular events associated with rofecoxib in a colorectal adenoma chemoprevention trial. The New England Journal of Medicine 352:1092–1102
9. Brown J, Grady D, Ouslander J et al for the Heart and Estrogen/progestin Replacement Study (HERS) Research Group 1999 Prevalence of urinary incontinence and associated risk factors in postmenopausal women. Obstetrics and Gynecology 94:66–70
10. Burt R W 2000 Colon cancer screening. Gastroenterology 119:837–853
11. Calle E E, Miracle-McMahill H L, Thun M J et al 1995 Estrogen replacement therapy and risk of fatal colon cancer in a prospective cohort of postmenopausal women. Journal of the National Cancer Institute 87:517–523
12. Cardozo L D, Rekers H, Tapp A et al 1993 Oestriol in the treatment of postmenopausal urgency: a multicentre study. Maturitas 18:47–53
13. Cauley J A, Robbins J, Chen Z et al 2003 Effects of estrogen plus progestin on risk of fracture and bone mineral density. The Women's Health Initiative randomized trial. The Journal of the American Medical Association 290:1729–1738
14. Centers for Disease Control and Prevention 1999 Screening for colorectal cancer. Morbidity and Mortality Weekly Report 48:116–121
15. Chlebowski R T, Wactawski-Wende J, Ritenbaugh C et al 2004 Estrogen plus progestin and colorectal cancer in postmenopausal women. The New England Journal of Medicine 350:991–1004
16. Derman R J, Dawood M Y, Stone S 1995 Quality of life during sequential hormone replacement therapy: a placebo-controlled study. International Journal of Fertility and Menopausal Studies 40:7–8
17. Eberhart C E, Coffrey R J, Radhika A et al 1994 Up-regulation of cyclooxygenase 2 gene expression in human colorectal adenomas and adenocarcinomas. Gastroenterology 107:1183–1188

18. Eriksen P S, Rasmussen H 1992 Low-dose 17 beta-oestradiol vaginal tablets in the treatment of atrophic vaginitis: a double-blind placebo-controlled study. European Journal of Obstetrics, Gynecology, and Reproductive Biology 44:137–144

19. Fantl J A, Bump R C, Robinson D et al 1996 Efficacy of estrogen supplementation in the treatment of urinary incontinence. The Continence Program for Women Research Group. Obstetrics and Gynecology 88:745–749

20. Fearon E R, Vogelstein B 1990 A genetic model for colorectal tumorigenesis. Cell 61:759–767

21. Fernandez E, La Vecchia C, Balducci A et al 2001 Oral contraceptives and colorectal cancer risk: a meta-analysis. British Journal of Cancer 84:722–727

22. Fraumeni J F, Lloyd J W, Smith E M et al 1969 Cancer mortality among nuns: role of marital status in etiology of neoplastic disease in women. Journal of the National Cancer Institute 42:455–468

23. Giovannucci E, Egan K M, Hunter D J et al 1995 Aspirin and the risk of colorectal cancer in women. The New England Journal of Medicine 333:609–614

24. Glare J (ed) 2003 West Midlands Medicines Information Service http://www.ukmicentral.nhs.uk/pressupp/costs/HT-bar.pdf

25. Grodstein F, Martinez M E, Platz E A et al 1998 Postmenopausal hormone use and risk for colorectal cancer and adenoma. Annals of Internal Medicine 128:705–712

26. Grodstein F, Newcomb P A, Stampfer M J 1999 Postmenopausal hormone therapy and the risk of colorectal cancer. A review and meta-analysis. The American Journal of Medicine 106:574–582

27. Haymarket Publishing Ltd. eMIMS. Monthly index of medical specialities: the definitive prescribing information system [online]. http//www.eMIMS.net (accessed 22 June 2004)

28. Hays J, Ockene J K, Brunner R L et al 2003 Effects of estrogen plus progestin on health-related quality of life. The New England Journal of Medicine 348:1839–1854

29. Hebert-Croteau N 1998 A meta-analysis of hormone replacement therapy and colon cancer in women. Cancer Epidemiology, Biomarkers & Prevention 7:653–659

30. Hendrix S L, Cochrane B B, Nygaard I E et al 2005 Effects of estrogen with and without progestin on urinary incontinence. The Journal of the American Medical Association 293:935–948

31. http://www.prb.org//Content/ContentGroups/Datasheets/wpds2002/2002_World_Population_Data_Sheet.htm

32. Hulley S, Furberg C, Barrett-Connor E et al 2002 Noncardiovascular disease outcomes during 6.8 years of hormone therapy. Heart and Estrogen/progestin Replacement Study follow-up (HERSII). The Journal of the American Medical Association 288:58–66

33. Iqbal M M 2000 Osteoporosis: epidemiology, diagnosis and treatment. Southern Medical Journal 93:2–18

34. Jackson S, Shepherd A, Brookes S et al 1999 The effect of oestrogen supplementation on post-menopausal urinary stress incontinence: a double-blind, placebo-controlled trial. British Journal of Obstetrics and Gynaecology 106:711–718

35. Jänne P A, Mayer R J 2000 Chemoprevention of colorectal cancer. The New England Journal of Medicine 342:1960–1968

36. Johannesson M, Johansson P-O, Kriström B et al 1993 Willingness to pay for antihypertensive therapy: further results. Journal of Health Economics 1993; 12:95–108

37. Ladabaum U, Chopra C L, Huang G et al 2001 Aspirin as an adjunct to screening for prevention of sporadic colorectal cancer: a cost-effectiveness analysis. Annals of Internal Medicine 135:769–781

38. Ladabaum U, Scheiman J M, Fendrick M 2003 Potential effect of cyclooxygenase-2-specific inhibitors on the prevention of colorectal cancer: a cost-effectiveness analysis. The American Journal of Medicine 114:546–554

39. Li C, Wilawan K, Samsioe G et al 2002 Health profile of middle-aged women. The Women's Health in the Lund Area (WHILA) study. Human Reproduction 17:1379–1385

40. McDonnell J, Redekop W K, van der Roer N et al 2001 The cost of treatment of Alzheimer's disease in the Netherlands: a regression-based simulation model. Pharmacoeconomics 19:379–390

41. McMichael A J, Potter J D 1980 Reproduction, endogenous and exogenous sex hormones, and colon cancer: a review and hypothesis. Journal of the National Cancer Institute 65:1201–1207

42. Mayne C J, Assassa R P 2004 Epidemiology of incontinence and prolapse. British

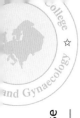

Journal of Obstetrics and Gynaecology 111 (Suppl 1):2–4

43. Moehrer B, Hextall A, Jackson S 2003 Oestrogens for urinary incontinence in women [Cochrane review]. Cochrane database of systemic reviews. 2003 Issue 2. Art. No: CD001405.D01:10.1002/1465 1858. CD001405

44. Müller A D, Sonnenberg A, Wasserman I H 1994 Diseases preceding colon cancer: a case-control study among veterans. Digestive Diseases and Sciences 39:2480–2484

45. Nanda K, Bastian L A, Hasselblad V et al 1999 Hormone replacement therapy and the risk of colorectal cancer: a meta-analysis. Obstetrics and Gynecology 93:880–888

46. Nelson H D, Humphrey L L, Nygren P et al 2002 Postmenopausal hormone replacement therapy. The Journal of the American Medical Association 288:872–881

47. Newcomb P A, Storer B E 1995 Postmenopausal hormone use and risk of large bowel cancer. Journal of the National Cancer Institute 87:1067–1071

48. Nygaard I, Turrey C, Burns T L et al 2003 Urinary incontinence and depression in middle-aged United States women. Obstetrics and Gynecology 101:149–156

49. Orsini L S, Rousculp M D, Long S R et al 2004 Health care utilization and expenditures in the United States: a study of osteoporosis-related fractures. Osteoporosis International 16:359–371 (epub ahead of print, 1 September 2004: available at: http://www.springerlink.com)

50. Pandit L, Ouslander J G 1997 Postmenopausal vaginal atrophy and atrophic vaginitis. The American Journal of Medical Sciences 314:228–231

51. Panidis D K, Matalliotakis I M, Rousso D H et al 2001 The role of oestrogen replacement therapy in Alzheimer's disease. European Journal of Obstetrics, Gynecology and Reproductive Biology 95:86–91

52. Persson J, Teleman P, Eten-Bergquist C et al 2002 Cost-analyses based on a prospective, randomized study comparing laparoscopic colposuspension with a tension-free vaginal tape procedure. Acta Obstericia et Gynecologica Scandinavica 81:1066–1073

53. Pfeilschifter J, Pientka L, Scheidt-Nave C 2003 Osteoporose in Deutschland 2003. Eine Bestandsaufnahme. Fortschritte der Medizin 123:42–43

54. Plumb J M, Guest J F 2000 Economic impact of tibolone compared with continuous-combined hormone replacement therapy in the management of postmenopausal women with climacteric symptoms in the UK. Pharmacoeconomics 18:477–486

55. Polder J J, Meerding W J, Bonneux L et al 2002 Healthcare costs of intellectual disability in the Netherlands: a cost-of-illness perspective. Journal of Intellectual and Disability Research 46:168–178

56. Polo-Kantola P, Erkkola R, Helenius H et al 1998 When does estrogen replacement therapy improve sleep quality? American Journal of Obstetrics and Gynecology 178:1002–1009

57. Population Reference Bureau 2004 World Population Data Sheet (http://www.prb.org/pdf04/04World DataSheet_Eng.pdf)

58. Potter J D, Bostick R M, Grandits G A et al 1996 Hormone replacement therapy is associated with lower risk of adenomatous polyps of the large bowel. The Minnesota Cancer Prevention Research Unit Case-Control Study. Cancer Epidemiology, Biomarkers & Prevention 5:779–784

59. Potter J D, Slattery M L, Bostick R M et al 1993 Colon cancer: a review of the epidemiology. Epidemiologic Reviews 15:499–545

60. Prihartono N, Palmer J R, Louik C et al 2000 A case-control study of use of postmenopausal female hormone supplements in relation to the risk of large bowel cancer. Cancer Epidemiology, Biomarkers & Prevention 9:443–447

61. Quievy A, Couturier F, Prudhon C et al 2001 Comparaison économique de deux techniques chirurgicales de traitement de l'incontinence urinaire d'effort chez la femme: technique de Burch contre techniqe TVT. Progrèsen Urologie 11:347–353

62. Randell A, Sambrook P N, Nguyen T V et al 1995 Direct clinical and welfare costs of osteoporotic fractures in elderly men and wo men. Osteoporosis International 5:427–432

63. Ray N F, Chan J K, Thamer M et al 1997 Medical expenditures for the treatment of osteoporotic fractures in the United States in 1995. Report from the National Osteoporosis Foundation. Journal of Bone and Mineral Research 12:24–35

64. Rote Liste 2005 Available at http://www.rote-liste.de

65. Ryan N, Rosner A 2001 Quality of life and costs associated with micronized progesterone and medroxyprogesterone acetate in hormone replacement therapy for

nonhysterectomized, postmenopausal women. Clinical Therapeutics 23:1099–1115

66. Samsioe G 1998 Urogenital aging: a hidden problem. American Journal of Obstetrics and Gynecology 178:S245–S249

67. Sandler R S, Galanko J C, Murray S C et al 1998 Aspirin and nonsteroidal anti-inflammatory agents and risk for colorectal adenomas. Gastroenterology 114:441–447

68. Sawyer N 2000 The state of affairs in Alzheimer's disease. Case Manager 11:61–68

69. Schaad M A, Bonjour J P, Rizzoli R 2000 Evaluation of hormone replacement therapy use by the sales figures. Maturitas 34:185–191

70. Selke B, Durand I, Marissal J P et al 2003 Coût du cancer colorectal en France en 1999. Gastroenterologie Clinique et Biologique 27:22–27

71. Semmens J P, Wagner G 1982 Estrogen deprivation and vaginal function in post-menopausal women. The Journal of the American Medical Association 248:445–448

72. Siris E, Adachi J D, Lu Y et al 2002 Effects of raloxifene on fracture severity in post-menopausal women with osteoporosis: Results from the MORE Study. Osteoporosis International 13:907–913

73. Solomon S D, McMurray J J, Pfeffer M A et al 2005 Cardiovascular risk associated with celecoxib in a clinical trial for colorectal adenoma prevention. The New England Journal of Medicine 352:1071–1080

74. Sonnenberg A 2002 Cost-effectiveness in the prevention of colorectal cancer. Gastroenterology Clinics of North America 31:1069–1091

75. Stürmer T, Glynn R J, Lee I M et al 1998 Aspirin use and colorectal cancer: post-trial follow-up data from the Physicians' Health Study. Annals of Internal Medicine 128:713–720

76. Suleiman S, Rex D K, Sonnenberg A 2002 Chemoprevention of colorectal cancer by aspirin. A cost-effectiveness analysis. Gastroenterology 122:78–84

77. Taketo M M 1998 Cyclooxygenase-2 inhibitors in tumorigenesis. Journal of the National Cancer Institute 90:1529–1536

78. Thom D 1998 Variation in estimates of urinary incontinence prevalence in the community. Effects of differences in definition, population characteristics, and study type. Journal of the American Geriatrics Society 46:473–480

79. Thomas M L, Xu X, Norfleet A M et al 1993 The presence of functional estrogen receptors in intestinal epithelial cells. Endocrinology 132:426–430

80. Thun M J, Namboodiri M M, Heath C W Jr 1991 Aspirin use and reduced risk of fatal colon cancer. The New England Journal of Medicine 325:1593–1596

81. Torgerson D J, Reid D M 1999 The pharmacoeconomics of hormone replacement therapy. Pharmacoeconomics 16:9–16

82. Townsend J 1998 Hormone replacement therapy: assessment of present use, costs, and trends. The British Journal of General Practice 48:955–958

83. Weber K, Hoffmann A, Leb G 1999 Therapie der Osteoporose: Strategien für eine individuelle Behandlung. Wiener Medizinische Wochenschrift 149:489–492

84. Wilson L, Brown J S, Shin G P et al 2001 Annual direct cost of urinary incontinence. Obstetrics and Gynecology 98:398–406

85. Wimo A, Winblad B, Aguera-Torres H et al 2003 The magnitude of dementia occurrence in the world. Alzheimer Disease and Associated Disorders 17:63–67

86. Wimo A, Winblad B, Engedal K et al 2003 An economic evaluation of donepezil in mild to moderate Alzheimer's disease. Results of a 1-year, double-blind, randomized trial. Dementia and Geriatric Cognitive Disorders 15:44–54

87. Wingo P A, Ries L A G, Rosenberg H M et al 1998 Cancer incidence and mortality, 1973–1995: a report card for the US. Cancer 82:1197–1207

88. Women's Health Initiative Steering Committee 2004 Effects of conjugated equine oestrogen in postmenopausal women with hysterectomy. The Women's Health Initiative randomized controlled trial. The Journal of the American Medical Association 291:1701–1712

89. World Health Organization 2001 Global burden of disease estimates: GBD 2001 estimates. Available at http://www3.who.int.-whosis/menu.cfm?path=evidence, burden_estimates&language=english (accessed 17 July 2002)

90. Writing Group for the Women's Health Initiative Investigators 2002 Risks and benefits of oestrogen plus progestin in healthy postmenopausal women. Principal results from the Women's Health Initiative randomized controlled trial. The Journal of the American Medical Association 288:321–333

91. Wuttke W, Weißlog D 1996 Das Klimak-
terium und seine Folgeerscheinungen: eine
Krankheitskostenstudie in der Bundesre-
publik Deutschland. In: Schindler A E (ed)
Menopause aktuell. Aesopus, Basel

92. Yang V W, Geiman D E, Hubbard W C
et al 2000 Tissue prostanoids as biomarkers
for chemoprevention of colorectal
neoplasia. Correlation between prostanoid
synthesis and clinical response in familial
adenomatous polyposis. Prostaglandins &
Other Lipid Mediators 60:83–96

93. Zandi P P, Carlson M C, Plassman B L et al
2002 Hormone replacement therapy and
incidence of Alzheimer's disease in older
women. The Cache County Study. The
Journal of the American Medical Association 288:2123–2129

94. Zethraeus N 1998 Willingness to pay for
hormone replacement therapy. Health
Economics 7:31–38

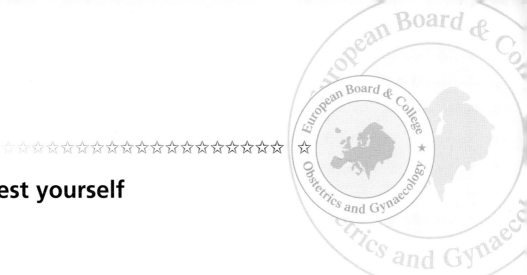

Test yourself

QUESTIONS

The Answers section begins on p. 295.

CHAPTER 1 ENDOCRINOLOGY OF THE MENOPAUSE

1. In menopausal women which pituitary hormone increases significantly in the first phase?
   a. LH;
   b. GnRH;
   c. inhibin-A;
   d. FSH;
   e. E_2.
2. In postmenopausal women the ovary is one of the major sources of:
   a. E_2;
   b. progesterone;
   c. E_1;
   d. DHEAS;
   e. androgens.
3. In which tissue does the conversion of androgens to oestrogens occur?
   a. muscles;
   b. ovaries;
   c. adrenal glands;
   d. adipose tissue;
   e. liver.
4. Which of the following hormones is exclusively produced by the adrenal glands?
   a. testosterone;
   b. dihydrotestosterone;
   c. DHEA;

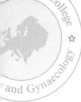
    d. DHEAS;

    e. andostenedione.

5. In postmenopausal women, thyroid anomalies:

    a. are more frequent than in men;

    b. increase with age;

    c. show symptoms similar to those of climacteric syndrome;

    d. correlate very little with ovarian function;

    e. all the above.

CHAPTER 2　MENOPAUSE-RELATED SYMPTOMS AND THEIR TREATMENT

NB More than one answer can be correct.

1. For which of the following symptoms is there scientific evidence to support a causal relationship with oestrogen deficiency:

    a. hot flushes;

    b. vaginal atrophy;

    c. depression;

    d. headache

    e. insomnia

2. For which of the following is oestrogen therapy indicated in peri- and postmenopausal women:

    a. night sweats;

    b. venous thrombosis;

    c. women with risk factors for ischaemic heart disease;

    d. women who have been operated on for breast cancer;

    e. vaginal dryness.

3. Which of the following statements are true?

    a. Vasomotor symptoms are experienced by 50–70% of peri- and post-menopausal women.

    b. Oestrogen receptors are found in the pelvic floor muscles.

    c. The female genital tract and urinary system have a common embryological origin.

    d. Lactobacilli predominate in the vaginal microenvironment of post-menopausal women.

    e. The prevalence of urinary tract infections decreases with increasing age after the menopause.

CHAPTER 3　MENOPAUSE, HORMONE REPLACEMENT THERAPY AND QUALITY OF LIFE

1. In which of the following countries are women (i) most and (ii) least aware of HRT?

    a. Germany;

    b. the UK;

   c. France;

   d. Spain.

2. Which of the following criteria should standardized menopause-specific scales satisfy?

   i. based on factor analysis;

   ii. consist of several subscales;

   iii. possess sound psychometric properties;

   iv. standardized using representative populations.

     a. i + iii;

     b. i + iv;

     c. all of them.

3. The Menopause Rating Scale has been linguistically validated in:

   a. four languages;

   b. six languages;

   c. eight languages;

   d. nine or more languages.

4. In Europe, what are the most frequently mentioned HRT benefits and risks?

   i. relief of hot flushes;

   ii. improvement of well-being;

   iii. risk of breast cancer;

   iv. increase of body weight;

   v. benefits the bones;

   vi. risk of thrombosis.

     a. i + ii + vi;

     b. iii + v + vi;

     c. all of them.

CHAPTER 4   INTERPRETING THE PLASMA LIPOPROTEIN PROFILE OF THE POSTMENOPAUSAL WOMAN

1. Which lipoproteins have been implicated in arterial disease?

   a. LDL;

   b. HDL;

   c. Lp(a);

   d. triglyceride-rich lipoproteins;

   e. all of the above.

2. Which lipoproteins are *not* affected by the menopause?

   a. LDL;

   b. HDL;

   c. Lp(a);

   d. triglyceride-rich lipoproteins;

   e. all of the above.

3. In general, which lipoproteins are *not* influenced by oral oestrogens?

   a. LDL;

   b. HDL;

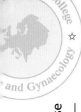

c. Lp(a);

d. triglyceride-rich lipoproteins;

e. all are influenced.

4. In general, which lipoproteins are *not* influenced by non-oral oestrogens?

a. LDL;

b. HDL;

c. Lp(a);

d. triglyceride-rich lipoproteins;

e. all are influenced.

5. Which lipoprotein is thought to be most involved in protecting HRT users from myocardial infarction?

a. LDL;

b. HDL;

c. Lp(a);

d. triglyceride-rich lipoproteins;

e. none of the above.

CHAPTER 5 THE EFFECT OF AGEING AND HORMONE REPLACEMENT THERAPY ON GLUCOSE METABOLISM

1. Among 60–70-year-old North American women, the metabolic syndrome is present in:

a. 10%;

b. 20%;

c. 30%;

d. more than 40%.

2. Which of the following is true about adiponectin?

a. It is an antiinflammatory cytokine.

b. It is produced by adipocytes.

c. It enhances insulin sensitivity.

d. All of the above.

3. Which of the following are not true? In animal studies, E_2;

a. enhances insulin secretion;

b. reduces insulin resistance;

c. leads to hyperglycaemia;

d. opposes natural progesterone.

4. In the PEPI trial's four arms, the following were given: CEE only; CEE + 2.5 mg continuous MPA daily; CEE + 10 mg sequential MPA in days 1–12; or CEE + 200 mg sequential micronized progesterone in days 1–12. Which arm had the best results in carbohydrate metabolism?

a. CEE;

b. CEE + progesterone;

c. CEE + cyclic MPA;

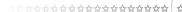

d. CEE + continuous MPA;

e. there was no difference.

CHAPTER 6   HORMONE REPLACEMENT THERAPY AND COAGULATION

1. Markers of activated coagulation are:
   a. fibrinonogen and factor VII;
   b. fibrinogen and prothrombin fragments 1 + 2;
   c. prothrombin fragments 1 + 2, thrombin–antithrombin complex and D-dimer;
   d. activated protein C resistance;
   e. tissue factor.
2. Haematologicical risk factors for venous thromboembolism are:
   a. antithrombin;
   b. antithrombin, protein C, protein S, activated protein C resistance and TFPI;
   c. fibrinogen;
   d. protein C;
   e. D-dimer.
3. Oral HRT is associated with:
   a. a decrease in prothrombin fragments 1 + 2;
   b. an increase in fibrinogen;
   c. an increase in protein C;
   d. an increased response to activated protein C;
   e. an increase in prothrombin fragments 1 + 2 and D-dimer.
4. Oral HRT is also associated with:
   a. acquired factor V Leiden mutation;
   b. acquired resistance to activated protein C;
   c. increased tissue factor pathway inhibitor and tissue factor;
   d. activation of the protein C–protein S anticoagulant pathway;
   e. reduced factor VII.
5. Transdermal HRT is associated with:
   a. marginal or no activation of coagulation;
   b. reduced activation of coagulation;
   c. increased levels of tissue factor pathway inhibitor;
   d. increased levels of factor VII;
   e. acquired resistance to activated protein C.

CHAPTER 7   CURRENT VIEWS ON HORMONE REPLACEMENT THERAPY AND CARDIOVASCULAR DISEASE

1. What is the approximate risk of dying from coronary heart disease in a 50-year-old Caucasian woman?
   a. 5%;
   b. 15%;

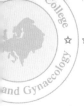
c. 20%;
d. 30%;
e. 45%.

2. In which situations do women have a greater risk than men of developing coronary heart disease?
   a. hypercholesterolaemia;
   b. severe obesity;
   c. hypertension;
   d. heavy smoking;
   e. diabetes.

3. Which is the most likely key factor for triggering the rupture of instable plaques?
   a. matrix metalloproteinases;
   b. PAI-I;
   c. C-reactive protein;
   d. platelet factor 6;
   e. none of the above.

4. Randomized controlled trials (RCTs) are considered the 'gold standard' but they are not problem free. Which of the following statements holds true for RCTs?
   a. They overestimate short-term results.
   b. Generally, they recruit a low-risk population.
   c. They are not truly population-based as they use specific exclusion criteria.
   d. They are not truly population-based as they use specific inclusion criteria.
   e. All of the above.

5. Hormone replacement therapy seems initially to increase the risk of coronary heart disease, followed by a decline. The reason for this is probably:
   a. that younger women have a decreased risk and older women an increased risk;
   b. the influence of progestogen;
   c. because of an initial increase in thromboembolism followed by the effects of reduced arteriosclerosis;
   d. an increase of triglycerides followed by a decrease in cholesterol;
   e. an increase in LDL also followed by an increase in HDL.

6. Coronary heart disease develops in women later than in men by:
   a. 5 years;
   b. 10 years;
   c. 15 years;
   d. 20 years.

7. The most common hypertension among postmenopausal women is:
   a. systolic;
   b. diastolic;
   c. both.

8. The lowest risk of venous thromboembolism is carried by:
   a. oral oestrogens;
   b. oral oestrogen–progestogen combination;
   c. raloxifene;
   d. transdermal oestrogen.

9. C-reactive protein:
   a. is a marker for coronary heart disease;
   b. is elevated during the transdermal application of HRT
   c. remains at the same level during oral HRT;
   d. all of the above.

CHAPTER 8   THE BIOLOGY AND CONSEQUENCES OF OSTEOPOROSIS

1. What kind of cells are found in bone?
   a. osteoblasts;
   b. osteoclasts;
   c. osteocytes;
   d. all of the above.
2. Which type of cell resorbs bone?
   a. osteoclasts;
   b. osteoblasts;
   c. osteocytes.
3. Which type of cell forms new bone?
   a. osteoclasts;
   b. osteoblasts;
   c. osteocytes.
4. The diagnosis of osteoporosis (T score):
   a. is only based on a bone mineral density measurement;
   b. is based on several risk factors.
5. Mortality is increased after:
   a. hip fractures;
   b. vertebral fractures;
   c. wrist fractures;
   d. a and b;
   e. b and c.
6. Which fractures are osteoporotic?
   a. hip;
   b. vertebral;
   c. wrist;
   d. pelvic;
   e. humeral;
   f. all of the above.

CHAPTER 9   THE EFFECT OF HORMONE REPLACEMENT THERAPY ON THE BONE

1. Which of the following is true about bone remodelling?
   a. The process only occurs before the menopause.
   b. The process only occurs after the menopause.

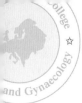
c. The process occurs after bone injury and in connection with metabolic bone diseases.

d. The process is coupled.

2. How does bone remodelling start?

a. by osteoblast activation;

b. by osteoclast activation;

c. by osteocyte activation;

d. by osteoblast/osteoclast inhibition.

3. How many phases are described for postmenopausal bone loss?

a. 1;

b. 2;

c. 3;

d. 4.

4. What is the primary action of HRT on bone?

a. It stimulates bone resorption.

b. It inhibits bone resorption.

c. It stimulates bone formation.

d. It inhibits bone formation.

5. What is characteristic about the effect on bone by oestrogen-like substances?

a. These substances have oestrogen agonist effects on bone.

b. These substances have oestrogen antagonist effects on bone.

c. These substances have combined oestrogen agonist–antagonist effect on bone.

d. These substances have no effect on bone.

CHAPTER 10   THE PREVENTION OF OSTEOPOROTIC FRACTURES

NB More than one answer can be correct.

1. Approximately how many new hip fractures are there worldwide every year?

a. 10 000.

b. 100 000.

c. 1 000 000.

d. 1 500 000.

2. Which of the following treatments have been demonstrated to reduce vertebral fractures?

a. calcitonin;

b. raloxifene;

c. aledronate;

d. aspirin.

3. Which of the following treatments have been shown to reduce non-vertebral fractures?

a. calcitonin;

b. aledronate;

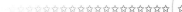

c. risedronate;

d. calcium;

e. risedronate.

4. Is it true that physical exercise has a balancing effect on bone turnover?

a. yes;

b. no.

5. Postmenopausal osteoporosis is associated with:

a. decreased bone resorption;

b. increased bone resorption;

c. increased bone turnover;

d. decreased bone mineral density.

CHAPTER 11   THE ACTION OF OESTROGENS IN THE BRAIN

NB More than one answer can be correct.

1. Which of the following describes the expression of oestrogen receptors in the brain?

a. developmentally regulated;

b. sexually dimorphic;

c. restricted to neurones;

d. regulated by oestradiol.

2. Which of the following describes the actions of oestradiol in the brain?

a. It is mediated exclusively by neurones.

b. It is restricted to the areas of the brain that are involved in sexual behaviour.

c. It is limited to the developmental period.

d. It is mediated in part by the activation of membrane signalling cascades.

3. Which of the following is/are included in the effects of oestradiol in the brain?

a. The activation of kinases.

b. The regulation of phosphatases.

c. The modulation of intracellular calcium levels.

d. The regulation of gene transcription.

4. The regulation of which of the following describes how oestradiol modulates the communication between brain cells?

a. The synthesis of neurotransmitters.

b. The expression of neurotransmitter receptors.

c. The activity of neurotransmitter receptors.

d. The transport of serotonin.

5. Which of the following is/are true about the brain?

a. The brain is unable to synthesize oestradiol under physiological condition.

b. The brain synthesizes oestradiol after injury.

c. The brain is unable to convert cholesterol into pregnenolone.

d. The brain expresses enzymes for steroid synthesis and metabolism.

285

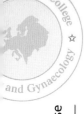
☆ ☆☆☆☆☆☆☆☆☆☆☆☆☆☆☆☆☆☆☆☆☆☆☆

CHAPTER 12   OESTROGENS, COGNITIVE FUNCTIONING AND DEMENTIA

NB More than one answer can be correct.

1. Which of the following describes how oestrogen affects brain function?
   a. by increasing serotonin levels;
   b. by increasing dopamine and noradrenaline levels;
   c. by decreasing the synthesis of acetylcholine;
   d. by increasing glutamate levels.
2. Cognitive impairment is associated with which of the following?
   a. Low levels of endogenous oestrogen.
   b. High levels of testosterone.
   c. Low levels of free thyroxine.
3. Which of the following describes the prevalence of Alzheimer's disease?
   a. 10% at the age of 65.
   b. 15% at the age of 85.
   c. Doubles every 5 years after the age of 65.
4. Which of the following describes ET/HRT?
   a. It alleviates the symptoms of Alzheimer's disease.
   b. It may aggravate the symptoms of Alzheimer's disease.
   c. It may prevent Alzheimer's disease.

CHAPTER 13   FEMALE SEX HORMONES, SLEEP AND MOOD

NB More than one answer can be correct.

1. Which of the following percentages shows the proportion of sleep complaints in 50–64-year-old women?
   a. 10%;
   b. 25%;
   c. 50%;
   d. 75%.
2. Complete the following sentence. Serotonin is an important sleep regulator and:
   a. its metabolism leads to increased and enhanced sleep;
   b. prevention of its synthesis leads to longer sleep;
   c. it affects the sleep stage;
3. Complete the following sentence. Sleep apnoea:
   a. occurs twice as often in men as in women;
   b. is improved by raising the oestrogen level;
   c. is due to upper airway obstruction.
4. Complete the following sentence. Lack of oestrogen:
   a. reduces the brain serotonin content;
   b. may affect the adrenergic and dopaminergic activities in the brain;
   c. does not affect cholinergic functions.

CHAPTER 14   SEXUALITY AND MENOPAUSE

1. Which is the most important factor influencing sexual health at menopause?
   a. physical health;
   b. mental health;
   c. partner;
   d. hormones;
   e. all of the above.
2. Which is the most relevant component of a normal sexual cycle response in women?
   a. the neuroendocrine system;
   b. neuroanatomical substrates;
   c. vascular supplies;
   d. the muscular system;
   e. all of the above.
3. In which condition has ET/AT been proven to be effective in improving sexual function?
   a. Only if it is administered transdermally.
   b. In surgical menopause.
   c. When sexual symptoms are diagnosed before menopause.
   d. In older women.
   e. None of the above.
4. Which is the simplest examination for determining vaginal oestrogenization?
   a. vaginal pH
   b. the karyopycnotic index
   c. genital blood flow
   d. plasma E_2 levels
   e. none of the above.
5. Are hormonal treatments the complete answer for postmenopausal women who experience sexual difficulties throughout the transition and beyond?
   a. Yes, they are the only answer.
   b. Counselling is the most important answer to women's sexual problems.
   c. Treating the partner is relevant.
   d. Psychoactive agents may be a solution.
   e. A balanced biopsychorelational perspective is mandatory.

CHAPTER 15   OESTROGENS AND THE LOWER UROGENITAL TRACT

1. When considering lower urinary tract function, which of the following increases with age?
   a. urinary flow rate;
   b. urine residual volume;
   c. uninhibited detrusor contractions;

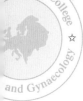
   d. functional bladder capacity;
   e. nocturnal fluid excretion;
   f. the ability to postpone voiding.
2. Which of the following are symptoms of urogenital ageing?
   a. vaginal dryness;
   b. recurrent urinary tract infections (UTIs);
   c. urogenital prolapse;
   d. superficial dyspareunia;
   e. urgency of micturition;
   f. urinary incontinence.
3. Complete the following sentence. Low-dose vaginal oestrogens:
   a. are effective in the management of urogenital ageing;
   b. are contraindicated with systemic HRT therapy;
   c. are possibly effective in the prevention of UTIs;
   d. should always be avoided in women with breast cancer;
   e. objectively improve the symptoms of stress incontinence;
   f. are more effective than systemic HRT in preventing recurrent UTIs.
4. Complete the following sentence. When considering postmenopausal lower urinary tract symptoms:
   a. 70% of women complain of urgency;
   b. 50% of women complain of stress incontinence;
   c. 20% of women complain of recurrent UTIs;
   d. frequency and urgency may be improved with topical oestrogens;
   e. oestrogens may subjectively improve stress incontinence;
   f. stress incontinence is more common than urge incontinence.

CHAPTER 16   HORMONE REPLACEMENT THERAPY: WHEN TO START, WHEN TO STOP?

1. Which of the following situations does the label HRT fit best?
   a. premature menopause;
   b. naturally occurring menopause.
2. Complete the following sentence. In a hysterectomized woman with an indication for HRT, the first choice is:
   a. oral continuous combined E + P;
   b. oral oestrogen;
   c. transdermal oestrogen;
   d. tibolone;
   e. vaginal oestrogen.
3. Complete the following sentence. When HRT is started after the menopause:
   a. it should continue for up to 5 years;
   b. it may continue beyond 5 years if its indication persists and if there are no developing contraindications;
   c. it should never last for more than 5 years.

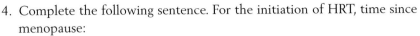

4. Complete the following sentence. For the initiation of HRT, time since menopause:
   a. is not important at all;
   b. is very important.
5. True or false: the primary prevention of cardiovascular diseases by oestrogen depends on the time of initiation of treatment?
   a. true;
   b. false.

CHAPTER 17   THE ADMINISTRATION AND DOSAGE OF OESTROGENS

1. Which of the choice of percentages completes this sentence. In post-menopausal women, a reduction of 50% in the oestrogen dose will reduce efficacy in vasomotor symptom relief by an average of:
   a. 10%;
   b. 25%;
   c. 50%;
   d. 75%.
2. Complete this paragraph. In a postmenopausal woman, treated with oral low-dose systemic oestrogen therapy, and who experiences adequate relief of her vasomotor complaints but insufficient relief of symptoms associated with urogenital atrophy, the doctor should first consider:
   a. stopping oral treatment and starting transdermal oestrogen application;
   b. stopping oral treatment and starting vaginal oestrogen application;
   c. combining oral treatment with vaginal oestrogen application;
   d. doubling the oral dosage.
3. Complete this sentence. In a postmenopausal woman, a reduction of 50% in the oestrogen dose will lead to:
   a. twice as many hip fractures;
   b. a reduction in bone mineral density comparable to untreated women;
   c. a 50% increase in bone mineral density;
   d. none of the above.
4. Complete this sentence. Compared to oral oestrogen administration, the transdermal route:
   a. has no effect on lipid concentrations;
   b. has no effect on C-reactive protein concentrations;
   c. increases resistance to activated protein C;
   d. increases homocysteine concentrations.
5. Complete this sentence. Compared to oral oestrogen administration, the transdermal route:
   a. helps with the prevention of osteoporotic fractures;
   b. helps with the prevention of colon cancer;
   c. helps with the prevention of Alzheimer's disease;
   d. none of the above.

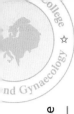
6. Complete this sentence. The Nurses' Health Study showed that low-dose oestrogen therapy (0.3 mg CEE) compared with the standard dosage of 0.625 mg:
   a. results in fewer strokes;
   b. results in more strokes;
   c. results in fewer coronary events;
   d. results in more coronary events.

CHAPTER 18   HOW TO SELECT PROGESTIN FOR HORMONE REPLACEMENT THERAPY

1. Which of the following is not a synthetic progestin?
   a. trimegestone;
   b. cyproterone acetate;
   c. progesterone;
   d. levonorgestrel;
   e. dianogest.
2. The effect of progestins are mediated by which of the following?
   a. oestrogen receptors;
   b. progesterone receptors;
   c. androgen receptors;
   d. glucocorticoid and mineralocorticoid receptors;
   e. all of them.
3. Progesterone has which of the following effects?
   a. moderate glucocorticoid and mineralocorticoid;
   b. oestrogenic;
   c. potent antiandrogenic
   d. potent androgenic;
   e. none of them.
4. Complete this sentence. The primary role of progestin in postmenopausal HRT is to:
   a. increase HDL cholesterol;
   b. provide endometrial protection;
   c. protect from breast cancer risk;
   d. produce endometrial disruption;
   e. provide ovarian protection.
5. Complete this sentence. In order to reduce the incidence of endometrial hyperplasia, we should prescribe progestin:
   a. 3–5 days per month;
   b. 5–7 days per month;
   c. 7–9 days per month;
   d. 9–11 days per month;
   e. 12 days or more per month.

CHAPTER 19   ANDROGEN REPLACEMENT THERAPIES FOR POSTMENOPAUSAL WOMEN

1. The peripherally most effective androgen is which of the following?
   a. testosterone;
   b. androstenedione;
   c. dihydrotestosterone;
   d. dihydroepiandrosterone.
2. DHEA originates mostly from which of the following?
   a. body fat;
   b. the ovaries and adrenals.
3. Which of the following is true about testosterone?
   a. It has a minimal effect on bone mineralization.
   b. It acts synergistically with oestrogens to prevent bone loss.
   c. It stimulates bone loss-opposing oestrogens.

CHAPTER 20   ALTERNATIVES TO OESTROGEN

1. Complete this sentence. Tibolone is indicated for:
   a. the treatment of climacteric complaints;
   b. the prevention and treatment of postmenopausal osteoporosis;
   c. the prevention of cardiovascular disease in postmenopausal women;
   d. a + b;
   e. a + b + c.
2. Complete this sentence. Tibolone:
   a. has no effect on endometrial tissue;
   b. has no effect on breast tissue;
   c. has no effect on lipid profile;
   d. a + b;
   e. a + c.
3. Complete this sentence. Tibolone:
   a. lowers triglyceride levels;
   b. increases triglyceride levels;
   c. lowers HDL cholesterol;
   d. a + c;
   e. b + c.
4. Complete this sentence. Raloxifene:
   a. may worsen hot flushes;
   b. increases bone mineral density in the spine;
   c. prevents vertebral fractures;
   d. lowers LDL cholesterol;
   e. all of the above.
5. Complete this sentence. Raloxifene:
   a. increases triglyceride levels;
   b. decreases breast cancer risk in postmenopausal women with osteoporosis;

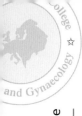

☆☆☆☆☆☆☆☆☆☆☆☆☆☆☆☆☆☆☆☆

  c. improves libido;
  d. increases HDL cholesterol;
  e. stimulates endometrial tissue.

CHAPTER 21   ALTERNATIVE MANAGEMENT OF THE FEMALE MENOPAUSE

1. Which of the following are important phyto-oestrogens?
   a. isoflavones;
   b. lignans;
   c. coumestans;
   d. a + b;
   e. all of the above.
2. Which of the following do isoflavones act through?
   a. oestrogen receptors;
   b. they have a direct action on tissue levels;
   c. they exert anti-oestrogenic properties with high level of endogenous oestradiol;
   d. a + b;
   e. All of the above.
3. Phyto-oestrogens act through which of the following?
   a. ER-α receptors;
   b. ER-β receptors;
   c. equally through both receptors;
4. Complete this sentence. Genistein:
   a. increases the synthesis of vitamin D;
   b. decreases the metabolism of vitamin D;
   c. does not affect the vitamin D level;
   d. a + b;
   e. All of the above.

CHAPTER 22   ENDOMETRIAL EFFECTS AND BLEEDING PATTERNS

1. Which of the following is the most common reason for bleeding disturbances in the perimenopausal period?
   a. endometrial cancer;
   b. anovulation;
   c. cervical dysplasia;
   d. infections.
2. The percentage risk for endometrial cancer to be the reason for postmenopausal bleeding is which of the following?
   a. 1%;
   b. 25%;
   c. 45%;
   d. 10%.

3. Which of the following statements, with regard to sequential oestrogen–progestogen therapy, is not true?
   a. It leads to withdrawal bleeding in more than 90% of women.
   b. The frequency of hyperplasia is negatively correlated to the duration of progestogen supplementation.
   c. The monthly blood loss during sequential therapy is less than 8 ml.
   d. There is no correlation between bleeding patterns and endometrial histopathology.
4. Which of the following is the most appropriate HRT for treatment of vasomotor symptoms in a woman 56 years of age who is 4 years into her menopause?
   a. progestogen-only;
   b. sequential oestrogen–progestogen;
   c. low-dose continuous combined;
   d. oestrogen-only.

CHAPTER 23   POSTMENOPAUSAL HORMONE REPLACEMENT THERAPY AND THE BREAST

1. Complete this sentence. Established hormone-related risk factors for breast cancer are:
   a. late age at menarche;
   b. early onset of menopause;
   c. postmenopausal obesity;
   d. all of the above.
2. Complete this sentence. The Women's Health Initiative study reported that after an average of 6.8 years of oestrogen therapy, breast cancer risk was:
   a. significantly increased (RR 1.77; 95% CI; range 1.59–2.01);
   b. not significantly decreased (RR 0.77; 95% CI; range 0.59–1.01);
   c. significantly decreased (RR 0.77; 95% CI; 0.59–0.99);
   d. all of the above are incorrect.
3. Complete this sentence. In breast tissue, in the luteal phase of the menstrual cycle:
   a. the mitotic rate increases;
   b. the apoptotic rate increases;
   c. the mitotic rate increases and the apoptotic rate increases;
   d. the mitotic rate decreases and the apoptotic rate decreases.
4. Complete this sentence. Mammographic breast density increases more during:
   a. combined oestrogen plus progestogen as compared with oestrogens alone;
   b. oestrogens alone compared with combined oestrogen plus progestogen;
   c. tibolone compared with combined oestrogen plus progestogen;
   d. all of the above are incorrect.

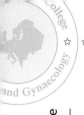

CHAPTER 24   THE USE OF HORMONE REPLACEMENT THERAPY IN EUROPE AND AROUND THE WORLD

NB More than one answer can be correct.
1. Which of the following is/are true about HRT use?
    a. It is mostly used to relieve vasomotor symptoms.
    b. Its use varies widely from 50% to 100%.
    c. It mostly occurs in women aged over 60 years.
    d. The dislike of withdrawal bleeds is a common reason for stopping HRT.
2. Which of the following is/are true about the characteristics of HRT users?
    a. A health user effect has been described.
    b. Oophorectomy reduces the risk of osteoporosis.
    c. Oophorectomized women have more hot flushes.
    d. HRT users tend to be more educated.
3. Which of the following is/are true about the decision-making process for the use of HRT?
    a. The physician's attitude to HRT does not influence the woman's use of it.
    b. The physician's sex does not influence the woman's use of HRT.
    c. Physician speciality is significantly associated with HRT use.
    d. Web-based information on HRT is all of a high quality.
4. Which of the following is/are true about the Women's Health Initiative study?
    a. It was a cohort study.
    b. It only studied oestrogen–progestin therapy.
    c. Using a global index, WHI investigators concluded that risks exceeded benefits of the combined regimen.
    d. The WHI has received little media attention.
5. Which of the following is/are true. Altered recommendations for HRT products include statements such as the following.
    a. The risk benefit is favourable for the treatment of menopausal symptoms.
    b. It is a first line in the prevention of osteoporosis for women aged over 50.
    c. Systemic HRT should be used throughout the rest of the woman's life.
    d. The lowest effective dose should be used.

CHAPTER 25   ECONOMIC ASPECTS IN THE MANAGEMENT OF THE MENOPAUSE

1. What is the root cause for the rising healthcare costs in developed countries?
    a. New (infectious) diseases such as HIV/AIDS and SARS.
    b. Increasing environmental stress (e.g. smog, ozone) causing more illness in the public.
    c. Rising travel activities resulting in a faster worldwide spread of pathogenic microorganisms.
    d. An increase in chronic diseases in an ever-ageing population with enhanced longevity.

2. Which diseases account for the largest amount of direct and indirect costs?
   a. Diseases of the urogenital tract.
   b. Cardiovascular and cerebrovascular diseases.
   c. Diseases of the musculoskeletal system.
   d. Vasomotor and psychological disorders.
3. Complete this sentence. Urinary incontinence is:
   a. a common, debilitating and costly disease in elderly women;
   b. a minor healthcare problem;
   c. a disease predominantly occurring in men;
   d. a disease generally caused by malformations of the urogenital tract.
4. What is the most cost-effective screening method for colorectal carcinoma?
   a. colonoscopy;
   b. flexible sigmoidoscopy;
   c. biopsy during colonoscopy;
   d. faecal occult blood testing.
5. Complete this sentence. A 1-month delay in nursing home placement results in cost savings of:
   a. €75 million per year;
   b. €350 million per year;
   c. €1.1 billion per year;
   d. €55 billion per year.

ANSWERS

Chapter 1   1d; 2e; 3d; 4d; 5e.
Chapter 2   1a, b, e; 2a, e; 3a, b, c.
Chapter 3   1(i) b (most aware 90%), (ii) d (least aware 41%); 2c; 3c; 4c.
Chapter 4   1e; 2b; 3e; 4c; 5e (as there is no evidence that HRT is better than placebo in terms of clinical outcomes).
Chapter 5   1d; 2d; 3a, b; 4e.
Chapter 6   1c; 2b; 3e; 4b; 5a.
Chapter 7   1d; 2e; 3a; 4e; 5c; 6b; 7a; 8d; 9a.
Chapter 8   1d; 2a; 3b; 4a; 5d; 6f.
Chapter 9   1d; 2a; 3b; 4b; 5a.
Chapter 10   1d; 2a, b, c; 3b, c; 4a; 5b, c, d.
Chapter 11   1a, b, d; 2d; 3a, b, c, d; 4a, b, c, d; 5b, d.
Chapter 12   1a, b; 2c (but 'a' is also possible); 3b, c; 4c.
Chapter 13   1b; 2b, c; 3a, c; 4a.
Chapter 14   1e; 2e; 3e; 4a; 5a.
Chapter 15   1b, c, e; 2a, b, c, d, e, f; 3a, c, f; 4b, c, d, e.
Chapter 16   1a; 2c; 3b; 4b; 5a.
Chapter 17   1a; 2c; 3d; 4b; 5d; 6a.
Chapter 18   1c; 2e; 3a; 4b; 5e.
Chapter 19   1c; 2b; 3b.
Chapter 20   1d; 2a; 3d; 4e; 5b.

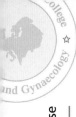

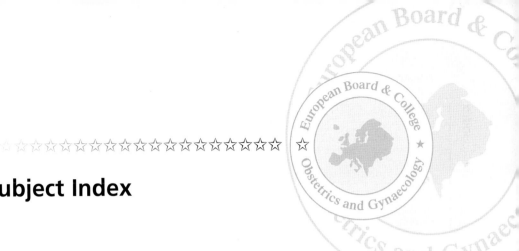

Subject Index

Notes: As the menopause is the main subject of this book, all index entries refer to the menopause unless otherwise indicated. Page numbers followed by 'f', 't' and 'b' refer to figures, tables and boxed material respectively.

Abbreviations used as subentries: hormone replacement therapy (HRT).

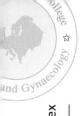

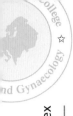

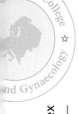

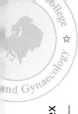

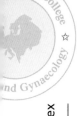

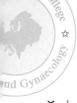